# Socio-Economic Burden of Disease:
# The COVID-19 Case

# Socio-Economic Burden of Disease: The COVID-19 Case

Editors

**Eduardo Tomé**
**Thomas Garavan**
**Ana Dias**

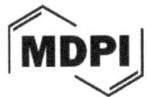

Basel • Beijing • Wuhan • Barcelona • Belgrade • Novi Sad • Cluj • Manchester

*Editors*

Eduardo Tomé
Universidade Lusófona
Lisboa
Portugal

Thomas Garavan
University College Cork
Cork
Ireland

Ana Dias
Universidade de Aveiro
Aveiro
Portugal

*Editorial Office*
MDPI
St. Alban-Anlage 66
4052 Basel, Switzerland

This is a reprint of articles from the Special Issue published online in the open access journal *Healthcare* (ISSN 2227-9032) (available at: https://www.mdpi.com/journal/healthcare/special_issues/socio-economic_burden_of_disease_covid-19_case).

For citation purposes, cite each article independently as indicated on the article page online and as indicated below:

Lastname, A.A.; Lastname, B.B. Article Title. *Journal Name* **Year**, *Volume Number*, Page Range.

ISBN 978-3-7258-0289-0 (Hbk)
ISBN 978-3-7258-0290-6 (PDF)
doi.org/10.3390/books978-3-7258-0290-6

© 2024 by the authors. Articles in this book are Open Access and distributed under the Creative Commons Attribution (CC BY) license. The book as a whole is distributed by MDPI under the terms and conditions of the Creative Commons Attribution-NonCommercial-NoDerivs (CC BY-NC-ND) license.

# Contents

About the Editors . . . . . . . . . . . . . . . . . . . . . . . . . . . . . . . . . . . . . . . . . . . . . . . . . . . vii

Preface . . . . . . . . . . . . . . . . . . . . . . . . . . . . . . . . . . . . . . . . . . . . . . . . . . . . . . . . . ix

**Abrar Almalki, Balakrishna Gokaraju, Yaa Acquaah and Anish Turlapaty**
Regression Analysis for COVID-19 Infections and Deaths Based on Food Access and Health Issues
Reprinted from: *Healthcare* 2022, 10, 324, doi:10.3390/healthcare10020324 . . . . . . . . . . . . . . . 1

**Timotej Jagrič, Dušan Fister and Vita Jagrič**
Reshaping the Healthcare Sector with Economic Policy Measures Based on COVID-19 Epidemic Severity: A Global Study
Reprinted from: *Healthcare* 2022, 10, 315, doi:10.3390/healthcare10020315 . . . . . . . . . . . . . . . 20

**Tienhua Wu**
Perception Bias Effects on Healthcare Management in COVID-19 Pandemic: An Application of Cumulative Prospect Theory
Reprinted from: *Healthcare* 2022, 10, 226, doi:10.3390/healthcare10020226 . . . . . . . . . . . . . . . 30

**Mohammed Arshad Khan, Md Imran Khan, Asheref Illiyan and Maysoon Khojah**
The Economic and Psychological Impacts of COVID-19 Pandemic on Indian Migrant Workers in the Kingdom of Saudi Arabia
Reprinted from: *Healthcare* 2021, 9, 1152, doi:10.3390/healthcare9091152 . . . . . . . . . . . . . . . 47

**Teresa Forte, Gonçalo Santinha and Sérgio A. Carvalho**
The COVID-19 Pandemic Strain: Teleworking and Health Behavior Changes in the Portuguese Context
Reprinted from: *Healthcare* 2021, 9, 1151, doi:10.3390/healthcare9091151 . . . . . . . . . . . . . . . 68

**Tinggui Chen, Jingtao Rong, Lijuan Peng, Jianjun Yang, Guodong Cong and Jing Fang**
Analysis of Social Effects on Employment Promotion Policies for College Graduates Based on Data Mining for Online Use Review in China during the COVID-19 Pandemic
Reprinted from: *Healthcare* 2021, 9, 846, doi:10.3390/healthcare9070846 . . . . . . . . . . . . . . . 83

**Yi-Man Teng, Kun-Shan Wu, Wen-Cheng Wang and Dan Xu**
Assessing the Knowledge, Attitudes and Practices of COVID-19 among Quarantine Hotel Workers in China
Reprinted from: *Healthcare* 2021, 9, 772, doi:10.3390/healthcare9060772 . . . . . . . . . . . . . . . 105

**Emily Chia-Yu Su, Cheng-Hsing Hsiao, Yi-Tui Chen and Shih-Heng Yu**
An Examination of COVID-19 Mitigation Efficiency among 23 Countries
Reprinted from: *Healthcare* 2021, 9, 755, doi:10.3390/healthcare9060755 . . . . . . . . . . . . . . . 118

**Rasha Itani, Mohammed Alnafea, Maya Tannoury, Souheil Hallit and Achraf Al Faraj**
Shedding Light on the Direct and Indirect Impact of the COVID-19 Pandemic on the Lebanese Radiographers or Radiologic Technologists: A Crisis within Crises
Reprinted from: *Healthcare* 2021, 9, 362, doi:10.3390/healthcare9030362 . . . . . . . . . . . . . . . 134

**Donglei Yu, Muhammad Khalid Anser, Michael Yao-Ping Peng, Abdelmohsen A. Nassani, Sameh E. Askar, Khalid Zaman, et al.**
Nationwide Lockdown, Population Density, and Financial Distress Brings Inadequacy to Manage COVID-19: Leading the Services Sector into the Trajectory of Global Depression
Reprinted from: *Healthcare* 2021, 9, 220, doi:10.3390/healthcare9020220 . . . . . . . . . . . . . . . 148

**Henry Asante Antwi, Lulin Zhou, Xinglong Xu and Tehzeeb Mustafa**
Beyond COVID-19 Pandemic: An Integrative Review of Global Health Crisis Influencing the
Evolution and Practice of Corporate Social Responsibility
Reprinted from: *Healthcare* **2021**, *9*, 453, doi:10.3390/healthcare9040453 . . . . . . . . . . . . . . . **166**

# About the Editors

**Eduardo Tomé**

Eduardo Tomé gained his PhD in Economics (2001), with a Thesis on the European Social Fund. Since then, he has worked in several Portuguese private universities. He has published over 50 papers in peer-reviewed Journals and presented 80 papers at international conferences. He has also authored seven book chapters, He was involved in organising and chairing 12 international conferences, of which he also co-edited the proceedings and edited four Special Issues in EJKM, EJTD and IJKBD. Since September 2020, he has worked at Universidade Lusófona in Lisbon, Portugal. His main interests are intangibles (human resources, knowledge management and intellectual capital), social policy and international economics (globalization and the European integration).

**Thomas Garavan**

Thomas Garavan is Professor of Leadership Practice in CUBS, UCC. He was recently listed in the Stanford University Science-Wide author citation indicators 2020 as one of the top 2% of academics in Economics and Business. He is a world leading expert in leadership development, learning and development and HRD. He has published 185 journal articles, 16 books, 26 book chapters and 6 monographs. He has published extensively in leading HRD journals including HRDQ, HRDR, ADHR and HRDI. He has also published extensively in the top four HRM journals: HRM (US) HRMJ, Personnel Review and IJHRM. In addition, he has published extensively in management journals including the International Journal of Management Reviews, European Management Review, Journal of Business Research, Tourism Management, Information Technology and People, International Small Business Journal, Thunderbird International Review and the Journal of Sleep Research and Business Ethics: A European Review. His most recent book publications include *Learning and Development in Organizations: A Systems-Informed Model of Effectiveness* (Palgrave), *Strategic Human Resource Management* (Oxford University Press), *Handbook of International Human Resource Development* (Edward Elgar) and *Global Human Resource Development* (Routledge). He is co-editor of the European Journal of Training and Development and Associate Editor of Personnel Review and is a member of the HRDQ, HRDI, HRDR, ADHR, HRMJ, International Journal of Training and Development and International Journal of Human Resource Management. He has extensive teaching experience with undergraduate, post-graduate and post-experience students, in addition to executive education and leadership development. He was recently elected to the Hall of Fame of the Academy of Human Resource Development, USA, and has won numerous awards for publication and journal editing.

**Ana Dias**

Ana Alexandra da Costa Dias has a PhD in Health Sciences and Technologies from the University of Aveiro (2015), a Masters in Innovation and Knowledge Management from the University of Aveiro (2005) and a degree in Management from the Institute of Superior, Financial and Fiscal Studies (1998). She has taught at the University of Aveiro since 2005 and is currently an Assistant Professor in the Department of Economics, Management, Industrial Engineering and Tourism (DEGEIT) at UA. She has been teaching the following subjects: Models and Business Processes, Organizational Behaviour and Organizational and Social Health Structures.

Her areas of interest focus on organizational models of health care provision and workflow management with applications in the health care sector and health policy.

She has participated in some UA research projects in collaboration with the social sector and the health sector, and she is author and co-author of scientific articles published in national and international journals and has several publications in national and international conference proceedings.

She also cooperates as a researcher with the research unit on Governance, Competitiveness and Public Policies (GOVCOPP).

# Preface

In 2020, the world was shaken by a very unexpected development, an unseen virus which could kill millions and spread without control. To reduce the impact of the pandemic and before the vaccine was created, lockdown and other safety measures were implemented. In this context, the socio-economic burden of the disease was, in our opinion, a major issue because we always considered that COVID-19 would have a hard impact on human beings and that that impact would be the most prominent effect of the pandemic. In consequence, when designing this Special Issue, we hoped to receive papers with "tales from the field" that would describe the mentioned socio-economic burden. Therefore, it was deeply rewarding to receive so many contributions of very good quality that ended up composing the Special Issue that is reprinted here.

This reprint includes the 11 papers that made the Special Issue on the socio-economic burden of the disease regarding the COVID-19 pandemic, published in the *Healthcare* journal in 2022.

These 11 papers provide a unique set of reflections regarding the pandemic and its consequences and should be read by everybody interested in the topic.

We sincerely thank all the authors and reviewers for the work they produced and we congratulate them for their success. We believe that this reprint of the Special Issue contributes to the understanding of the major consequences of COVID-19 in society. Crucially, the reprint includes papers on global perspectives but also national cases and also sector-specific cases. Finally, we hope the legacy of this volume will be long-lasting and that the papers it contains will be quoted and cited for many years to come.

**Eduardo Tomé, Thomas Garavan, and Ana Dias**
*Editors*

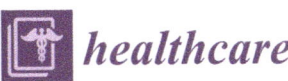

Article

# Regression Analysis for COVID-19 Infections and Deaths Based on Food Access and Health Issues

Abrar Almalki [1,*], Balakrishna Gokaraju [1], Yaa Acquaah [1] and Anish Turlapaty [2]

1. Computational Science and Engineering, North Carolina A&T University, Greensboro, NC 27411, USA; bgokaraju@ncat.edu (B.G.); ytacquaah@aggies.ncat.edu (Y.A.)
2. Department of Electronics and Communication Engineering, Indian Institute of Information Technology, Sri City 517 646, India; anish.turlapaty@iiits.in
* Correspondence: aaalmalki@aggies.ncat.edu

**Abstract:** COVID-19, or SARS-CoV-2, is considered as one of the greatest pandemics in our modern time. It affected people's health, education, employment, the economy, tourism, and transportation systems. It will take a long time to recover from these effects and return people's lives back to normal. The main objective of this study is to investigate the various factors in health and food access, and their spatial correlation and statistical association with COVID-19 spread. The minor aim is to explore regression models on examining COVID-19 spread with these variables. To address these objectives, we are studying the interrelation of various socio-economic factors that would help all humans to better prepare for the next pandemic. One of these critical factors is food access and food distribution as it could be high-risk population density places that are spreading the virus infections. More variables, such as income and people density, would influence the pandemic spread. In this study, we produced the spatial extent of COVID-19 cases with food outlets by using the spatial analysis method of geographic information systems. The methodology consisted of clustering techniques and overlaying the spatial extent mapping of the clusters of food outlets and the infected cases. Post-mapping, we analyzed these clusters' proximity for any spatial variability, correlations between them, and their causal relationships. The quantitative analyses of the health issues and food access areas against COVID-19 infections and deaths were performed using machine learning regression techniques to understand the multi-variate factors. The results indicate a correlation between the dependent variables and independent variables with a Pearson correlation $R^2$-score = 0.44% for COVID-19 cases and $R^2 = 60\%$ for COVID-19 deaths. The regression model with an $R^2$-score of 0.60 would be useful to show the goodness of fit for COVID-19 deaths and the health issues and food access factors.

**Keywords:** COVID-19; GIS; machine learning; regression; North Carolina; Gilford County

## 1. Introduction

An outbreak is announced as a pandemic when it spreads in a large geographical area, infects, and results in mortality for a high number of people, and all of that is caused by a virus that is a subtype of a current virus [1]. The first pandemic recorded was in 1580 [1]. Before 1889, pandemics' patterns show a 50–60-year cycle, while, after 1889, a 10–40-year cycle is shown, with the possibility of shortening [1]. Unfortunately, nothing has been done to change this pandemic pattern in the last century [1].

Research indicates that the current outbreak started to spread between people in late November to December 2019 [2]. On 31 December, 27 cases were recorded of unknown diseases [2]. The recent outbreak was identified on 7 January 2020, a virus called SARS-CoV-2, which is caused by the beta coronavirus and attaches to the lower respiratory census tract [2]. On 18 January, the cases spread around the country regarding the travel for the Chinese Lunar New Year [3]. The government started to lock down the city of

**Citation:** Almalki, A.; Gokaraju, B.; Acquaah, Y.; Turlapaty, A. Regression Analysis for COVID-19 Infections and Deaths Based on Food Access and Health Issues. *Healthcare* **2022**, *10*, 324. https://doi.org/10.3390/healthcare10020324

Academic Editor: Francesco Faita

Received: 24 December 2021
Accepted: 28 January 2022
Published: 8 February 2022

**Publisher's Note:** MDPI stays neutral with regard to jurisdictional claims in published maps and institutional affiliations.

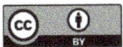

**Copyright:** © 2022 by the authors. Licensee MDPI, Basel, Switzerland. This article is an open access article distributed under the terms and conditions of the Creative Commons Attribution (CC BY) license (https://creativecommons.org/licenses/by/4.0/).

Wuhan, considered as ground zero, and closed all routes to the province [3]. The origin of the cases was connected to visiting the Wuhan's Huanan Seafood market [2]. All the cases were related to traveling from Wuhan until 2 February 2020 [3]. Later, the cases spreaded all over the world and to the United States of America. The first case in the United States was recorded on 20 January 2020 [4]. By October 2021, the United States recorded 44,518,018 total cases and 716,370 total deaths [4].

The Chinese government reacted to the spread of COVID-19 by restricting people's movement, mandatory masks, and monitoring machines [5]. Internationally, the responses included things such as social distancing, vaccines, and disinfecting hands to control the spread [6]. The Center of Disease Control CDC in the United States reacted to the pandemic by advising mask use, requiring negative tests for people to enter the US from a foreign country, and collecting contact information from passengers to minimize incoming infection cases [7]. However, the World Health Organization recommendations of face masks and sanitizer were difficult to enforce in low-income countries in Africa because of poor facilities and low access to equipment [8].

Investigating the factors or variables associated with a pandemic is essential to understand its spread. In the case of this pandemic, investigating the COVID-19 spread in relation to food access distribution, income, population density, health issues, and poverty is associated with future pandemic recovery plans and prevention. Food access would be limited by a stay-at-home order, curfew, and social distance rule. At the same time, population density or human traffic in public places, such as food outlets, would increase the chance of infection. Food access in urban areas is a critical factor for human survival. Equal distribution of food outlets supports healthy and active life in communities, while unequal distribution may have a negative impact on people's health and result in a higher incidence of diabetes and other health risks. Analyzing food distribution is a multi-variate problem as it depends on various factors of influence ranging from income to demography [9]. More variables, such as income levels, affect people's ability to buy food and access transportation for takeout. Health issues and chronic diseases may be affected by the pandemic conditions and the consequences associated with weakened immunity and infections.

A healthy life and well-being are some of the United Nations goals and strategies, especially the Sustainable Development Goals SDG 3.3, which aims to end pandemics by 2030 [3]. However, the spread of a new virus threatens this goal [3] because this pandemic is not the first and will not be the last, and the frequency of these pandemics might increase as influenza mutates every cold season to form a new strain. Investigating the current stage of the pandemic and its adverse effects helps us as humans to prepare for future pandemics.

## 2. Literature Review

Scientists have documented outbreaks and pandemics and analyzed them to limit their negative influence. Previous pandemics, such as malaria and H1N1, affected human health and life. In a study by Malik & Abdalla, they mapped the spread of H1N1 by using spatiotemporal analysis. The study analyzed the spatial spread and spatial–temporal distribution with the factors of population density and international flights from Mexico [10]. The second study indicates the use of spatiotemporal analysis to map the H1N1 outbreak [11]. The study found that the virus infections did not spread much as clusters between the first and third weeks but increased to larger clusters in the sixth week [12]. These clusters started to converge further from week six to eighteen, and then started to decline in week 22 [12]. There have been some studies on pre-existing health risks and their susceptibility to higher infection rates during epidemics. One study presented the effect of obesity on influenza infection duration and concluded that obesity extended the shedding duration by 42% for influenza and by 43% for influenza-H1N1 [13].

Since COVID-19 was announced as a pandemic on March 11 2020, scientists started to study and analyze the spread of the virus and its associated factors. Several studies focused on the global scale, while other studies investigated smaller scales and examined specific variables' correlation to COVID-19 [14]. In a study, the authors presented the sectors that were disrupted globally, namely: tourism, restaurants, leisure, entertainment, travel, sports, etc. [15]. Another study presented the comparison between developed and developing countries, where increased COVID-19 cases and deaths were present in developed countries compared to developing countries [14].

Pandemic spread and prediction could be analyzed by several methods, including the Geographic Information System (GIS) and machine learning (ML). The GIS is an effective tool for visualizing the spread of cases with spatial reference maps, time, location, and other overlaying techniques. The role of GIS is clear in mapping cases, mapping case clusters, mapping the outbreak spread, and helping decision-makers act [16]. The geospatial analysis of GIS on COVID-19 was mostly on five topics, which are spatial–temporal analysis, health and social geography, environmental variables, data mining, and web-based mapping [17]. As an example, GIS can be used for dashboard tracing, which was applied for the first time at John Hopkins University [18]. Another use of GIS was applied by the World Health Organization to illustrate confirmed cases and deaths [9]. More examples are in the HealthMap by the Boston Children's Hospital, USA [19]. A study proved the effectiveness of ML models on outbreak predictions by applying multi-layered perceptron MLP and Adaptive Network-based Fuzzy Inference System ANFIS [20].

Currently, GIS is a useful tool for mapping cases and deaths, spreading, and predicting the future spread for health authorities regarding taking necessary and precise action on future outbreaks. The use of GIS is critical during the pandemic and post-pandemic for policymakers to make decisions on developing surveillance tracking systems for controlling and preventing future pandemics [18]. South Korea shows the best example of creating a web-GIS tracking for its pandemic tracking system by tracing cases and highly infected sites [21]. The application of the GIS into the South Korean method provided a decision-making tool on updated tracking and predicted the needed procedures [22]. Given this orientation, another study investigated the outbreak spree by applying the five GIS model sizes in the United States [23]. It investigated the differences in using different size modeling from local to global and applied those methods on four variables, black female populations, income, household income, and percentage of nurse practitioners [23].

More tools on the analysis of COVID-19 cases and spreads included statistical regression models. These models have been used to investigate the fluctuation in cases and then connect that to variables. A study presented the investigation in Germany on the spike and decrease in COVID-19 cases in the first two months of the pandemic and found increases and decreases in cases, and these changes on carve may be by variables that need to be studied [24]. More investigation on the correlation of COVID-19 with other variables, such as health issues, is critical around the world. The importance of cholesterol and its relation to the virus entering human cells is illustrated in a study, and lower cholesterol helps clear the virus sooner and limit infections [25]. High blood pressure recorded a correlation with a reduction in lung function [26].

The correlation of COVID-19 with variables has been investigated by several regression models as an efficient method. More specifically, research on the correlation with health issues has been applied and presents a correlation to various health issues. A multivariable linear regression analysis on global data of COVID-19 cases and deaths recorded a high correlation of cases and deaths with high cholesterol and high body mass [14]. Moreover, the correlation is stronger in the younger population [14]. An analysis in the United Kingdom on people's body mass and COVID-19 hospitalization by applying logistic regression demonstrated higher hospitalization for people with obesity [27]. Further, a study conducted by penalized logistic regression models proved that hypertension illustrates a correlation to COVID-19 cases and mortality [28]. Nevertheless, moderate blood pressure is considered a dramatic factor in patient survival and limiting organ damage [28]. COVID-19 affects people's health, and that effect may be more severe on people with health conditions. A study presented a regression analysis on patients' clearance after being affected with COVID-19 and concluded that more days are recorded for people suffering from high cholesterol and diabetes [29]. Additionally, a study presented a positive correlation between COVID-19 and population density in India by computational correlation coefficient models [30].

The analysis of the geographical spread of a virus provides a tool for decision-making and long-term management for outbreaks [21]. Mapping the data based on normality would show a visualization, followed by normalizing data, such as showing the percentage based on every 100,000 people [31]. A recent study on the environmental effects of COVID-19 spread took place in China to analyze the effects of temperature and humidity [3]. The results illustrated the relationship between infected cases and weather, where low humidity supported the suitability and spread of the virus [24]. Moreover, strong cases showed a temperature range of 10 °C to 20 °C [3]. Furthermore, a higher number of cases were shown in economically developed cities, such as Beijing, and lower cases in less developed cities, such as Lhasa, which could be due to air pollution, geographical location, or population density [3]. Moreover, a study in Malaysia discussed that tourism was affected badly by the outbreak and, in turn, affected the economy and financial development [32].

Additional variables, such as income, were investigated in various geographical locations. An investigation in Spain demonstrated the negative correlation of the mean income to COVID-19 cases spread, where more cases spread in lower mean income districts because of low access to health care, lack of awareness, and poverty rates [33]. More specifically, low median income districts had 2.5 times higher cases than higher than mean income districts in Spain [33]. More studies presented the correlation of income to COVID-19 cases and deaths and its influence on food security. For instance, researchers in Kenya analyzed surveys on COVID-19 influence and concluded that low-income households that depend on labor jobs are more vulnerable to food insecurity due to financial shock [34]. More specifically, during the pandemic, people in low-income neighborhoods spent more time at work than those in high-income neighborhoods due to labor shortages [35].

COVID-19 has a long-term influence on food security and impacted a population increase of 17 million Americans in 2020 compared to 2018 [36]. Despite the increase in food insecurity, the pandemic has had a dramatic influence on the increase in children classified as having food insecurity by 3% more in 2020 than in 2017 [37]. Hence, the U.S government increased the free food programs in nation-wide K–12 public schools.

In Brazilian data studies, the investigations found a positive correlation to different socio-economic variables, such as population density, and negative correlation to social isolation rates, which proves the importance of social distancing enforcement [38]. Another investigation was done in India by statistical analysis called Pearson's correlation coefficient [39]. A positive correlation between people density and COVID-19 cases was presented in five states. A statistical analysis recorded a correlation of COVID-19 with the number of tests and population density [39]. More variables, such as public transportation, were investigated for the correlation to COVID-19 cases and deaths. A statistical analysis recorded a correlation of COVID-19 with the number of tests and population density [40]. Regarding another study, a positive correlation was presented between public transportation sites, such as airports and train stations, and COVID-19 cases, in which the people living less than 25 miles from transportation spots showed higher cases than people living more than 50 miles away [41]. This was further supported by another study on the spatial distribution of COVID-19 cases in China, describing the possibility of transportation influence on the spread between neighborhoods [42].

The demographic variables were also investigated in several studies. A study that took place in the United States analyzed the cases and death numbers of COVID-19 and concluded that African Americans have the highest rates because of their low income, low access to transportation, and the high rate of chronic diseases, such as diabetes and obesity [43]. Also, the study recorded the vulnerability of the Hispanic community on the age of to the pandemic because of their high uninsured status rate, high chronic diseases, language barrier, and their immigration status [10].

Researchers indicate that there is a lack of application of GIS on pandemic spreads and more application is needed [12]. There is a need for more GIS analysis on the outbreak with different variables. Further research is needed to investigate more variables, such as food access, in the United States [11]. The proposed study illustrates the investigation of the spatial distribution of COVID-19 cases and deaths in Guilford County and examines the possibility of correlation with specific variables in food access and health risks. This study investigates variables such as health issues, income, food outlets and access areas, population density, and poverty rates. This study is applying technology by exploring machine learning models' efficiency to analyze the pandemic distribution.

The research questions in this study are:

1. Is it possible that COVID-19 cases and deaths in geospatial distribution are associated with food outlets and restaurants distribution?
2. Can other variables illustrate a geospatial correlation with COVID-19 cases and deaths?
3. How can machine learning discover a higher quantitative statistical correlation of COVID-19 cases and deaths against various independent variables?
4. Do the machine learning results concur with the GIS regression results?

Our contributions in this study are:

1. Investigated the geospatial association of COVID-19 cases and deaths to food outlets distribution
2. Examined the dependency of various socio-economic and health risk variables on COVID-19 cases and deaths
3. Applied ML techniques to investigate the statistical association between COVID-19 cases and deaths to other variables

## 3. Study Area and Materials

This study took place in Guilford County (Figure 1) in the state of North Carolina, with an area of 645.70 square miles and a population of 537,174 [44]. The county population consisted of 35.4% black, 49.4% is white, 5.3% Asian, 8.4% Hispanic, and 1.5% other [44]. The county took steps to maintain people's health and wellness. Mandatory face masks were officially announced starting from 5 PM on Jun 26, 2020 [45]. Guilford County issued a "stay at home" order for transportation on April 17, 2020 [46]. In June, the county announced 5 testing sites spread around the county [46]. The county has three zip code areas with a high cluster of cases, and they are 27,405, 27,407, and 27,406 [47]. By October 14, 2021, North Carolina recorded 1,436,699 total cases [4]. The datasets were obtained from the health department in Guilford County.

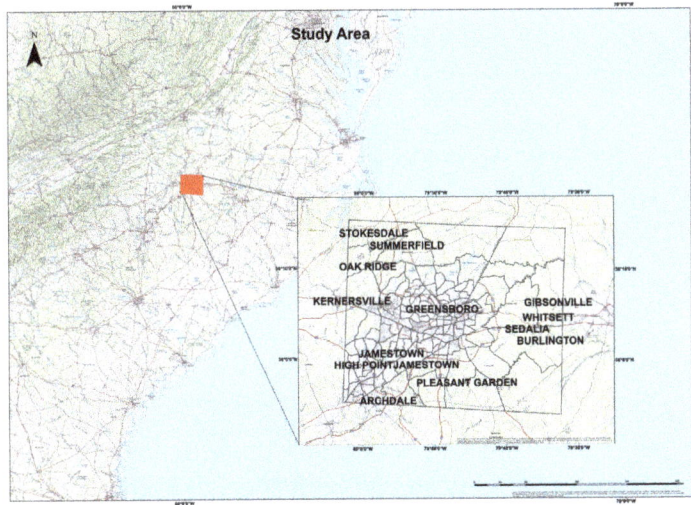

**Figure 1.** Study area.

## 4. Methods and Results

This study adopted a spatial-based and machine learning regression method to analyze the correlation between COVID-19 cases, deaths, and independent variables. The spatial method was applied to analyze the correlation and to present it visually on maps with variation of correlation degree. ML regression model is a strong tool that could be used for different topics and purposes, and the cause and analysis is one of them. Moreover, applying several models to compare results is important to find the most suitable model for this study and document it. In this study, the authors used ArcGIS-ArcMap software version 10.3 for GIS analysis and Jupiter software to apply the regression analysis. The method (Figure 2) applied used GIS tools for spatial and Sci-Kit Learn software libraries for machine learning regression, respectively. The GIS regression methods applied four models: the scatterplot matrix graph, spatial autocorrelation (Moran's I), ordinary least squares (OLS), and the geographically weighted regression. The ML regression method applied four models, and they are linear multioutput regression, K-nearest neighbors of multioutput regression, random forest of multioutput regression, and support vector regression. These models were applied to analyze the correlation between dependent (COVID-19 cases and deaths) and independent variables (med-income, poverty rate, population density, high blood pressure, high cholesterol, obesity, number of healthy food outlets, and number of healthy food outlets).

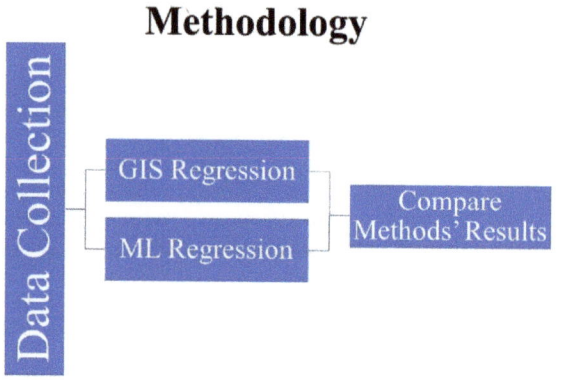

**Figure 2.** Methodology graph.

*4.1. GIS Methods*

These maps in Figures 3 and 4 present the COVID-19 cases and deaths. In Figure 3, higher numbers of cases are presented in dark blue color. The lowest COVID-19 infections are in the downtown of Greensboro, where it has fewer residential homes than businesses, and the highest are located outside of Greensboro in Summerfield, Gibsonville, Sedalia, Burlington, and Pleasant Garden. In Figure 4, the highest numbers of deaths are ranging between 22 and 33 per each census tract, displayed in blue color, and the lowest numbers of deaths are given 0 to 3 per each census tract in yellow color. The COVID-19 deaths low numbers are reported in Greensboro and the high mortality reported out of the city. An observation from this distribution could be about people's education and the mask enforcement in large stores or offices. After that, scatterplot matrix graph in Figure 5 presents the interaction between COVID-19 cases and independent variables. The graph illustrates some positive and negative correlations and no correlation. Positive correlations include obesity with poverty and high blood pressure. Negative correlation is presented between obesity and med-income variables. However, there is no apparent strong correlation observed between COVID-19 cases and other variables through this scatter matrix visualization.

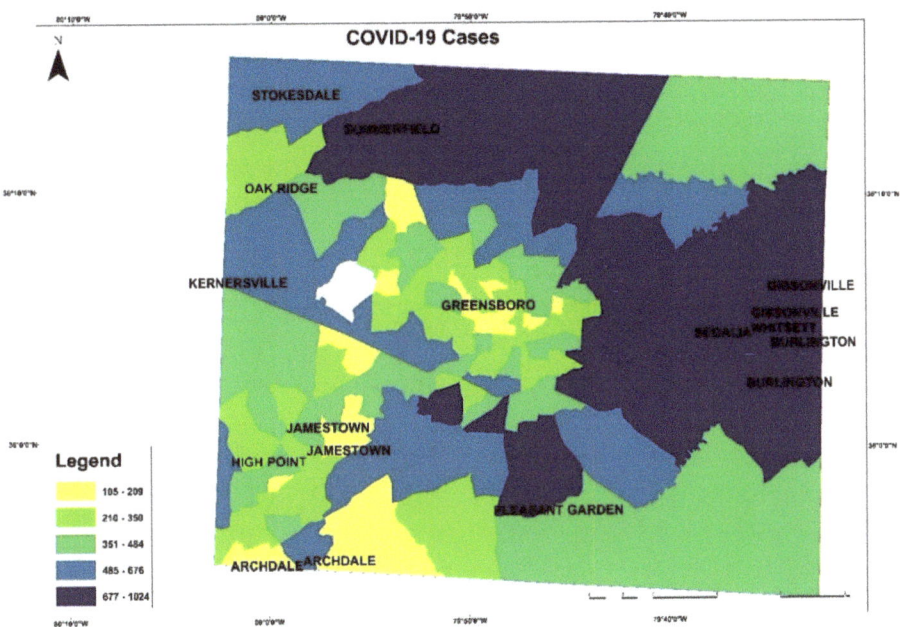

Figure 3. COVID-19 cases in Guilford County.

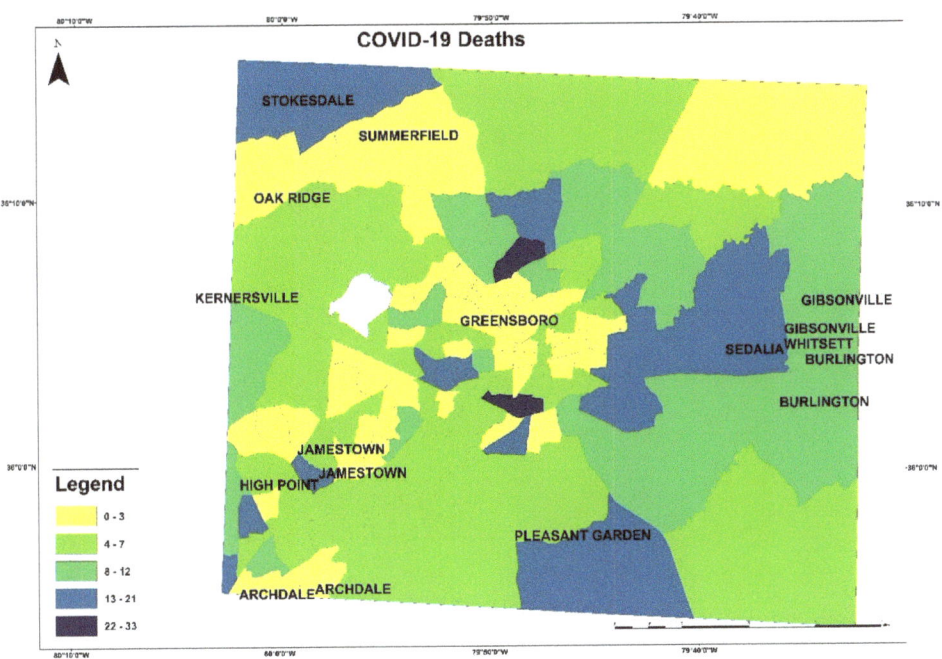

Figure 4. COVID-19 deaths distribution.

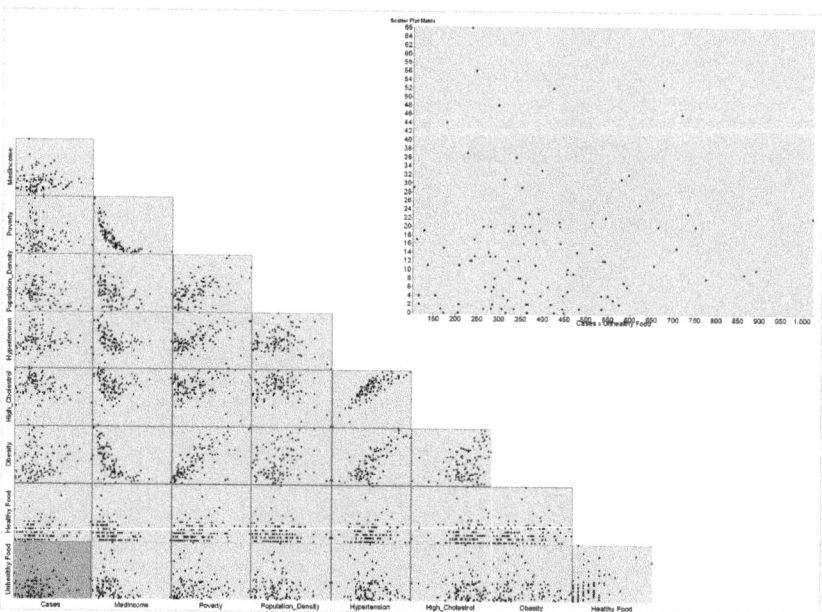

**Figure 5.** Scatterplot matrix graph using cases as dependent variable.

The scatterplot matrix graph is also applied to COVID-19 deaths as a dependent variable. The graph (Figure 6) also presents no correlation between COVID-19 deaths and variables. Negative correlations are presented between med-income and poverty and obesity.

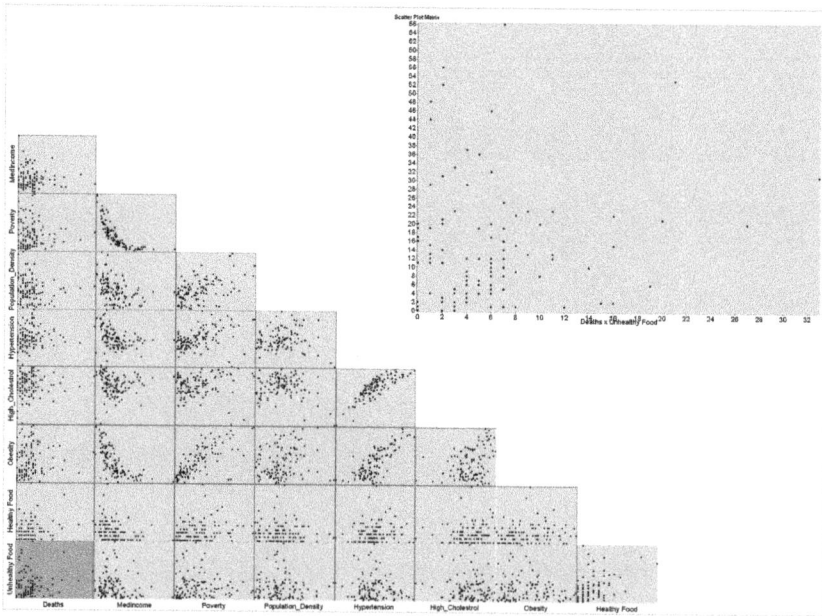

**Figure 6.** Scatterplot matrix graph using deaths as dependent variable.

After that, we applied the spatial autocorrelation (Moran's I) to find the cluster of cases and deaths on some census tracts. The spatial autocorrelation is applied by this equation:

$$I = \frac{n}{S_0} \frac{\sum_{i=1}^{n} \sum_{j=1}^{n} W_{i.j} Z_i Z_j}{\sum_{i=1}^{n} Z_i^2} \qquad (1)$$

In Equation (1) $Z_i$ is the deviation of an attribute for feature $i$ from its mean ($X_i - \overline{X}$). The $W_{i.j}$ is the spatial weight between feature $I$ and $j$, and $n$ is equal to the total number of features. The $S_0$ is the aggregate of all spatial weight. After applying the equation, results are presented in Figures 7 and 8. Figure 7 illustrates that COVID-19 cases are significantly clustered in Guilford County, which means there is high dependency of output and independent input variables.

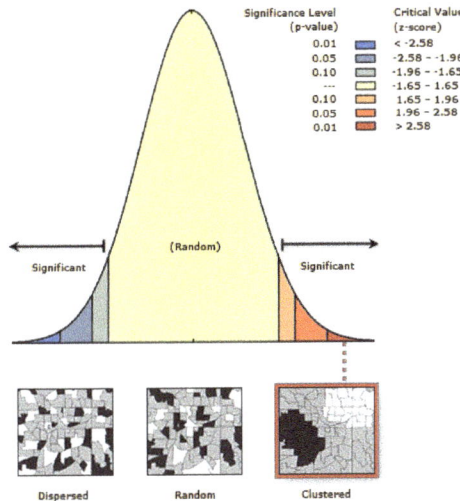

**Figure 7.** Spatial autocorrelation for COVID-19 cases.

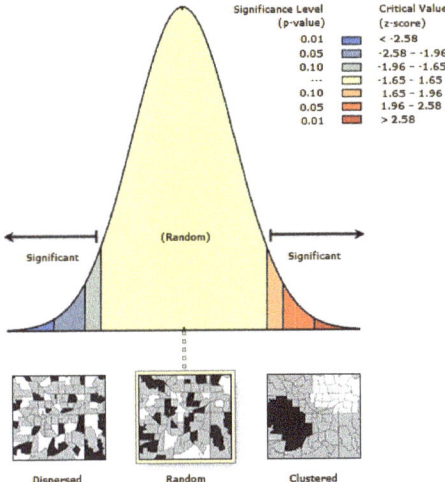

**Figure 8.** Spatial autocorrelation for COVID-19 deaths.

In Figure 8, the spatial autocorrelation concluded that the cluster of COVID-19 deaths is a result of random chance, which encourages the investigation further on different variables. The Moran's summary of COVID-19 cases and deaths by the Moran's I spatial autocorrelation is in Table 1 below.

**Table 1.** OLS results for COVID-19 cases and deaths.

| Measures | COVID-19 Cases | COVID-19 Deaths |
| --- | --- | --- |
| Moran's Index | 0.118617 | 0.005965 |
| Expected Index | −0.009259 | −0.009259 |
| Variance | 0.000575 | 0.000551 |
| Z-score | 5.3314423 | 6.48788 |
| *p*-value | 0.000000 | 0.516475 |

Next, local Moran's was applied based on this formula:

$$I_i = \frac{X_i - \overline{X}}{S_i^2} \sum_{j=1, j \neq i}^{n} w_{i.j}(x_j - \overline{X}) \qquad (2)$$

In Equation (2), $n$ is the total number of features, and $X_i$ is the attribute for feature $i$. Moreover, $w_{i.j}$ is the spatial weight between feature $i$ and $j$. The output of this equation is presented in Figures 9 and 10. Figure 9, the local Moran's on COVID-19 cases, presents tracts with high case numbers and its correlation with a high number and percentage of variables in the south of Greensboro and east of Guilford County. The pink patch represents high cases of COVID-19 with an increase in variables. The red patch represents high cases and low variables correlation. The blue patch illustrates tract with low cases number with low variables in Greensboro downtown. In Figure 10, the local Moran's on COVID-19 deaths is presented with the correlation of variables in each tract. The red patch represents high mortality with low correlation with variables, and the pink patch represents high mortality number with high variables in the north of Greensboro.

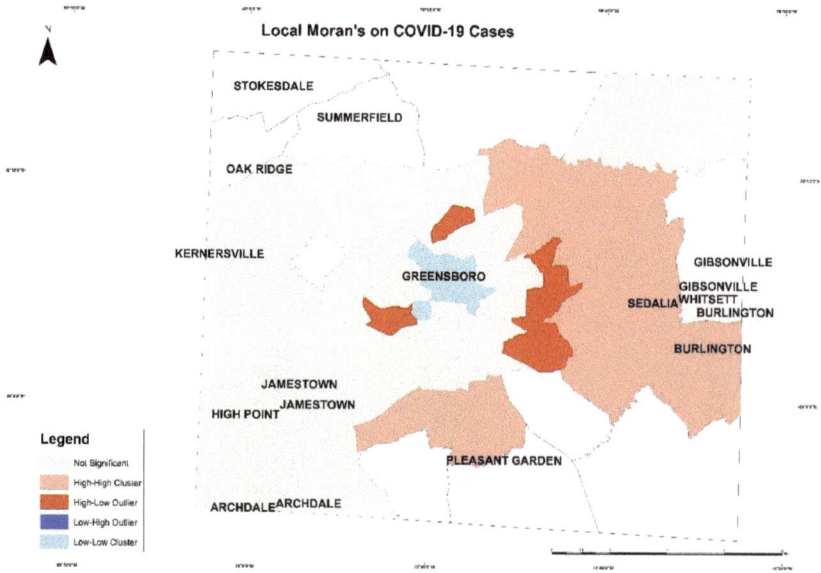

**Figure 9.** The local Moran's on COVID-19 cases in Guilford County.

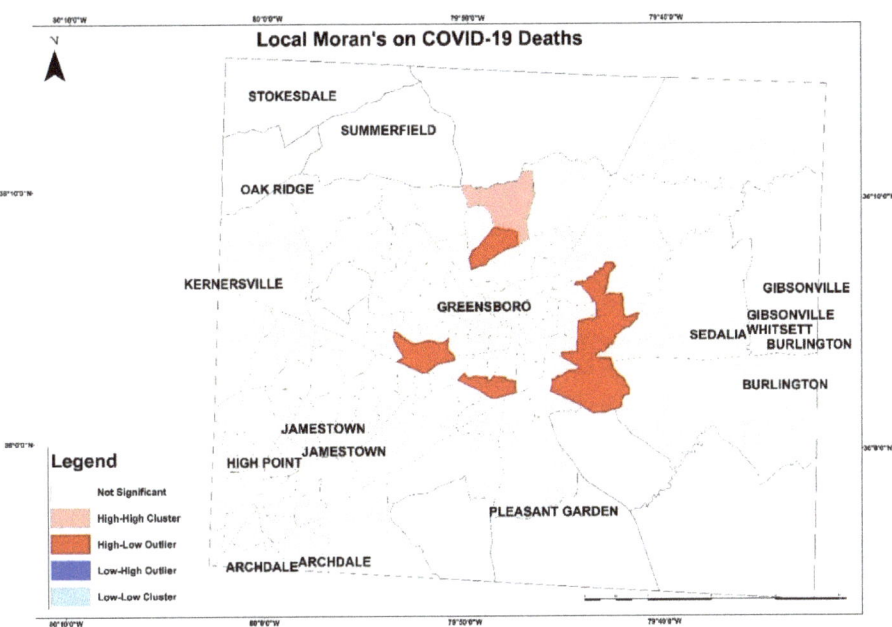

**Figure 10.** The local Moran's on COVID-19 deaths in Guilford County.

Then, OLS was applied to examine dependent and independent variables. OLS is a linear regression to perform a prediction or detect relationship between dependent and independent variables. We examine COVID-19 cases as a dependent variable with all independent variables. This OLS model uses the equation below:

$$Y = \beta_0 + \beta_1 X_1 + \beta_2 X_2 + \beta_n X_n + \varepsilon \qquad (3)$$

where Y is the dependent variables, β is coefficients, X is explanatory or independent variables, and ε is random error. In Figure 11, red patches represent areas with higher COVID-19 cases than the model predicted, and the blue shaded census tracts illustrate areas with lower COVID-19 cases than the model expected. In this model, the multiple R square was 0.358946, and the adjusted R-square was 0.307662. The Akaike's information criterion (AICc) was 1412.247528. The joint F-statistic was 0.000000, which was a significant result. The Jarque–Bera statistic [g] was 1.511785, which indicates that the independent variables have an influence on the dependent variable. The joint Wald statistic [e] was significant and computed as 0.000000. The Keonker (BP) statistics, which determine if the independent variables have a consistent relationship to the dependent variable, was 0.009854, also significant, but the relationship is not consistent.

In Figure 12, red patches represent areas with higher COVID-19 deaths than the model predicted, and the blue shaded illustrates areas with lower COVID-19 deaths than the model predicted. In this model, the multiple R square was 0.159614, and the adjusted R-square was 0.092383. The Akaike's information criterion (AICc) was 685.908921. Joint F-statistic was 0.021994, which was a significant result. The joint Wald statistic [e] was 0.000000 as a significant result. The Keonker (BP) statistics determine if the independent variables have a consistent relationship to the dependent variable, and it was 0.388493, which was not significant. The Jarque–Bera statistic [g] was 0.000000, which is significant and means the model is biased and needs further investigation.

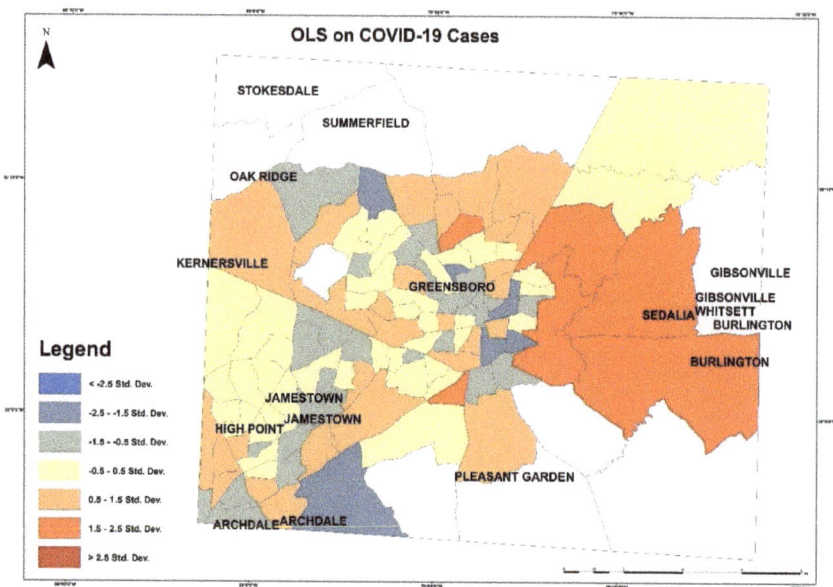

**Figure 11.** OLS on COVID-19 cases in Guilford County.

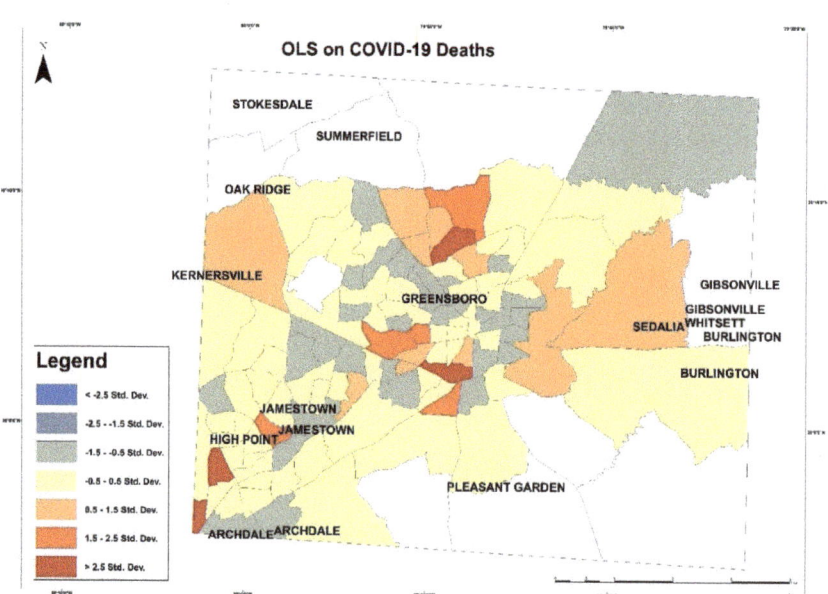

**Figure 12.** OLS on COVID-19 deaths in Guilford County.

Based on the independent variables' coefficient of the OLS, variables with higher coefficients than 7.5 will be applied in the GWR. These variables are high cholesterol, high blood pressure, and healthy food outlets. In Figures 13 and 14 GWRs were applied on COVID-19 cases and deaths to visualize the correlation with independent variables by applying this equation:

$$y = \mathcal{B}_0 + \mathcal{B}_1 x + \mathcal{E} \qquad (4)$$

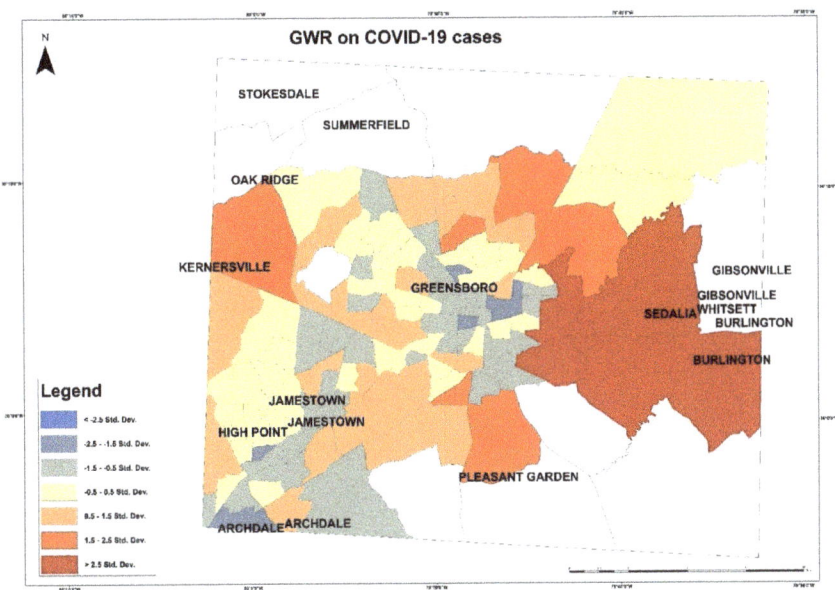

**Figure 13.** Geographically weighted regression on COVID-19 cases.

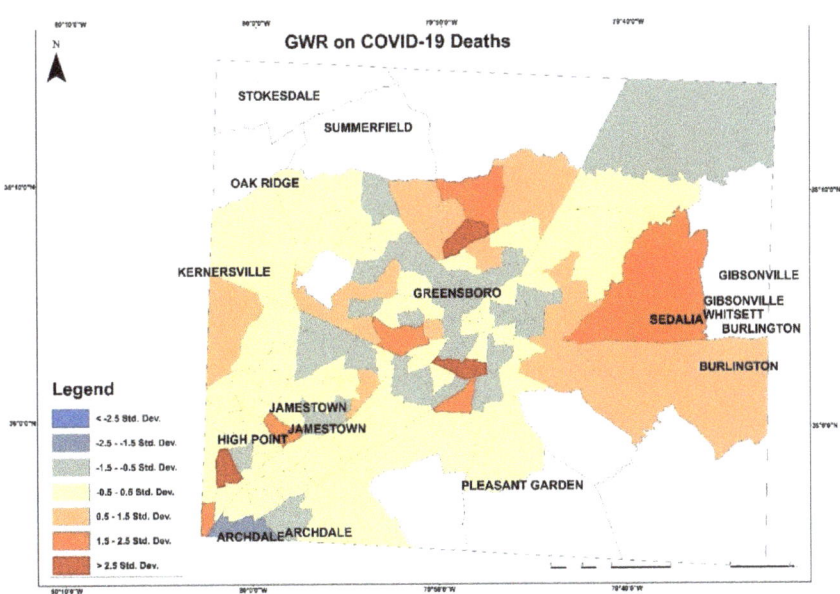

**Figure 14.** Geographically weighted regression on COVID-19 deaths.

In this equation above, the coefficient $\beta_1$ illustrates the increase in y because of one-unit increase in $x$. This map shows less tract with high correlation and more with medium correlation. In Figure 13, the map presents the correlation between the dependent and independent variables. Red patches, which represent high correlation, are in east of Gilford County in the tracts 012803, 015300, and 017200. In Figure 14, the map presents the correlation of COVID-19 deaths with variables (high cholesterol, high blood pressure, and health food outlets) and presents correlation degrees in color shades. The highest correlation of COVID-19 deaths with the variables is presented on the tracts 015703, 012604, and 013700.

*4.2. ML Regression Results and Discussion*

This study adopted machine learning techniques to investigate the correlation by applying both linear and nonlinear regression models. Linear, multi-output linear, random forest, and K-nearest neighborhood regression models were applied to investigate the data. All models investigate all variables at the same time, but linear regression investigates single output at a time. These four models were applied to evaluate their results. These models are predicting the values of the dependent variables, such as COVID-19 cases and COVID-19 deaths, with the correlation of independent variables of med-income, poverty rate, population density, number of healthy food outlets, and number of un-healthy food outlets. The dataset was divided into 80% training and 20% testing for multioutput model development. The training set contained eighty-seven (87) observations and twenty-two (22) observations in the testing set, and two different metrics: root mean square (RMS) and R-squared ($R^2$), which were used to evaluate the models developed. The implementation of multioutput and multiple linear regression models were done with the Sklearn package in Python and MATLAB 2020a, respectively. The default parameters for the multioutput regression models were used in Table 2.

Table 2. Regression models' parameters.

| Model | Parameters |
| --- | --- |
| Linear Regression Model | copy_X = True,fit_intercept = True,n_jobs = None,normalize = False. |
| Random Forest Regression Model | bootstrap = True,ccp_alpha = 0.0,critrion = 'mse',max_depth = None,max_features = 'ato',max_leaf_nodes = None,max_saples = None,min_impurity_decrease = 0.0,min_imprity_split = None,min_samples_leaf = 1,min_samples_split = 2,min_weight_fraction_leaf = 0.0,n_estimtors = 100,n_jobs = None,oob_score = False,random_state = None,verbose = 0, warm_start = False) |
| K-Nearest Neighbor Regression Model | lgorithm':'auto','leaf_size':30,'metric':'minkowski','metric_params': None, 'n_jobs': None,'n_neighbors': 5, 'p': 2, 'weights': 'uniform' |

The equation below is derived in the linear regression model. In the equation, coefficients of variables were computed based on the linear regression model.

$$Y = 0.53 + 0.194 \times 1 - 0.251X_2 + 0.887X_3 - 0.915X_4 - 0.0996X_5 + 0.315X_6 - 0.026X_7 \quad (5)$$

The degree of linear association between all variables is computed by the Pearson correlation coefficient ($R^2$)-scores in the correlation matrix heatmap format in Figure 15. The results could be read in three directions: R values close to 1 show a positive relationship, and R values close to −1 illustrate negative relationships, but results close to zero have no linear relationships. It can be observed in the heatmap (Figure 13) that there is a positive correlation between obesity and poverty ($R^2$ = 0.74). There is a high positive correlation between high cholesterol and high blood pressure ($R^2$ = 0.82). Furthermore, there is a positive correlation between obesity and high blood pressure ($R^2$ = 0.77). Moreover, there is a strong negative correlation between obesity and med-income ($R^2$ = −0.7), and a negative correlation between income and poverty ($R^2$ = −0.75). There is no correlation between COVID-19 cases and health issues (obesity, high cholesterol, and high blood pressure). Moreover, there is no correlation between unhealthy food outlets, healthy food outlets, and health issues.

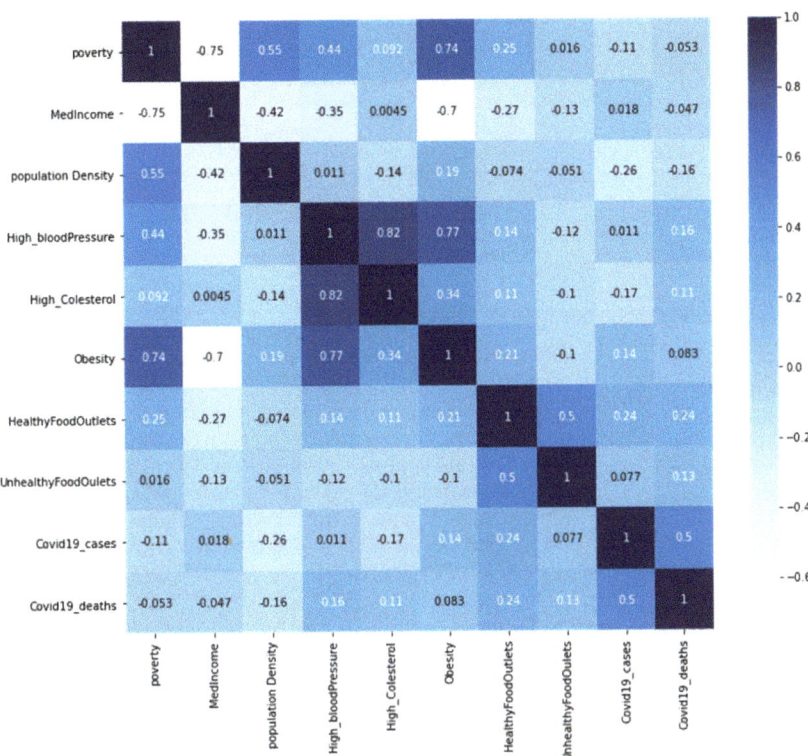

**Figure 15.** Correlation matrix with heatmap.

From the tables' results below (Tables 3 and 4), the authors applied and compared the regression models results. The COVID-19 cases as a dependent variable have the highest value of $R^2$-score as 45% by the application of linear regression for multioutput regression model, and COVID-19 deaths had a higher value of 60% by the application of support vector regression model. The high correlation $R^2$-scores of COVID-19 deaths and variables were also presented by the GIS spatial autocorrelation as clustered distribution in Figure 7. These regression models' results indicate that independent variables (med-income, poverty rate, population density, number of healthy food outlets, and number of unhealthy food outlets) have more influence on the dependent variable COVID-19 deaths than COVID cases.

**Table 3.** R-square value of regression models.

| | Root Mean Square Error | |
|---|---|---|
| Models | CVID-19 Cases | COVID-19 Deaths |
| Linear regression for multioutput Regression | 0.146 | 0.141 |
| K-nearest neighbors for multioutput regression | 0.208 | 0.147 |
| Random forest for multioutput regression | 0.186 | 0.175 |
| Support Vector Regression | 0.168 | 0.127 |

**Table 4.** Root square error (RMSE) values of regression models.

| Models | Correlation Coefficient | |
|---|---|---|
| | CVID-19 Cases | COVID-19 Deaths |
| Linear regression for multioutput regression | 0.446 | 0.508 |
| K-nearest neighbors for multioutput regression | −0.085 | 0.466 |
| Random forest for multioutput regression | 0.137 | 0.239 |
| Support Vector Regression | 0.290 | 0.601 |

The application of the multiple linear regression models considered the two dependent variables (COVID-19 cases and deaths). The support vector regression model was applied to examine all the data and errors within the threshold. In Figure 16, the predicted trends for dependent variable COVID-19 deaths are presented against the original trend values. Both trends, match the peaks and troughs well overall, showing similar behavior. However, the residual errors seem to vary both on the positive and negative side of the trend. The test data are kept out of the sample. The significance of Figure 11 is that the prediction trend is matching the peaks and troughs present in the original trend of number of COVID cases well (ground-truth). There are still many residual gaps between the original and predicted values, but the trend was predicted well overall. This figure coincides well with the $R^2$-coefficient of 0.60 for number of COVID-19 deaths.

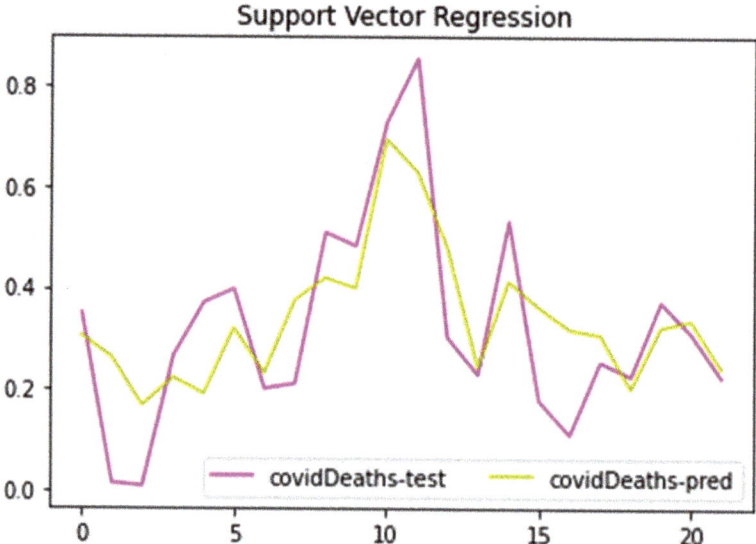

**Figure 16.** Support vector regression model.

## 5. Conclusions

This study implemented GIS and machine learning techniques on COVID-19 data in 109 census tracts in Guilford County to investigate any correlation between the spread of the pandemic and social–economic, food access, and health issues variables. The GIS and machine learning methods were applied to examine the datasets and compare their results regarding if they are equivalent or different.

The GIS results illustrate the distribution of the variables where COVID-19 cases have a cluster in Guilford County, while COVID-19 deaths have no cluster. The cases cluster was biased and indicated more investigation of independent variables. COVID-19 deaths presented a *p*-value at 0.00000, which indicates a 99% confidence that independent dose had no influence on the distribution. Moreover, the COVID-19 infection cases $p$-value result was 0.516475, and that indicates less than 90% confidence that independent variables do not influence the distribution. The OLS results did not a indicate high influence of the independent variables on the dependents. The R-square of the influence of the independent variables on COVID-19 cases is only 35%. It also indicated only 9% on COVID-19 deaths. These percentages are low, and we suggest more investigation and including more variables.

The application of four spatial regression models indicates some influence on the independent variables. The heat map presented a weak correlation between the dependent and independent variables. There was a positive but not strong correlation between the dependent variables COVID-19 cases and deaths, which means deaths increase where cases are high. However, there were several strong negative correlations between income and two variables (poverty and obesity), but there was a positive correlation between poverty and obesity. More correlations between the independent variables are clear in a positive correlation of high blood pressure with obesity and high cholesterol. These independent variables do not show direct impacts on the dependent variables, but they affect people's health, which could make them control variables. For example, poverty led to unhealthy diet, which affects people's immune system, and the presence of two health issues in a community makes them more vulnerable to health issues and risks. The highest R-square for COVID-19 cases was 60% by support vector regression and for COVID-19 death; the highest R-square was 44% by the linear regression for multioutput regression. These numbers are not high for correlation, which indicates an unclear influence of the independent variables on the dependent variables.

The machine learning results take the same direction as the GIS results, correlation between variables or independent variables. The study illustrates the need for future investigation on the spread of COVID-19 infections and deaths in Guilford County. Further study may include the distribution of more health issues, such as autoimmune diseases, to investigate more correlations to COVID-19 infections. Further analysis would require more datasets or a larger geographical scale.

In future, this study would examine several variables exclusively independent in the regression model and investigate the feature engineering in machine learning to increase the $R^2$-score. Other independent variables would be related to the distribution of health centers, religion, and public transportation stops and routes. These data could be obtained from the transportation department and state health department. This study has a data limitation. The study area has 118 census tracts but only 107 census tracts had all the data variables recorded. That affected the results because more data would show more correlation and distribution analysis. More data would provide a clearer picture of the analysis to examine the issues on a state level, which includes many counties, and to analyze patterns and compare the counties.

**Author Contributions:** Conceptualization, B.G. and A.A.; methodology, A.A., Y.A. and B.G.; software, Y.A. and A.A.; validation, B.G.; formal analysis, A.A. and Y.A.; investigation, A.A.; resources, B.G.; data curation, B.G., A.A., B.G., and Y.A.; writing—original draft preparation, A.A.; writing—review and editing, A.A., B.G. and A.T.; visualization, A.A, Y.A.; supervision, B.G.; project administration, A.A. and B.G.; funding acquisition, A.A., B.G. All authors have read and agreed to the published version of the manuscript.

**Funding:** This research is sponsored by North Carolina Dept. of Environmental Quality, (NCDEQ), Center for Energy Research and Technology (CERT), Visualization and Computation Advancing Research Center (ViCAR), and Computational Data Science and Engineering Department at NC A&T State University.

**Informed Consent Statement:** Not applicable.

**Data Availability Statement:** Data such as income and food access were downloaded from the USDA Food Desert Locator Map website at https://www.ers.usda.gov/data-products/food-access-research-atlas/go-to-the-atlas.aspx (accessed on 28 October 2019).

**Acknowledgments:** We thank King Abdulaziz University for the financial support of the first author's degree. We thank Mark Smith from the Health Department in Guilford County, Greensboro, NC for providing the preliminary datasets on health statistical records and other data. The authors also sincerely acknowledge the Health Surveillance and Analysis Unit of the Guilford County Department of Health and Human Services, Division of Public Health as a source as well as the NC Electronic Disease Surveillance System (NC EDSS) of NC DHHS for providing datasets.

**Conflicts of Interest:** The authors declare no conflict of interest.

## References

1. Potter, C.W. A history of influenza. *J. Appl. Microbiol.* **2001**, *91*, 572–579. [CrossRef] [PubMed]
2. Sohrabi, C.; Alsafi, Z.; O'Neill, N.; Khan, M.; Kerwan, A.; Al-Jabir, A.; Agha, R. World Health Organization declares global emergency: A review of the 2019 novel coronavirus (COVID-19). *Int. J. Surgery* **2020**, *76*, 71–76. [CrossRef] [PubMed]
3. Xu, H.; Yan, C.; Fu, Q.; Xiao, K.; Yu, Y.; Han, D.; Wang, W.; Cheng, J. Possible environmental effects on the spread of COVID-19 in China. *Sci. Total Environ.* **2020**, *731*, 139211. [CrossRef] [PubMed]
4. "COVID Data Tracker". Centers for Disease Control And Prevention, 2021. Available online: https://covid.cdc.gov/covid-data-tracker/?CDC_AA_refVal=https%3A%2F%2Fwww.cdc.gov%2Fcoronavirus%2F2019-ncov%2Fcases-updates%2Fcases-in-us.html#cases_casesper100klast7days (accessed on 1 December 2021).
5. Bo, W.; Ahmad, Z.; Alanzi, A.R.; Al-Omari, A.I.; Hafez, E.; Abdelwahab, S.F. The current COVID-19 pandemic in China: An overview and corona data analysis. *Alex. Eng. J.* **2021**, *61*, 1369–1381. [CrossRef]
6. Pan, L.; Wang, J.; Wang, X.; Ji, J.S.; Ye, D.; Shen, J.; Li, L.; Liu, H.; Zhang, L.; Shi, X.; et al. Prevention and control of coronavirus disease 2019 (COVID-19) in public places. *Environ. Pollut.* **2021**, *292*, 118273. [CrossRef] [PubMed]
7. Centers for Disease Control and Prevention. CDC COVID-19 Global Response. 2022. Available online: https://www.cdc.gov/ (accessed on 23 January 2022).
8. Donde, O.O.; Atoni, E.; Muia, A.W.; Yillia, P.T. COVID-19 pandemic: Water, sanitation and hygiene (WASH) as a critical control measure remains a major challenge in low-income countries. *Water Res.* **2021**, *191*, 116793. [CrossRef] [PubMed]
9. Almalki, A.; Gokaraju, B.; Mehta, N.; Doss, D.A. Geospatial and Machine Learning Regression Techniques for Analyzing Food Access Impact on Health Issues in Sustainable Communities. *ISPRS Int. J. Geo-Information* **2021**, *10*, 745. [CrossRef]
10. Gil, R.M.; Marcelin, J.R.; Zuniga-Blanco, B.; Marquez, C.; Mathew, T.; A Piggott, D. COVID-19 Pandemic: Disparate Health Impact on the Hispanic/Latinx Population in the United States. *J. Infect. Dis.* **2020**, *222*, 1592–1595. [CrossRef]
11. Malik, A.; Abdalla, R. Mapping the impact of air travelers on the pandemic spread of (H1N1) influenza. *Model. Earth Syst. Environ.* **2016**, *2*, 1–15. [CrossRef]
12. Lee, S.S.; Wong, N.S. The clustering and transmission dynamics of pandemic influenza A (H1N1) 2009 cases in Hong Kong. *J. Infect.* **2011**, *63*, 274–280. [CrossRef] [PubMed]
13. Maier, E.H.; Lopez, R.; Sanchez, N.; Ng, S.; Gresh, L.; Ojeda, S.; Burger-Calderon, R.; Kuan, G.; Harris, E.; Balmaseda, A.; et al. Obesity Increases the Duration of Influenza A Virus Shedding in Adults. *J. Infect. Dis.* **2018**, *218*, 1378–1382. [CrossRef] [PubMed]
14. Sarmadi, M.; Ahmadi-Soleimani, S.M.; Fararouei, M.; Dianatinasab, M. COVID-19, body mass index and cholesterol: An ecological study using global data. *BMC Public Heal.* **2021**, *21*, 1–14. [CrossRef]
15. Priyadarshini, I.; Mohanty, P.; Kumar, R.; Son, L.H.; Chau, H.T.M.; Nhu, V.-H.; Ngo, P.T.T.; Bui, D.T. Analysis of Outbreak and Global Impacts of the COVID-19. *Health* **2020**, *8*, 148. [CrossRef] [PubMed]
16. Bhatia, A.; Kumar, M.; Magotra, R. *Role of GIS in Managing COVID-19*; NISCAIR-CSIR: New Delhi, India, 2020.
17. Franch-Pardo, I.; Napoletano, B.M.; Rosete-Verges, F.; Billa, L. Spatial analysis and GIS in the study of COVID-19. A review. *Sci. Total Environ.* **2020**, *739*, 140033. [CrossRef]
18. Ahasan, R.; Hossain, M.M. Leveraging GIS Technologies for Informed Decision-making in COVID-19 Pandemic. *SocArXiv* **2020**, preprint.
19. Boulos, M.N.K.; Geraghty, E.M. Geographical tracking and mapping of coronavirus disease COVID-19/severe acute respiratory syndrome coronavirus 2 (SARS-CoV-2) epidemic and associated events around the world: How 21st century GIS technologies are supporting the global fight against outbreaks and epidemics. *Int. J. Health Geogr.* **2020**, *19*, 1–12.
20. Ardabili, S.; Mosavi, A.; Ghamisi, P.; Ferdinand, F.; Varkonyi-Koczy, A.; Reuter, U.; Rabczuk, T.; Atkinson, P. COVID-19 Outbreak Prediction with Machine Learning. *Algorithms* **2020**, *13*, 249. [CrossRef]
21. Rezaei, M.; Nouri, A.A.; Park, G.S.; Kim, D.H. Application of Geographic Information System in Monitoring and Detecting the COVID-19 Outbreak. *Iran. J. Public Heal.* **2020**, *49*, 114–116. [CrossRef] [PubMed]
22. Rosenkrantz, L.; Schuurman, N.; Bell, N.; Amram, O. The need for GIScience in mapping COVID-19. *Heal. Place* **2020**, *67*, 102389. [CrossRef] [PubMed]
23. Mollalo, A.; Vahedi, B.; Rivera, K.M. GIS-based spatial modeling of COVID-19 incidence rate in the continental United States. *Sci. Total Environ.* **2020**, *728*, 138884. [CrossRef] [PubMed]
24. Küchenhoff, H.; Günther, F.; Höhle, M.; Bender, A. Analysis of the early COVID-19 epidemic curve in Germany by regression models with change points. *Epidemiol. Infect.* **2021**, *149*, e68. [CrossRef] [PubMed]

25. Radenkovic, D.; Chawla, S.; Pirro, M.; Sahebkar, A.; Banach, M. Cholesterol in Relation to COVID-19: Should We Care about It? *J. Clin. Med.* **2020**, *9*, 1909. [CrossRef] [PubMed]
26. Vicenzi, M.; Di Cosola, R.; Ruscica, M.; Ratti, A.; Rota, I.; Rota, F.; Bollati, V.; Aliberti, S.; Blasi, F. The liaison between respiratory failure and high blood pressure: Evidence from COVID-19 patients. *Eur. Respir. J.* **2020**, *56*, 2001157. [CrossRef] [PubMed]
27. Hamer, M.; Gale, C.R.; Kivimäki, M.; Batty, G.D. Overweight, obesity, and risk of hospitalization for COVID-19: A community-based cohort study of adults in the United Kingdom. *Proc. Natl. Acad. Sci. USA* **2020**, *117*, 21011–21013. [CrossRef]
28. Caillon, A.; Zhao, K.; Klein, K.O.; Greenwood, C.M.T.; Lu, Z.; Paradis, P.; Schiffrin, E.L. High Systolic Blood Pressure at Hospital Admission Is an Important Risk Factor in Models Predicting Outcome of COVID-19 Patients. *Am. J. Hypertens.* **2021**, *34*, 282–290. [CrossRef] [PubMed]
29. Ding, X.; Zhang, J.; Liu, L.; Yuan, X.; Zang, X.; Lu, F.; He, P.; Wang, Q.; Zhang, X.; Xu, Y.; et al. High-density lipoprotein cholesterol as a factor affecting virus clearance in covid-19 patients. *Respir. Med.* **2020**, *175*, 106218. [CrossRef] [PubMed]
30. Bhadra, A.; Mukherjee, A.; Sarkar, K. Impact of population density on Covid-19 infected and mortality rate in India. *Model. Earth Syst. Environ.* **2021**, *7*, 623–629. [CrossRef] [PubMed]
31. Adams, A.; Li, W.; Zhang, C.; Chen, X. The disguised pandemic: The importance of data normalization in COVID-19 web mapping. *Public Heal.* **2020**, *183*, 36–37. [CrossRef]
32. Shakeel, S.; Hassali, M.A.A.; Naqvi, A.A. Health and Economic Impact of COVID-19: Mapping the Consequences of a Pandemic in Malaysia. *Malays. J. Med Sci.* **2020**, *27*, 159–164. [CrossRef] [PubMed]
33. Baena-Díez, J.M.; Barroso, M.; Cordeiro-Coelho, S.I.; Díaz, J.L.; Grau, M. Impact of COVID-19 outbreak by income: Hitting hardest the most deprived. *J. Public Heal.* **2020**, *42*, 698–703. [CrossRef] [PubMed]
34. Kansiime, M.K.; Tambo, J.A.; Mugambi, I.; Bundi, M.; Kara, A.; Owuor, C. COVID-19 implications on household income and food security in Kenya and Uganda: Findings from a rapid assessment. *World Dev.* **2021**, *137*, 105199. [CrossRef]
35. Jay, J.; Bor, J.; Nsoesie, E.O.; Lipson, S.K.; Jones, D.K.; Galea, S.; Raifman, J. Neighbourhood income and physical distancing during the COVID-19 pandemic in the United States. *Nat. Hum. Behav.* **2020**, *4*, 1294–1302. [CrossRef]
36. Gundersen, C.; Hake, M.; Dewey, A.; Engelhard, E. Food insecurity during COVID-19. *Appl. Econ. Perspect. Policy* **2021**, *43*, 153–161. [CrossRef]
37. Ahn, S.; Norwood, F.B. Measuring Food Insecurity during the COVID-19 Pandemic of Spring 2020. *Appl. Econ. Perspect. Policy* **2021**, *43*, 162–168. [CrossRef]
38. Nakada, L.Y.K.; Urban, R.C. COVID-19 pandemic: Environmental and social factors influencing the spread of SARS-CoV-2 in São Paulo, Brazil. *Environ. Sci. Pollut. Res.* **2021**, *28*, 40322–40328. [CrossRef] [PubMed]
39. Arif, M.; Sengupta, S. Nexus between population density and novel coronavirus (COVID-19) pandemic in the south Indian states: A geo-statistical approach. *Environ. Dev. Sustain.* **2021**, *23*, 10246–10274. [CrossRef] [PubMed]
40. Budhwani, K.I.; Budhwani, H.; Podbielski, B. Evaluating Population Density as a Parameter for Optimizing COVID-19 Testing: Statistical Analysis. *Jmirx Med.* **2021**, *2*, e22195. [CrossRef] [PubMed]
41. Gaskin, D.J.; Zare, H.; Delarmente, B.A. Geographic disparities in COVID-19 infections and deaths: The role of transportation. *Transp. Policy* **2021**, *102*, 35–46. [CrossRef]
42. Kang, D.; Choi, H.; Kim, J.-H.; Choi, J. Spatial epidemic dynamics of the COVID-19 outbreak in China. *Int. J. Infect. Dis.* **2020**, *94*, 96–102. [CrossRef]
43. Kullar, R.; Marcelin, J.R.; Swartz, T.H.; Piggott, D.A.; Macias Gil, R.; Mathew, T.A.; Tan, T. Racial disparity of Coronavirus Disease 2019 in African American communities. *J. Infect. Dis.* **2020**, *222*, 890–893. [CrossRef] [PubMed]
44. U.S. Census Bureau QuickFacts: Guilford County, North Carolina. 2020. Available online: http://www.census.gov/quickfacts/guilfordcountynorthcarolina (accessed on 18 August 2020).
45. How will North Carolina's Face Mask Requirement be Enforced? 2020. Available online: https://www.wcnc.com/article/news/health/coronavirus/how-will-north-carolina-mask-mandate-be-enforced/275-03964fa3-2c39-4c2c-a2e8-44d17d5a0cfa (accessed on 18 August 2020).
46. Our County | Guilford County, NC. 2020. Available online: https://www.guilfordcountync.gov/our-county (accessed on 17 August 2020).
47. Guilford County's Zip Codes with Highest Number of COVID-19 Cases. 2020. Available online: https://myfox8.com/news/coronavirus/guilford-countys-zip-codes-with-highest-number-of-covid-19-cases/ (accessed on 17 August 2020).

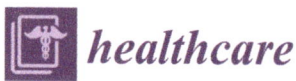

Article

# Reshaping the Healthcare Sector with Economic Policy Measures Based on COVID-19 Epidemic Severity: A Global Study

Timotej Jagrič, Dušan Fister and Vita Jagrič *

Institute of Finance and Artificial Intelligence, Faculty of Economics and Business, University of Maribor, Razlagova 14, SI-2000 Maribor, Slovenia; timotej.jagric@um.si (T.J.); dusan@dusanfister.com (D.F.)
* Correspondence: vita.jagric@um.si

**Abstract:** Governments around the world are looking for ways to manage economic consequences of COVID-19 and promote economic development. The aim of this study is to identify the areas where the application of economic policy measures would enhance the resilience of societies on epidemic risks. We use data on the COVID-19 pandemic outcome in a large number of countries. With the estimation of multiple econometric models, we identify areas being a reasonable choice for economic policy intervention. It was found that viable remediation actions worth taking can be identified either for long-, mid-, or short-term horizons, impacting the equality, healthcare sector, and national economy characteristics. We suggest encouraging research and development based on innovative technologies linked to industries in healthcare, pharmaceutical, and biotech, promoting transformation of healthcare systems based on new technologies, providing access to quality healthcare, promoting public healthcare providers, and investing in the development of regional healthcare infrastructure, as a tool of equal regional development based on economic assessment. Further, a central element of this study, i.e. the innovative identification matrix, could be populated as a unique policy framework, either for latest pandemic or any similar outbreaks in future.

**Keywords:** COVID-19 pandemic; healthcare sector transformation; research and development; artificial intelligence; economic development; health system resilience

Citation: Jagrič, T.; Fister, D.; Jagrič, V. Reshaping the Healthcare Sector with Economic Policy Measures Based on COVID-19 Epidemic Severity: A Global Study. *Healthcare* **2022**, *10*, 315. https://doi.org/10.3390/healthcare10020315

Academic Editors: Eduardo Tomé, Thomas Garavan and Ana Dias

Received: 16 November 2021
Accepted: 2 February 2022
Published: 7 February 2022

**Publisher's Note:** MDPI stays neutral with regard to jurisdictional claims in published maps and institutional affiliations.

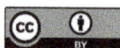

**Copyright:** © 2022 by the authors. Licensee MDPI, Basel, Switzerland. This article is an open access article distributed under the terms and conditions of the Creative Commons Attribution (CC BY) license (https://creativecommons.org/licenses/by/4.0/).

## 1. Introduction

The COVID-19 pandemic is a case of a health-triggered economic crisis resulting in a simultaneous health and economic crisis [1]. Besides the healthcare sector operating on its limits, there is not a single economic sector left not being impacted by COVID. The measures to slow-down or control the spread of virus impacted the daily life of households and, what is more, caused economic costs. The closures of public life and constrains on people's mobility caused many businesses to lose revenue in the sort-run and are fearing the loss of customers due to changed consumers' habits in the middle- and long run. There were disrupted supply chains causing delay in production and delivery of goods [2]. Besides the initial economic shock, together with simultaneous demand and supply disruptions, the COVID-19 pandemic was of a size not experienced before, and economic consequences could even lead to long-lasting declines in global economic output [3].

Not all applied measures turned out to be effective. As reported by Berry [4], for the first wave of the pandemic the effects of shelter-in-place (SIP) orders did not exhibit a detectable impact on disease spread or COVID-19 caused deaths.

As seen by Sagan et al., 2021 [5], for the case of four European countries, and similarly in many countries, there were expensive but effective measures in containing the spread of the virus, such as the lockdown measures. The applied measures have hidden the insufficiency and the unpreparedness of the healthcare systems to manage the health crisis.

Traditional measures to tackle epidemics, although efficient (e.g., quarantine, social distancing, mobility restrictions, economic lockdown, etc.), have, in modern societies, two main problems: the discussion on restricting human rights, and immense financial burden.

Regarding the discussion on human rights, there are already several findings. Protecting public health requires prioritizing the common good and broader societal implications over individual autonomy and the interest of an individual. Further, protecting an individual's health also includes preventing him from contacting diseases, resulting in long-term interests prevailing over short-term interests. Therefore, public health policies are designed in line with the view that human health is given priority over human rights, as stated by Chia and Oyeniran in 2020 [6]. Besides the negative impact of applied measures against the spread of the virus on human rights, these was also an undesirable effect on the security of food and water, as reported for the African region by Boretti [7]. Further, common measures in the epidemic were not sustainable [7]. The evidence reported by Huffstetler et al. [8] on public health actions across six geographic regions shows an impact on distinct human rights and on civil, political, economic, and social rights that underlie public health. Additionally, Huffstetler et al. [8] found disproportion in effect on the human rights of particular groups, such as women and minority populations.

Undoubtedly, COVID-19 patients filled the healthcare capacities and caused access and quality of healthcare to worsen for many other patients, which can be seen in greater numbers of avoidable deaths caused by diagnostic delays. Apart from great human loss, diagnostic delays also bring economic consequences, as shown in the case of England by Gheorghe et al. [9]. Authors estimate productivity losses of GBP 104 million over 5 years, and this figure only reflects the first epidemic wave caused by additional excess cancer deaths due to diagnostic delays [9].

The economic cost of the pandemic, consequently, was urging for reasonable measures to promote economic recovery. Guerrieri et al. [10] argue that economic shocks associated with the COVID-19 epidemic may be a kind of a supply shock that triggers changes in aggregate demand larger than the shocks themselves. Due to healthcare sector capacity limits, urgent measures were applied, many of them harming the economy. In cases of less prepared health systems, governments had to apply stricter confinement measures and higher levels of stringency in the confinement measures, which have larger negative, socio-economic effects [11]. Therefore, more resilient healthcare systems should be developed in the future to be better prepared to handle public health crises.

Empirical results indicate that short-term economic losses were greater where less fiscal stimulus was implemented, and where monetary policy easing was limited [10]. We argue that economic policy measures for successful recovery should take into account characteristics of economic sectors. In the economic ecosystem, the healthcare sector plays an important role. The economic impact and economic characteristics of the healthcare sector were broadly explored in the literature [12–17].

Further, the literature on the economic consequences of the COVID-19 pandemic is broad and thorough [3,4,9,11,18–26]. Economic downturn of one country, e.g., the U.S., will have different spill-over effects on other economic ecosystems, e.g., the European Union, as suggested by Wang and Han [18]; no economy is isolated due to global interconnections and thus cannot avoid the economic impact of the pandemic from abroad (Chudik et al. [3]). Additionally, destabilised and disrupted supply chains due to the COVID-19 pandemic might have secondary ripple effects on other economies [23]. The literature reports on the relationship between pollution and COVID-19 related deaths while economic growth has contributed to build-up of pollutants [21].

Empirical findings have shown that healthcare sectors have large and positive macroeconomic impacts on domestic economy (e.g., Stuckler et al. [27]). The economic impact is often above the average of national economy, suggesting that this sector is a more favourable choice for economic policy. Findings also indicate (Jagrič et al. [16]) that additional spending for healthcare services stimulates the creation of jobs across the national economy and that creating jobs in the economy is higher in less developed economies. Investments into healthcare in regions (or countries) with lower regional GDP per capita will promote equality, stimulate regional output, diminish regional unemployment, and increase income levels. Investments into less developed regions suggest higher multiplicative effects, suggesting the use of investment into regional healthcare sectors as a tool for equal regional development.

Although healthcare spending has been growing for decades in a large number of countries, there were attempts to cut the costs, especially in times of public finance constraints. Empirical data and the literature give grounds to believe this strategy does not bring the desired result in either the economic perspective, as austerity measures do not promote but rather harm the recovery (Darvas et al. [14]), nor in the health outcomes, as the avoidable mortality can be affected. A study by Arcà et al. [28] reveals that, even in countries with relatively low avoidable mortality, spending cuts in healthcare can hurt survival. Furthermore, the procyclicality matters, as reducing procyclicality of government health expenditure by keeping them in bad times may generate substantial health gains (Liang and Tussing [29]).

The literature extensively explores economic effects of the pandemic along with the policy measures to reduce them and the damage to the national and global economy. These measures arise from monetary, macroprudential, and fiscal policies. Applied policies include relief measures, recovery policies, and international coordination measures and are stated to reduce the consequences independently or as a combined mix of measures [19]. However, while such a research approach explores policy options to act against the consequences of an economic crisis caused by the pandemic, our approach is innovative in moving the perspective to the options of economic policy to reduce contributing factors of the severity of the pandemic outcome. The present study is thus original in the following ways. While the economic literature often takes the perspective of empirically exploring an individual determinant or some determinants which are ex-ante, selected based on theoretical grounds and the impact on the health outcomes during a specified time frame, we take an innovative point of view. We await to identify areas where an impact on the health outcomes in the case of the COVID-19 pandemic originated and can be affected by economic policy measures in the short- or long-term perspective to enhance reliance to possible future health crisis.

The paper is organized as follows. After highlighting the relevant economic characteristics and exploring grounds for economic recovery in the first section, we present the data sources and methods used in the study. Next, Section 3 gives technical results and their interpretation regarding the research question. Finally, Sections 4 and 5 complete with the discussion and conclusions, respectively.

## 2. Materials and Methods

Although the COVID-19 epidemic is not yet over, already a lot of data is made available by statistical offices, international organizations, national governments and their public health institutes, and many other organizations. Initially, we have collected 171 data variables for 197 countries, from 2017 to 2020, to ensure that, in some minor cases where the most current data were not available, the latest possible data, or an estimation, were taken. Collected data considered economic, infrastructure, cultural, health, and other areas. Economic variables were obtained from World Bank Open Data (https://data.worldbank.org/, accessed on 10 December 2020), IMF's World Economic Outlook Database (https://www.imf.org/en/Publications/WEO/weo-database/2020/October, accessed on 10 December 2020), Trading Economics portal (https://tradingeconomics.com/indicators, accessed on 10 December 2020), and FDI Attractiveness Index website (Ben [30], accessed on 10 December 2020) (http://www.fdiattractiveness.com/ranking-2020/, accessed on 10 December 2020). Infrastructure variables were fetched from Enerdata (https://yearbook.enerdata.net/, accessed on 10 December 2020) and ITU (https://www.itu.int/en/ITU-D/Statistics/Pages/stat/default.aspx, accessed on 10 December 2020), while other relevant cultural variables from Wikipedia, ETH's KOF (https://kof.ethz.ch/en/forecasts-and-indicators/indicators/kof-globalisation-index.html, accessed on 10 December 2020) (Gygli et al. [31] and Dreher [32]), and Google Mobility (GM) website (https://www.google.com/covid19/mobility/, accessed on 10 December 2020). As GM data were reported as high frequency (daily) data, basic transformation for integration with the low-frequency data (others) were necessary. First, the average values of GM data during the first corona-virus outbreak (1 March–1 May 2020) and during the second outbreak (last two months prior to 6th December 2020) were calculated. Two vectors of six categories (retail and recreation, supermarket and pharmacy, parks, public transport, workplaces, and residential) were built in this way.

Next, the average between the two built vectors was taken to form a single, consolidated, composite indicator. There, it was found that the retail and recreation category showed as most relevant here. Variables on health outcomes were obtained from WHO's Global Health Observatory data repository https://apps.who.int/gho/data/node.main (accessed on 10 December 2020) and Nextstrain https://nextstrain.org/ncov/global (Hadfield et al. [33], accessed on 10 December 2020). These were also categorized as high frequency data (number of infected, dead, and recovered people and number of clade mutations) and were recorded at the day of beginning the research, i.e., 10th December. Again, these required specialized treatment, such that composite indicators were built. The rest of the variables came from a consolidated web portal, Our World in Data https://ourworldindata.org/charts (accessed on 10 December 2020), which holds datasets of different data providers. After building a complete (consolidated) dataset as a combination of high and low frequency data, missing data were found such that cleaning of dataset was necessary. Two versions of reduced datasets were generated. In the first, there were data for 78 countries with 11 variables altogether. In the second, by reducing the number of countries, 13 more variables could be included. The list of the explanatory variables is as follows and can be divided into several groups: virus characteristics (COVID-19 cases—cumulative total, COVID-19 virus clade 20A, and COVID-19 virus clade 20B), population characteristics (share of population older than 65, share of the population living in urban areas, mean BMI (male and female)), equality characteristics (female employment-to-population ratio and Gini index of consumption), healthcare sector characteristics (share of public healthcare sector and the Healthcare Access and Quality Index), national economy characteristics (GDP per capita and PPP, i.e., constant 2011 international $, High-Tech export (share of manufactured exports), FDI country attractiveness, and share of the agriculture sector), and cultural characteristics (Google mobility measures). Additionally, as dummy variables, we included the world regions. Both reduced datasets were generated to the best extent, compromising the number of variables and number of countries to have a good mix of high- and low-income countries. Finally, all the variables were standardized before use in models by subtracting the mean and dividing by the standard deviation.

As the dependent variable we used data on the number of COVID-19 deaths from WHO's COVID-19 Dashboard as the variable indicating the severity of the COVID-19 epidemic outcome in an individual country. All gathered data was prepared in pre-processing step (e.g., logarithmic transformation) and analyzed in order to prepare for estimation of regression models. In the first two models, the least squares method was used. In the third one, the Huber-White-Hinkley estimator was used. We used software package EViews 10+ (Enterprise Edition, 64-bit, IHS Global Inc., Irvine, CA, USA, 2018) for the model estimation.

A limitation to the study has to be noted here. Although we have taken unified data sources across countries, different inconsistencies in the methodology of collecting data can be found, e.g., number of dead due to COVID-19 (as a main source of implication) is not uniquely defined across countries. The full extent of COVID-19 outcome will be possible to be evaluated when all statistical data in full range and reliability will be available.

## 3. Results

Based on empirical evidence, we considered estimations on multiple regression models to draw an integral framework for identification of areas, where the determinants of severity of COVID-19 outcome came from. Although the results depend on the limited selection of countries and variables, both logarithm–linear and linear–linear models suggested reasonably-connoted connections. Multiple models were estimated instead of one, and composite indicators were used. Despite this fact, signs on regression coefficients stayed consistent for explanatory variables that appear in more than one model. The integral framework comprises three models and unites the findings altogether. This is presented in Figure 1. We chose the presented three models over other experimental models as they at best met the criteria of high explanatory power, expressed by high levels of coefficient of determination (R-squared). However, the ability to further improve the study's econometric quality was impacted by our research aim of including the biggest possible number of countries and the widest possible selection of the explanatory variables. Nevertheless, the final models exhibit high values of R-squared, especially due to the fact that we are dealing with cross-section and highly heterogeneous data.

| | Model 1 LOG(Deaths - cumulative total) | | Model 2 Deaths - cumulative total | | Model 3 Deaths - cumulative total | | Areas of possible policy measures | Types of possible policy measures |
|---|---|---|---|---|---|---|---|---|
| Covid 19 outcome variable | | | | | | | | |
| Determinants of the Covid 19 outcome | Coefficient | Prob. | Coefficient | Prob. | Coefficient | Prob. | | |
| South America | -1.381*** | | | | | | Regional characteristics | No policy measures possible |
| Africa | -1.856*** | | | | | | | |
| Asia | -1.894*** | | -0.639* | | -0.7105* | | | |
| Oceania | -3.360*** | | -2.828*** | | -4.8998*** | | | |
| Covid 19 Cases - cumulative total | 0.307*** | | | | | | Virus characteristics | No policy measures possible |
| Covid 19 virus clade _20A | 0.024 | | 0.030 | | 0.4856 | | | |
| Covid 19 virus clade _20B | 0.250* | | 0.240* | | 0.6210*** | | | |
| Share of population older than 65 | -0.587** | | | | | | Population characteristics | Long- and mid-term policy measures possible |
| Share of the population living in urban areas | 1.713*** | | | | 2.0748** | | | |
| Mean BMI (male and female) | | | 3.872** | | 9.9473*** | | | |
| Female employment-to-population ratio | -1.266*** | | | | | | Equality characteristics | Long-, mid-, and short-term policy measures possible |
| Gini index of consumption | | | -1.814** | | -3.9628*** | | | |
| Share of public health care sector | | | -0.478* | | -0.9352** | | Health sector characteristics | Long-, mid-, and short-term policy measures possible |
| Healthcare Access and Quality Index | | | | | -3.9142** | | | |
| GDP per capita, PPP (constant 2011 international $) | | | -0.393* | | | | National economy characteristics | Long-, mid-, and short-term policy measures possible |
| High-Tech export (share of manufactured exports) | | | -0.350** | | -0.7123*** | | | |
| FDI country attractiveness | | | 5.063*** | | 6.7496*** | | | |
| Share of the agriculture sector | -0.393* | | | | | | | |
| Google mobility measures | | | 0.451*** | | 0.4016*** | | Cultural characteristics | Short-term policy measures possible |
| Constant | 0.101 | | -5.472*** | | -11.4865*** | | | |
| Sample | 78 | | 61 | | 61 | | | |
| R-squared | 0.734 | | 0.664 | | 0.7918 | | | |
| F-statistic | 16.538*** | | 8.794*** | | 15.2122*** | | | |
| Method | Least Squares | | Least Squares | | Huber-White-Hinkley estimator | | | |

Complexity of possible policy measures

**Figure 1.** '*' = p-value lower than 0.10, '**' = p-value lower than 0.05, '***' = p-value lower than 0.01. Economic policy framework for determining pandemic outbreak measures. Source: own calculations and figure presentation.

In this research, there was a challenge of heteroscedasticity. In the modelling phase, we controlled for the heteroscedasticity by different approaches reflected in the three models. In the first, we chose to use the logarithmic value of the dependent variable. In the third, we took another approach, namely, a heteroscedasticity robust estimator: Huber–White–Hinkley estimator. For a benchmark, we did not apply any adjustments in the second model due to the heteroscedasticity.

When interpreting the results, another fact should be taken into account, namely the possible presence of multicollinearity. In the initial modelling step, multicollinearity has impacted the selection of explanatory variables severely. After the selection, we empirically found that a possible threat of multicollinearity was still indicated in the model. Namely, some of the regression coefficients exposed the signs (connotations, i.e., −/+) opposite as expected, which we interpreted exclusively as a consequence of multicollinearity. Still, we followed a common econometric rule that a multicollinearity is not a reason for omitting the model.

There were dummy variables included in the models for regions that statistically significantly deviated from the global average. We believe this is due to the huge differences in the initial position at the beginning of the epidemic in individual countries. However, when considering the robust estimator, the only significant results remain the dummies for Asia and Oceania, where very restrictive measures against the spread of the virus were applied.

The results on the estimated econometric models reveal some interesting findings. Among contributing factors to a more severe epidemic outcome, higher population mobility, a higher level of the population living in urban areas, a weaker physical condition of the population, and the openness of the economy all featured. On the other hand, a positive impact came from a higher share of the primary economic sector in the ecosystem structure (agriculture) and high economic development measured as High-Tech export. Additionally, the importance of public healthcare was revealed, as better healthcare access and quality notably contributed to a more favourable epidemic outcome.

The results suggest there are multiple areas which determined the severity of the COVID-19 outcome in individual countries:

- regional characteristics;
- virus characteristics;
- population characteristics;
- equality characteristics;
- healthcare sector characteristics;
- national economy characteristics;
- cultural characteristics.

When examining the areas closely, the overall analysis of all three models suggests that there are three groups of factors which influence the outcome of the pandemic in individual countries. In regards to the economic policy, these groups differ and can be listed as follows:

- areas where factors cannot be influenced by economic policy measures;
- areas where factors can be influenced by long- and mid-term policy measures;
- areas where factors can also be influenced with short-term policy measures and prompt results are possible.

The analysis of the framework reveals that economic policy measures cannot influence the regional characteristics, e.g., where the individual country is placed, as well as the virus characteristics, e.g., virus clade present in the particular country. The other two groups of factors are relevant for the economic policy, as they might be influenced by long, mid-, and short-term policy measures. The area of population characteristics could be addressed with mid- and long-term measures, and could be directed to the population structure, ranging from living conditions such as urbanization up to ageing structure or physical characteristics of the population. The group of measures, likely to be less complex than those previous, would be long-, mid-, and short-term policy measures and would aim to favourably enhance the equality characteristics of the society. The understanding of equality, in this sense, is broad and includes the gender impact, the labour market conditions, and the distribution of wealth, also on the regional level.

The next area of possible economic policy measures would be undertaken aiming at changes of the healthcare sector characteristics. These can be impacted with combination of long-, mid-, and short-term measures, therefore it also includes structural characteristics of the sector, including the capacity, quality, and accessibility of the services. The area of characteristics of the healthcare sector includes the structure according to the public and private share of the healthcare sector. The results are in favour of a larger share of the public healthcare sector.

Our results also indicate that the characteristics of national economy had an impact on the severity of the pandemic outcome. By economic characteristics, not only the level of economic development measured by e.g., GDP per capita is meant, but the structure of the economy, namely the sectoral structure, is encountered. The level of innovation and structural changes will be at the forefront of this area of economic policy measures.

Furthermore, short-term policy measures could influence the area of cultural characteristics, among which the mobility of the population is limited. The complexity of measure will gradually increase. The less complex measures will be applied at the area of population characteristics, while the most complex measures are expected to be applied at the area of national economy characteristics and the cultural characteristics.

Based on empirical findings, we propose a mix of possible economic policy measures directly or indirectly linked to the healthcare sector. This includes promoting public healthcare, ensuring crisis capacities, and access to quality healthcare. On the other hand, state and obligatory health insurance premiums should also account for individuals' decisions, resulting in higher healthcare costs, e.g., non-vaccination once a vaccine is available. Alternatively, participation in healthcare costs for non-vaccinated could be applied and used to finance scaling-up the capacities. To encourage a resilient economy for the future, economic policy must implement policy measures, based on empirical findings on characteristics of economic structures and multiplicative effects as well as actual lessons learned from the economic consequences of COVID. Furthermore, it has been argued that standard fiscal stimulus might be less effective than normally expected due to muted Keynesian multiplier feedback (Guerrieri et al. [10]). Additionally, as indicated in the literature (Bekö et al. [15]), the impact of the healthcare sector seems to remain stable throughout the business cycle, which suggests the predictability of economic measures.

In the end, economic recovery is costly. Instead of burdening future generations due to higher public debt, financing sources should be at the cost of individuals who behave opportunistically in the epidemic crisis. State sovereignty includes fiscal measures; therefore, finding these additional sources in a form of a COVID-19 tax could be justified.

## 4. Discussion

As with any study, the limitations have to be considered for proper interpretation of the results. In this study, limitations arise from two perspectives: the data and the methods. Although we have taken unified data sources across countries, we found inconsistencies in their data collection approaches, e.g., number of deaths due to COVID-19 is not uniquely defined across countries. Further, the data availability was limited in the sense that for an individual variable for some countries there were missing values. Consequently, it has led to the trade-off between a larger number of variables or a larger number of included countries. The results are thus impacted by the choice we made in this perspective and might differ from models, where we would either include fewer explanatory variables but even more countries or contrary, more explanatory variables, and fewer countries. Further, regarding the study design, standard testing of policy impact (e.g., treatment effect models, but also Granger causality test) was according to the nature, quality, and availability of data not possible to apply. Additionally, because the pandemic and the applied measures have not yet come to an end, other econometric approaches as what we went for did not seem reasonable in our case. Again, we tried to make the study as broad as possible (in the number of countries included and in the range of variables included), which also impacted the possibilities of applied econometric approaches.

The obtained scientific implications thus are based on a starting period of the COVID-19 pandemic. Later, it will be possible to evaluate the full extent of the dependencies analysed here in relation to COVID-19, once all statistical data in full range and reliability is be available.

The study gives several scientific implications. We found that multiple factors, which determined the severity of the COVID-19 outcome in individual countries, arise from regional, virus, population, equality, healthcare sector, national economy, and cultural characteristics.

Along with the scientific implications presented in detail in the results section, another important finding was revealed by this study, namely the relevance of high-frequency data. In our study, we used Google mobility data as one explanatory variable, but many more could be relevant in the future. High-frequency data, in general, emerged as a result of the use of modern information technologies. However, two aspects of their applicability in science have to be given attention: first, appropriate methodological approaches capable of dealing with such data, and secondly, the availability of the data to the scientific community.

Next, we turn to the economic policy framework, which is serving as an identification matrix for policy implications. We identified several areas that could be relevant for the severity of the epidemic outcome. This section discusses several ideas that suggest economic policy measures to impact the severity of the epidemic outcome favourably.

Our results suggest that national economy characteristics matter; thus, we discuss the policy measures which would address them. The GDP per capita and high-tech export could be influenced. Financial data show that the healthcare sectors' stocks outperformed most others. The research and development in the healthcare sector industry promotes a high level of innovation which not only contributes to the affordable healthcare, but promotes economic development with high value-added and creates jobs for highly skilled professionals. Encouraging investments in innovative industries (healthcare, pharmaceutical, biotech, and associated industries) could thus be a good way to influence the variables which are found in the group "national economy characteristics" in our framework.

Next, we argue that post COVID-19 investments should encourage R&D in artificial intelligence (AI). Innovation and transformation accelerate economic growth and promote resilient economic systems. AI can already be applied as the first stage in diagnosing less severe cases, thereby releasing capacities (AbuShaban [2]). Investing in AI in the healthcare sector will have huge spill over effects, as this means investment into AI professionals, companies developing AI solutions, and implementation of these solutions in other sectors, making the economy future-ready. Promoting R&D in AI and AI usage in healthcare could have a favourable impact on the variables in the groups "national economy characteristics" as well as "health sector characteristics". Additionally, AI can be seen as a convenient tool for stipulation of a healthy lifestyle (in smart watches, sensors, and wearables), which importantly lowers COVID-19 severity (we noticed a significant connection between physical condition measured by BMI and cumulative total).

We further discuss the measures aiming to change the characteristics of the healthcare sector, especially due to the high relevancy of the regression variable "Healthcare Access and Quality Index" ($-3.9142$ **), as indicated in the third model of the variable. Additionally, the framework from this study indicates that the private–public healthcare matters. As the healthcare sector must be part of the critical infrastructure, the government and the private sector should establish a relationship between each other to encourage the necessary cooperation (see also AbuShaban [2]). Networks of regional providers are more critical to community recovery than centres.

Public healthcare providers are more suitable to provide sufficient backup capacities in areas which are not profitable. If public healthcare providers operate in profitable healthcare services, profits can be used for covering losses from operating in non-profitable services. For example, reserving and maintaining capacities for national medical emergencies is costly and does not gain profits.

Transformation of healthcare systems with more flexibility can contribute to provide access to quality healthcare. Both flexibility in physical capacities (AbuShaban [2]) and medical staff flexibility (Ferreira et al. [34], Casha and Casha [35]) should thus be addressed.

The healthcare sector of many countries is suffering from medical stuff shortages resulting from emigration of medical professionals (Ferreira et al. [34], Casha and Casha [35]). We argue that there is the need to design policy measures that mitigate the intention of healthcare professionals to emigrate. Temporary deficits on the labour markets can be solved by encouraging short-term medical staff mobility. Long-term shortages should be addressed by economic policy measures. However, one must notice that mobilities in general are not appreciated, as the "Google mobility measures" exposes positive regression coefficients.

Additionally, we suggest reconsidering "state aid" in industries that negatively affect health and environment in any economic policy action. Therefore, capital injection measures should be considered in industries according to economic, environmental, and health criteria. This would have long-term effects on health and environment and would make economies more resilient to future disruptions while also contributing to equity.

## 5. Conclusions

In this study, we support the thesis that innovative measures of economic policy should be applied in the after-COVID-19 period. These measures should differ from traditional ones, be applied in advance of an epidemic, and thus to support economic and social ecosystems to become more resistant to current and future epidemic crises. Many of the proposed measures directly or indirectly concern the healthcare systems and healthcare sector, aiming to impact its characteristics, such as public-vs-private healthcare or the access and quality of the healthcare provided. Economic policy measures could thus promote new technologies in healthcare, sectoral staff flexibility, or reinforce decentralised (regional) public health services providers. A central element of this study, the innovative identification matrix, which combines unbiased econometric results with remediation, could be populated as a unique policy framework, either for latest pandemic or any similar outbreaks in future. However, such a policy framework is not only to be used for identifying pandemic outcomes, but also when the final data on the pandemic outbreak outcomes become available, to make accurate and reliable predictions of the effect on individual economic, health, and social life factors. In the end, its application in policy design could contribute to modern societies' efforts on equality, human rights, and social cohesion.

We suggest further research on this topic. With the passage of time, the data on the longer time frame of the COVID-19 pandemic period will be available. This would enable a panel-based econometric approach instead of a cross-sectional one. In doing so, both the range of included characteristics of the countries and the genetic changes of the virus could improve the model and reveal new dependencies in the examined countries' characteristics to the severity of the pandemic. Additionally, as we discussed the scientific potential of high-frequency data, future research could include them in investigations. The latter would enable the detailed study of interaction between high-frequency data variables and the genetic profile of the virus.

**Author Contributions:** Conceptualization, T.J.; methodology, T.J.; software, T.J. and D.F.; validation, T.J. and D.F.; formal analysis, T.J. and D.F.; resources, D.F.; data curation, D.F.; writing—original draft preparation, V.J.; writing—review and editing, T.J. and V.J.; visualization, T.J.; and supervision, T.J. All authors have read and agreed to the published version of the manuscript.

**Funding:** The authors acknowledge the financial support from the Slovenian Research Agency (Research core funding No. P5-0027).

**Institutional Review Board Statement:** Not applicable.

**Informed Consent Statement:** Not applicable.

**Data Availability Statement:** Publicly available datasets from multiple sources were analysed in this study. The data can be found here: [https://data.worldbank.org/, https://www.imf.org/en/Publications/WEO/weo-database/2020/October, https://tradingeconomics.com/indicators, http://www.fdiattractiveness.com/ranking-2020/, https://yearbook.enerdata.net/, https://www.itu.int/en/ITU-D/Statistics/Pages/stat/default.aspx, https://kof.ethz.ch/en/forecasts-and-indicators/indicators/kof-globalisation-index.html, https://www.google.com/covid19/mobility/, https://apps.who.int/gho/data/node.main, https://nextstrain.org/ncov/global, https://ourworldindata.org/charts], all accessed on 10 December 2020.

**Conflicts of Interest:** The authors declare no conflict of interest. The funders had no role in the design of the study; in the collection, analyses, or interpretation of data; in the writing of the manuscript, or in the decision to publish the results.

## References

1. Lytras, T.; Tsiodras, S. Lockdowns and the COVID-19 pandemic: What is the endgame? *Scand. J. Public Health* **2021**, *49*, 37–40. [CrossRef] [PubMed]
2. AbuShaban, Y. COVID-19 to Transform Healthcare Investment. 2020. Available online: https://www.meed.com/covid-19-impact-healthcare-investment (accessed on 11 December 2020).
3. Chudik, A.; Mohaddes, K.; Pesaran, M.H.; Raissi, M.; Rebucci, A. A counterfactual economic analysis of Covid-19 using a threshold augmented multi-country model. *J. Int. Money Financ.* **2021**, *119*, 102477. [CrossRef]
4. Berry, C.R.; Fowler, A.; Glazer, T.; Handel-Meyer, S.; MacMillen, A. Evaluating the effects of shelter-in-place policies during the COVID-19 pandemic. *Proc. Natl. Acad. Sci. USA* **2021**, *118*, e2019706118. [CrossRef]
5. A reversal of fortune: Comparison of health system responses to COVID-19 in the Visegrad group during the early phases of the pandemic. *Health Policy* **2021**, in press.
6. Chia, T.; Oyeniran, O.I. Human health versus human rights: An emerging ethical dilemma arising from coronavirus disease pandemic. *Ethics. Med. Public Health* **2020**, *14*, 100511. [CrossRef] [PubMed]
7. Boretti, A. COVID-19 lockdown measures as a driver of hunger and undernourishment in Africa. *Ethics. Med. Public Health* **2021**, *16*, 100625. [CrossRef]

8. Huffstetler, H.E.; Williams, C.R.; Meier, B.M. Human rights in domestic responses to the COVID-19 pandemic: preliminary findings from a media-coverage database to track human rights violations. *Lancet Glob. Health* **2021**, *9*, S16. [CrossRef]
9. Gheorghe, A.; Maringe, C.; Spice, J.; Purushotham, A.; Chalkidou, K.; Rachet, B.; Sullivan, R.; Aggarwal, A. Economic impact of avoidable cancer deaths caused by diagnostic delay during the COVID-19 pandemic: A national population-based modelling study in England, UK. *Eur. J. Cancer* **2021**, *152*, 233–242. [CrossRef]
10. Guerrieri, V.; Lorenzoni, G.; Straub, L.; Werning, I. *Macroeconomic Implications of COVID-19: Can Negative Supply Shocks Cause Demand Shortages?* Technical Report; National Bureau of Economic Research: Cambridge, MA, USA, 2020. [CrossRef]
11. Aristodemou, K.; Buchhass, L.; Claringbould, D. The COVID-19 crisis in the EU: The resilience of healthcare systems, government responses and their socio-economic effects. *Eurasian Econ. Rev.* **2021**, *11*, 251–281. [CrossRef]
12. Medeiros, J.; Schwierz, C. *Efficiency Estimates of Health Care Systems*; Technical Report 549; Directorate General Economic and Financial Affairs (DG ECFIN); European Commission: Brussels, Belgium, 2015.
13. Cylus, J.; Papanicolas, I.; Smith, P.C. *Health Policy Series No. 46 Health System Efficiency How to Make Measurement Matter for Policy and Management*; World Health Organization; Regional Office for Europe: Copenhagen, Denmark, 2016; pp. 115–138.
14. Darvas, Z.; Moës, N.; Myachenkova, Y.; Pichler, D. *The Macroeconomic Implications of Healthcare*; Technical Report 11; Bruegel Policy Contribution. 2018. Available online: https://www.bruegel.org/wp-content/uploads/2018/08/PC-11_2018_cover.pdf (accessed on 12 December 2020).
15. Bekő, J.; Jagrič, T.; Fister, D.; Brown, C.; Beznec, P.; Kluge, H.; Boyce, T. The economic effects of health care systems on national economies: an input-output analysis of Slovenia. *Appl. Econ.* **2019**, *51*, 4116–4126. [CrossRef]
16. Jagrič, T.; Brown, C.; Boyce, T.; Jagrič, V. The impact of the health-care sector on national economies in selected European countries. *Health Policy* **2021**, *125*, 90–97. [CrossRef] [PubMed]
17. Gutiérrez-Hernández, P.; Abásolo-Alessón, I. The health care sector in the economies of the European Union: An overview using an input–output framework. *Cost Eff. Resour. Alloc.* **2021**, *19*, 1–22. [CrossRef]
18. Wang, Q.; Han, X. Spillover effects of the United States economic slowdown induced by COVID-19 pandemic on energy, economy, and environment in other countries. *Environ. Res.* **2021**, *196*, 110936. [CrossRef] [PubMed]
19. Padhan, R.; Prabheesh, K. The economics of COVID-19 pandemic: A survey. *Econ. Anal. Policy* **2021**, *70*, 220–237. [CrossRef] [PubMed]
20. Morgan, A.K.; Awafo, B.A.; Quartey, T. The effects of COVID-19 on global economic output and sustainability: Evidence from around the world and lessons for redress. *Sustain. Sci. Pract. Policy* **2021**, *17*, 77–81. [CrossRef]
21. Magazzino, C.; Mele, M.; Sarkodie, S.A. The nexus between COVID-19 deaths, air pollution and economic growth in New York state: Evidence from Deep Machine Learning. *J. Environ. Manag.* **2021**, *286*, 112241. [CrossRef] [PubMed]
22. Ludvigson, S.C.; Ma, S.; Ng, S. COVID-19 and the Costs of Deadly Disasters. *AEA Pap. Proc.* **2021**, *111*, 366–370. [CrossRef]
23. Goel, R.K.; Saunoris, J.W.; Goel, S.S. Supply chain performance and economic growth: The impact of COVID-19 disruptions. *J. Policy Model.* **2021**, *43*, 298–316. [CrossRef]
24. Das, S.; Wingender, P.; Barrett, P.; Pugacheva, E.; Magistretti, G. After-Effects of the COVID-19 Pandemic: Prospects for Medium-Term Economic Damage. *IMF Work. Pap.* **2021**, *2021*, 1. [CrossRef]
25. Buera, F.; Fattal-Jaef, R.; Hopenhayn, H.; Neumeyer, P.A.; Shin, Y. *The Economic Ripple Effects of COVID-19*; Technical Report; National Bureau of Economic Research: Cambridge, MA, USA, 2021. [CrossRef]
26. Milani, F. COVID-19 outbreak, social response, and early economic effects: A global VAR analysis of cross-country interdependencies. *J. Popul. Econ.* **2021**, *34*, 223–252. [CrossRef]
27. Stuckler, D.; Reeves, A.; McKee, M. Social and economic multipliers: What they are and why they are important for health policy in Europe. *Scand. J. Public Health* **2017**, *45*, 17–21. [CrossRef] [PubMed]
28. Arcà, E.; Principe, F.; Van Doorslaer, E. Death by austerity? The impact of cost containment on avoidable mortality in Italy. *Health Econ.* **2020**, *29*, 1500–1516. [CrossRef] [PubMed]
29. Liang, L.L.; Tussing, A.D. The cyclicality of government health expenditure and its effects on population health. *Health Policy* **2019**, *123*, 96–103. [CrossRef] [PubMed]
30. Ben Jelili, R. Does foreign direct investment affect growth in MENA countries? A semi-parametric fixed-effects approach. *Middle East Dev. J.* **2020**, *12*, 57–72. [CrossRef]
31. Gygli, S.; Haelg, F.; Potrafke, N.; Sturm, J.E. The KOF Globalisation Index-revisited. *Rev. Int. Organ.* **2019**, *14*, 543–574. [CrossRef]
32. Dreher, A. Does globalization affect growth? Evidence from a new index of globalization. *Appl. Econ.* **2006**, *38*, 1091–1110. [CrossRef]
33. Hadfield, J.; Megill, C.; Bell, S.M.; Huddleston, J.; Potter, B.; Callender, C.; Sagulenko, P.; Bedford, T.; Neher, R.A. NextStrain: Real-time tracking of pathogen evolution. *Bioinformatics* **2018**, *34*, 4121–4123. [CrossRef]
34. Ferreira, P.L.; Raposo, V.; Tavares, A.I.; Correia, T. Drivers for emigration among healthcare professionals: Testing an analytical model in a primary healthcare setting. *Health Policy* **2020**, *124*, 751–757. [CrossRef]
35. Casha, A.; Casha, R.; Azzopardi Muscat, N. Moving health professionals as an alternative to moving patients: The contribution of overseas visiting medical specialists to the health system in Malta. *Health Policy* **2020**, *124*, 519–524. [CrossRef]

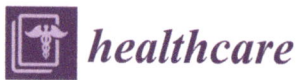 

Article

# Perception Bias Effects on Healthcare Management in COVID-19 Pandemic: An Application of Cumulative Prospect Theory

Tienhua Wu

Department of Management, Air Force Institute of Technology, Kaohsiung 82047, Taiwan; 9428901@nkust.edu.tw

**Abstract:** Coronavirus disease 2019 (COVID-19) has posed severe threats to human safety in the healthcare sector, particularly in residents in long-term care facilities (LTCFs) at a higher risk of morbidity and mortality. This study aims to draw on cumulative prospect theory (CPT) to develop a decision model to explore LTCF administrators' risk perceptions and management decisions toward this pandemic. This study employed the policy Delphi method and survey data to examine managers' perceptions and attitudes and explore the effects of sociodemographic characteristics on healthcare decisions. The findings show that participants exhibited risk aversion for small losses but became risk-neutral when considering devastating damages. LTCF managers exhibited perception bias that led to over- and under-estimation of the occurrence of infection risk. The contextual determinants, including LTCF type, scale, and strategy, simultaneously affect leaders' risk perception toward consequences and probabilities. Specifically, cost-leadership facilities behave in a loss-averse way, whereas hybrid-strategy LTCFs appear biased in measuring probabilities. This study is the first research that proposes a CPT model to predict administrators' risk perception under varying mixed gain–loss circumstances involving considerations of healthcare and society in the pandemic context. This study extends the application of CPT into organizational-level decisions. The results highlight that managers counteract their perception bias and subjective estimation to avoid inappropriate decisions in healthcare operations and risk governance for a future health emergency.

**Keywords:** coronavirus disease 2019 (COVID-19); healthcare decisions; perception bias; attitude; long-term care facilities (LTCFs); cumulative prospect theory (CPT)

Citation: Wu, T. Perception Bias Effects on Healthcare Management in COVID-19 Pandemic: An Application of Cumulative Prospect Theory. *Healthcare* **2022**, *10*, 226. https://doi.org/10.3390/healthcare10020226

Academic Editors: Eduardo Tomé, Thomas Garavan and Ana Dias

Received: 13 December 2021
Accepted: 14 January 2022
Published: 25 January 2022

**Publisher's Note:** MDPI stays neutral with regard to jurisdictional claims in published maps and institutional affiliations.

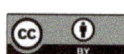

**Copyright:** © 2022 by the author. Licensee MDPI, Basel, Switzerland. This article is an open access article distributed under the terms and conditions of the Creative Commons Attribution (CC BY) license (https://creativecommons.org/licenses/by/4.0/).

## 1. Introduction

Identified as a pandemic by the World Health Organization (WHO) in January 2020, coronavirus disease 2019 (COVID-19) remarkably affected the healthcare sector and rapidly evolved into a global emergency [1,2]. This disease is harmful to all populations, particularly individuals residing in long-term care facilities (LTCFs) who require specialized medical care and life support [2,3]. LTCF residents are a vulnerable population group at a higher risk of susceptibility and mortality from COVID-19 than younger population groups [4–6]. The high morbidity and mortality of COVID-19 presents challenges for surveillance systems and infection prevention and control (IPC) and causes severe damage to safety, healthcare provision, and administrative operations in LTCFs, leading to higher reported deaths compared to younger population groups [7,8].

Since this public health emergency was identified, governments and institutions have released guidelines or implemented regulations to meet the demands of LTCFs while mitigating the impacts of the crisis [1,5]. However, considerable health, psychology, and socioeconomic damage highlight the existence of managerial problems at the system and facility levels [4,9–11]. The European Centre for Disease Prevention and Control (ECDC) [7] suggests that the lack of unique surveillance systems, differences in testing strategies and capacities, and LTCF staff's abilities are the main factors contributing to facility-wide outbreaks. Renda and Castro [10] note that the reasons underlying this emergency are insufficient investments and fragmented efforts in governing low-risk, high-consequence events such as COVID-19. D'Adamo et al. [4] also suggest that governments underscore coronavirus disease risk spreading among elderly LTCF populations. Healthcare leaders' responses to the threat of COVID-19 remain weak and differ across facilities.

This outbreak should have been predicted and avoided given the sufficient experience and knowledge learned from SARS or H1N1; however, it was underestimated or even ignored by decision-makers in the COVID-19 context [10,11]. The decisions for mitigating the impacts of the pandemic on healthcare operations may include risk assessment and response [12], medical supplies and inventory management [13], or comprehensive preparedness and contingency plans [14]. Notably, since decision-makers are risk-sensitive, their attitudes affect strategy selection and implementation [15]. Liu et al. [16] argue that emergency choice problems are complicated because of the evolution of disaster scenarios and the uncertain information. Indeed, the rapidly changing situations make clinical and care management decisions complex [4,17]. If managers have a bias that prevents them from making decisions effectively and efficiently, devastating health and economic outcomes may result [4].

The abovementioned discussion emphasizes human factors in making decisions related to care provision and risk practices. The extant literature inadequately addresses this issue. To bridge this research gap, the following research questions arise:

RQ 1: How do administrators in LTCFs define and evaluate unprecedented adverse events such as COVID-19?

RQ 2: How do administrators' cognitive heuristics and risk-related behaviors influence their decisions in response to the pandemic?

RQ 3: If administrators have biases, what factors contribute to these biases, and how can these biases be adjusted to ensure effective decision-making under risk?

This study uses infection risk in the ongoing COVID-19 pandemic affecting healthcare operations in LTCFs as the research setting. To respond to the research questions, this study first conducts the policy Delphi method of data collection to explore varying LTCF administrators' risk perceptions and attitudes regarding COVID-19 and contextual factors affecting healthcare management. Then, this study draws on cumulative prospect theory (CPT) to build a model examining how risk perceptions and attitudes of managers impacted their decision in detecting, evaluating, and managing risk during the outbreak. CPT has been widely applied in studying individuals' behaviors and choices under various risk contexts [18,19]. Last, based on policy Delphi results and a literature review [20–25], this study identifies and incorporates individual and organizational variables in the proposed model to examine bias effects on healthcare management decisions by the survey data. The results contribute to the literature by proposing a CPT decision-making model to capture managers' risky choice behaviors when facing an unprecedented outbreak. The present study also helps practitioners examine bias effects of individual and organizational factors on decisions, better plan proper countermeasures in healthcare management decisions, and reorient risk practices in the post-COVID-19 period.

This study proceeds as follows: Section 2 provides a literature review on the impacts of the pandemic on LTCFs, CPT, and factors affecting healthcare decisions. Section 3 presents the methods and decision tasks, a CPT-based decision model, and a regression model for sociodemographic factors. This study then provides the results regarding administrators' perceptions and attitudes toward infection risk and the distortive effects of individual and organizational factors on managers' decisions. This study discusses the results in Section 5 and summarizes the implications in Section 6.

## 2. Literature Review

### 2.1. Research on the Impact of COVID-19 and Policy Delphi Method

The literature highlights that COVID-19 has dramatically impacted long-term care facilities (LTCFs), a specific group of facilities in the healthcare sector [1,7]. LTCFs care for people with physical, mental, intellectual, or sensory disabilities who require specialized medical care and life support. Given physical or mental disabilities and a high probability of infection clusters, residents are particularly vulnerable populations who suffer the worst consequences from this infection [1,6,7]. Evidence reports that the deaths of residents in many EU countries correspond to 30~60% of the total COVID-19 deaths [7,26], and half of the infected people in LTCFs in the United States are asymptomatic, making it difficult to estimate the numbers of residents and staff affected by COVID-19 [27]. Such situations may result from underestimating the coronavirus risk [4,8] or failures at the systems level [9].

In response, managers and staff require additional preparedness in terms of workforce capacity, resources, care planning, and organizational efforts to reduce safety damage while sustaining healthcare operations [1,7,28]. However, these requirements post many decision nodes that require accurate responses by healthcare personnel to achieve transmission mitigation. For example, D'Adamo et al. [4] suggest that managers and staff require awareness of ongoing situations, appropriate managerial behaviors, containment strategies, and decisions on all levels of governance. Leite et al. [29] emphasize the importance of dealing with the operational dilemma of capacity and demand when the infection curve is generated. Bhaskar et al. [13] and Kuo et al. [14] stress managers' efforts and responsiveness of organizations in governing their medication supply and contingency plans to reduce damages. Therefore, the current pandemic has exposed the vital roles of human factors and managers' risky behaviors in clinical and managerial decisions in the current and post-COVID-19 period [7,12].

This indicates a need for healthcare personnel to generate viewpoints on contextual factors affecting decisions under COVID-19 risk. In the healthcare setting, the literature highlights the benefit of the policy Delphi method for generating ideas through structured, critical collective debate within a group of anonymous experts [30–32]. For example, Paraskevas and Saunders [33] highly recommend using the policy Delphi to generate options regarding organizational crisis signals detection and suggest alternative courses of action for consideration. Meskell et al. [32] suggest affordance of the policy Delphi method in nursing research, which identifies best practices in the clinical role of nurse lecturers by examining stakeholders' perceptions. Despite the weaknesses such as inconsistent execution process and incomplete data [30,31], De Loë et al. [30] note that the policy Delphi method is well suited for inquiry into complex problem areas with multiple perspectives solutions with no one clear normative solution. Thus, this study employed the policy Delphi method to understand LTCF managers' perceptions of this unprecedented risk.

*2.2. Cumulative Prospect Theory and Its Applications*

To explain variations that cannot be predicted by rational decision theory, Kahneman and Tversky [34] and Tversky and Kahneman [35] proposed prospect theory (PT) and CPT. PT and CPT used the value function (VF) and the probability weighting function (PWF) to observe individuals' risky choice behaviors such as reference dependence, loss aversion, diminishing sensitivity, and probability weighting. These behaviors may result in irrationality, cognitive bias, and nonlinear transformation in a decision, leading to a situation in which risks may not be appropriately predicted, evaluated or managed [19]. In CPT, the VF relates to the subject's irrational valuation of money, i.e., the nonlinear perception of the action monetary spending. The function in VF is asymmetric and exhibits risk aversion behavior if it is steeper for significant losses than it is for small losses. The PWF measures the likelihood of event occurrence on the perceived money prospects. The PWF carries the nonlinear transformation from objective to subjective probabilities for each individual [18,19,34–36]. Individuals, constrained to cognitive limitations, are usually challenged to rationalize the fair value of probabilistic events. Thus, biased individuals tend to overweight low probabilities and underweight high probabilities.

CPT has been widely applied in a variety of contexts, including economics and business [18,37–39], public emergencies and catastrophic events [16,40], and the healthcare domain [41–43]. The goals of all of the studies above are to further study human agents' risk-related behaviors in uncertain environments and their decisions regarding risky choices, which help managers adjust their choices to manage risks [16,39]. Given the importance of agents' risk-related behavior in COVID-19 control, this research extends prior work by proposing a CPT decision-making model to capture managers' risky choice behaviors when facing this unprecedented outbreak.

*2.3. Factors Affecting Healthcare Decisions*

Scholars [20–25] have highlighted the significance of individual and organizational variables in framing, assessing, and managing risks. The literature addresses the vital roles of individual factors such as personal characteristics and expert knowledge elicitation [20], domain experience [21], or gender equity [22] in decisions under risk. Concerning organizational variables, March and Shapira [23] suggest that managers' decisions are particularly affected by their attention to critical performance targets. McNamara and Bromiley [24] find that factors such as organizational standardization or pressure for profitability appeared to influence executives' assessment of risky decisions. Additionally, Cagliano et al. [20] note that errors may have roots grounded in people highly influenced by the working environment and the organizational processes.

During the COVID-19 pandemic, studies have shown that human errors have contributed to disease spread within and between LTCFs. For example, policymakers and healthcare personnel failed to identify outbreaks earlier [7,10], attended to infections with limited IPC training and equipment [7,26,27], and underestimated the transmissibility rate and disease burden [4,7]. Leite et al. [29] acknowledge that healthcare organizations must face varying difficulties in managing COVID-19 demand, such as lack of system thinking in decision-making or staff issues regarding numbers and safety concerns. Variations in personnel's risk perception are the primary sources that result in their different risk-taking behavior in response to infection risk [21]. Thus, the individual difference in healthcare decisions under risk warrant additional research in the context of this unexpected, severe pandemic.

While the WHO and CDC (Centers for Disease Control and Prevention) provide IPC guiding principles for LTCF stakeholders, they do not consider differences in organizational features and capacities, the health conditions of residents, the staff's abilities, or their resource supply models. Actual measures and actions may depend on different regions and facilities [44]. In the hospital setting, the extant literature identifies that organizational variables, such as strategy types [45–47] or business environments and contexts [48,49], affect managerial decisions and performance. Similarly, organizational characteristics and strategy types of LTCFs should be considered in managers' decision-making, given the complex political, legal, societal, business, and financial environments created by COVID-19. Based on the abovementioned discussion, this study thus focuses on six factors: gender, job title, funding status, LTCF type, facility scale, and strategy in influencing decision-making that benefit better planning of proper clinical and managerial countermeasures in the light of future health emergencies.

## 3. Methodology

This study employed a multi-methods approach. First, a two-round policy Delphi technique was used to explore information about risk management faced by LTCFs during the COVID-19 pandemic and design decision tasks for the CPT decision model. Second, drawing on CPT, this study proposed a decision model to examine managers' perceptions and attitudes toward pandemics and a regression model to explore the effects of sociodemographic characteristics on healthcare decisions. Last, the survey method was utilized to examine the models above to gain advanced knowledge of human biased effects on decision making and provide countermeasure suggestions.

*3.1. Decision Task Design and Factors Using Policy Delphi Method*

The policy Delphi method uses iterative stages of exploring the broadest range of insights or revealing possible opposing positions on an issue rather than generating consensus among anonymous panelists [30,50], and it is a reliable means because of its four primary characteristics: anonymity, iteration with controlled feedback of group opinion, statistical aggregation of group response, and expert input [51]. Meskell et al. [32] suggest that the policy Delphi technique is highly recommended in a healthcare setting because healthcare organizations are hierarchically structural, and junior personnel tend to avoid challenging their superiors' opinions. Moreover, the policy Delphi technique aims to draw out the different views and is a tool for analyzing complex issues [50]. The COVID-19 emergency is a complicated issue in which evaluation and responses to this adverse event vary among various LTCF stakeholders in vastly different IPC conditions and disrupt resource supply and logistics. Therefore, in the COVID-19 context, the policy Delphi is a suitable method for understanding varying LTCF administrators' risk perceptions to design decision tasks to examine individual and organizational factors in influencing managers' healthcare decisions.

The policy Delphi is a multiphase process. This method includes six phases: formulation of the issues, exposing the options, determining initial positions on the issues, exploring the obtaining of the reasons for disagreements, evaluating the underlying reasons, and re-evaluation the options [50]. The first three phases deal primarily with statements, arguments, and comments on an issue from varying perspectives of participants [32,33,50]. The fourth and fifth phases focus on assessment and justifications, and the last phase is to re-evaluate the alternatives with acceptability or feasibility [32,33,50].

This study used two Delphi rounds conducted from June to November 2020. Following the research of De Loë et al. [30] and Meskell et al. [32], interviewees were recruited by two principles: whether interviewees were knowledgeable about healthcare operations and supply strategies and had decision-making authority with pandemic risk. Interviewees were informed to (1) generate ideas about risk management for COVID-19 and (2) act as representatives of their facilities rather than as individual anonymous interviewees. After explaining the details associated with research aims and procedures, seven interviewees were recruited, and all maintained participation in the subsequent rounds. Data were collected using face-to-face interviews, providing opportunities for LTCF representatives to express the different views of the COVID-19 pandemic from their facilities' perspectives [51].

*3.2. CPT Decision Model and Measurement of Prospect Values*

PT and CPT suggest that in a choice process, individuals first edit the available options as prospects that are a representation of outcomes and probabilities, evaluate the edited prospects, and eventually choose the one with the highest value as jointly determined by the VF and the PWF [34,35]. The VF relates a subject's nonlinear perception of monetary spending. This CPT model used VFs to describe subjects' valuation of money on infection cluster losses derived from the entrance of possible infected or asymptomatic agents [35]. The PWF measures the likelihood of event occurrence on perceived monetary prospects. Probabilities represented the risk associated with the entrance of possibly infected or asymptomatic stakeholders. Participants' attitudes toward these probabilities were shown by CPT's PWFs [35].

Complementing the straightforward expected utility theory, CPT incorporates human bias into utility functions $v(\cdot)$ and $w(\cdot)$, as shown in (1). The model parameters are estimated by an intermediate measure of certainty equivalent ($CE$):

$$v(CE) = w(p)v(X) + (1 - w(p))v(Y) \qquad (1)$$

The procedure involves collecting individuals' responses and performing nonlinear regression on the curves of $v(\cdot)$ and $w(\cdot)$. The functional forms are employed according to the suggestion of [35]:

$$v(X) = -\lambda(-X)^{\alpha}, \text{ for } X < 0, \text{ and,} \qquad (2)$$

$$w(p) = p^{\beta} / \left(p^{\beta} + (1-p)^{\beta}\right)^{1/\beta}. \qquad (3)$$

To estimate model parameters $\alpha$ and $\beta$ in (2) and (3), this study solved nonlinear regression (1) by the Markov Chain Monte Carlo (MCMC) method. The MCMC technique has the advantage of numerical stability, statistical accuracy, and computational efficiency in handling significant problems. This study used the MCMC method to estimate posterior probabilities of the target parameters $\alpha$ and $\beta$ in a solver of OpenBugs 3.2.3, a publicly available MCMC software. In contrast to previous studies in iterative approximating approaches [16,35,52,53], this study used the nonlinear fitting and obtained the posterior probability $p(\alpha, \beta | CE, v, w)$ based on likelihood functions $(p(v|\alpha), p(w|\beta))$. In nonlinear regression, it is unnecessary to assume Gaussian distribution for any error terms.

This study rewrote (1) into an indexed form (4) with corresponding sampling sets. For individual $i$, $j$-th loss probability $p_j$, and $k$-th loss value $X_k$, this study fitted the model with an additional error term $\epsilon$ in CPT Equation (4):

$$v\left(CE_{ijk}\right) = w(p_j)v(X_k) + w(1-p_j)v(0) + \epsilon. \quad (4)$$

Equation (4) can be explained as a respondent facing situations in decision Tasks. The first loss value is USD 10,000 ($X_1 = 10{,}000$), and the first loss probability is 1% ($p_1 = 0.01$). Because the choice of investment is either $X_1$ or nothing, the alternative to $X_1$ is 0. The CE value is USD 1000 ($CE_{111} = 1000$). This study tentatively assumed the error term to be Gaussian, and it turned out to be well represented in the simulation of the MCMC iterations.

This study also explored the roles of individual and organizational variables in influencing agents' risky choice behaviors. To address this research aim, this study used a regression analysis technique involving six sociodemographic variables: gender, job title, the funding status of the organization, LTCF type, facility scale, and organizational strategy type. This study estimated the model as follows and used $\theta_1 \sim \theta_6$ to represent the six factors above, respectively.

$$v(X) = -\lambda(-X)^\alpha, w(p) = p^\beta / \left(p^\beta + (1-p)^\beta\right)^{1/\beta}, \quad (5)$$

$$\alpha = \gamma_0 + \sum_{i=1}^{6} \gamma_i \theta_i + \eta, \quad (6)$$

$$\beta = \xi_0 + \sum_{i=1}^{6} \xi_i \theta_i + \zeta, \quad (7)$$

where $\gamma, \xi$ are the regression coefficients and $\eta, \zeta$ are the regression errors. The $\alpha$ parameter values for the factor coefficients represent the effects of individual and organizational variables on the VFs of respondents, whereas the values of the $\beta$ parameter show factor effects on the PWFs.

### 3.3. Survey Method

The survey was conducted from February to April 2021. This study first contacted the potential long-term care organizations in Taiwan via telephone to ask whether they were willing to participate in this study. Next, this study mailed paper questionnaires regarding organization strategy and decision tasks in the Appendix A to participating facilities and asked administrators to respond to the survey. Concerning strategy, participants were asked to indicate on a seven-point scale the extent to which, compared with other LTCFs, their care services (1) provided innovative, differentiated, diverse, and large-scale services/programs and (2) engaged in a cost-efficient analysis of equipment and resources, facilities, workforce, and services and programs. This study received the questionnaires by mails, and there were no personal identification data on the paper questionnaires. A total of 327 questionnaires as a sample size were used to examine the CPT decision models. According to the definition of LTCF types by ECDC [44], participants' facilities were three types: general nursing homes, residential homes, and mixed LTCFs. Table 1 provides the sample characteristics. Respondents who gave a higher sum value on engaging in innovative services were the differentiation group, comprising approximately 43.8% of the participating facilities. Participants who indicated a higher sum value on performing cost control were assigned to the cost-leadership group; 25% of all respondents were from cost-leadership organizations. Approximately 31.2% of organizations were hybrid organizations whose sum values were between cost-leadership and differentiation groups.

**Table 1.** Demographics of the participants.

| Variables | Items | Frequency | Percent |
|---|---|---|---|
| Gender | Male | 123 | 37.6 |
|  | Female | 204 | 62.4 |
| Job title | Facility administrator | 102 | 31.2 |
|  | Healthcare/Medical administrator | 225 | 68.8 |
| Funding status | Public | 61 | 18.7 |
|  | For-profit | 266 | 81.3 |
| LTCF type | General nursing homes | 61 | 18.7 |
|  | Residential homes | 102 | 31.2 |
|  | Mixed LTCFs | 164 | 50.1 |
| Facility scale | Less than 99 beds | 82 | 25.1 |
|  | 100~399 beds | 164 | 50.1 |
|  | More than 400 beds | 81 | 24.8 |

Note: LTCF: long-term care facilities.

## 4. Results

### 4.1. Policy Delphi Results

The first round was designed to incorporate phases 1–3 of the design suggested by Turoff and Linstone [50]: formulation of issues, exposing the options, and determining initial positions on the issues. In the first round, this study reviewed the relevant literature: CPT, the study of Guo, et al. [39], and IPC guidance released by the WHO and ECDC for questions and preliminary IPC decision tasks. Interviewees provided their views on pandemic perceptions, contextual factors, critical agents, and occurrences and impacts of this virus transmission. Interviewees agreed that possible infected agents' movement and health conditions, such as residents, staff, and visitors, should be screened daily to effectively identify new infections and prevent further spread [1,4]. They also suggested that pre-symptomatic or asymptomatic cases are hard to identify but remarkably contribute to disease transmission [26,27]. Similar to situations in Europe [44], interviewees emphasized re-assessing workplace risk under occupational safety and health legislation and therefore need to find a way to minimize the workload for facilities while achieving an acceptable cost–benefit ratio. Moreover, they pointed out that an additional burden for environmental cleaning, waste management, and daily reporting depends on LTCF types and scale and challenges administrators and healthcare staff. Except for mandatory IPC regulations, interviewees' actions to IPC practices widely differed, and organizational factors could determine the extent to which a facility engages in healthcare operations to control COVID-19 risk. Overall, data revealed the facility's weakness to IPC practices and the gaps regarding workforce and resource capacities and demand [29].

Interviewees in the second round aimed to gain an advanced understanding of views that emerged from round one [32,51] and helped modify preliminary IPC decision tasks for a survey purpose. This round focused on exploring and obtaining the reasons for disagreements and evaluating the underlying reasons suggested by Turoff and Linstone [50]. Due to high transmissibility rates, possibly infected and asymptomatic stakeholders were identified and monitored as these cases had varying possibilities to enter facilities and cause different degrees of impact. Interviewees noted that infection control would add a significant burden that might be difficult to fulfill without additional financial and medical resource provision or affecting primary care. They thus modified monetary amounts of decision tasks representing facilities' investment in IPC practices and the consequences of confirmed cases and infection clusters. Meanwhile, interviewees also modified the risk probabilities regarding the entrance of possibly infected or asymptomatic stakeholders. To evaluate the effects of facilities' strategies, interviewees agreed to adopt the measurements from the study of Kumar and Subramanian [46] to identify the extent to which LTCFs use cost, differentiation, or hybrid strategies to provide healthcare services.

The decision task questionnaire was refined in the second round then mailed to survey respondents to rank preference on decision tasks as phase 6 of Turoff and Linstone [50]. The questionnaire has two task circumstances, in which possibly infected or asymptomatic stakeholders enter facilities, leading to varying degrees of losses represented by monetary values. To avoid losses, managers make a risky choice by transforming the representation of the entrance occurrence probabilities with loss outcomes.

Taking Task 1 as an example, the entrance probability of a possibly infected stakeholder is assumed to increase from 1% (i.e., one possible agent among 100 agents who entered facilities) to 3%, 10%, 30%, and then 90%. The entrance of possible cases lead to losses in the amounts of USD 10,000, 40,000, 70,000, 100,000, or 130,000 (Scenarios 1.1~1.5, respectively). In response, numerous choices regarding investment in IPC activities, ranging from USD 1000, 3000, 10,000, 30,000, or 100,000, are offered. In each loss scenario of Task 1, administrators' decisions depend on how they edit numerous possibilities and losses under risks and evaluate and select the preferred investment choices in an essential, continuing manner. Similarly, each manager is asked to complete decision Task 2 where the entrance occurrence of asymptomatic stakeholders with different possibilities (i.e., from 0.1% up to 9%) leads to tremendous financial losses, ranging from USD 0.2 to 1.4 million (Scenarios 2.1~2.5). The amount of IPC investment includes five choices: USD 10,000, 30,000, 100,000, 300,000, or 1,000,000. The manager is also asked to assess and choose the acceptable amounts of IPC investments under different probabilities for each loss scenario 2.1~2.5 of Task 2.

Figure 1 shows the scenarios of the decision tasks in the questionnaire. The upward one depicts scenario 1.1 of Task 1, and the downward one is for scenario 2.1 of Task 2. Scenarios 1.1~1.5 are the same except that the loss amount increases from USD 40,000, 70,000, 100,000, to 130,000. Similarly, the loss scenarios of 2.2~2.5 are the same except the questionnaire indicates various loss amounts: USD 500,000, 800,000, 1,100,000, or 1,400,000. Every participant makes decisions in five scenarios of each task based on their perceived probabilities and impacts of outcomes. Given the cognitive limitation and varying perceptions of COVID-19, managers' risky choices could be observed and modeled in a CPT-based decision model.

*4.2. Estimation Results of Risk Perception and Attitude*

The survey data were used to examine the two CPT functions: the VF and the PWF. The technique is a nonlinear fitting procedure. For each decision task, participants edited choice problems and selected their preferred 25 CEs for 25 different combinations of possibilities and loss outcomes. First, this study examined the validity of a CPT model, separately fitted the function parameters for each task using the MCMC method, performed 320,000 iterations in the MCMC procedure, and discarded the data of the first 6000 iterations. As shown in Figure 2, the probabilities of the parameters such as $\lambda$, $\alpha$, $\beta$, and $\epsilon$ approximately fit a Gaussian distribution. Table 2 exhibits the results of the nonlinear fitting. The mean of the error term $\epsilon$ in the CPT equation is $8.657 \times 10^{-7}$; all Monte Carlo errors are less than 0.025, suggesting that the proposed CPT model is acceptable.

| 1.1 US$ 10,000 loss scenario / IPC Investments / Probabilities of entrance of a possibly infected agent | 100,000 (US $) | 30,000 | 10,000 | 3 000 | 1 000 |
|---|---|---|---|---|---|
| 1% | ☐ | ☐ | ☐ | ☐ | ☐ |
| 3% | ☐ | ☐ | ☐ | ☐ | ☐ |
| 10% | ☐ | ☐ | ☐ | ☐ | ☐ |
| 30% | ☐ | ☐ | ☐ | ☐ | ☐ |
| 90% | ☐ | ☐ | ☐ | ☐ | ☐ |

| 2.1 US$ 200,000 loss scenario / IPC Investments / Probabilities of entrance of an asymptomatic agent | 1,000,000 (US $) | 300,000 | 100,000 | 30,000 | 10,000 |
|---|---|---|---|---|---|
| 0.1% | ☐ | ☐ | ☐ | ☐ | ☐ |
| 0.3% | ☐ | ☐ | ☐ | ☐ | ☐ |
| 1% | ☐ | ☐ | ☐ | ☐ | ☐ |
| 3% | ☐ | ☐ | ☐ | ☐ | ☐ |
| 9% | ☐ | ☐ | ☐ | ☐ | ☐ |

**Figure 1.** Decision Tasks 1 and 2 under various loss scenarios. The upward one is for scenario 1.1 of Task 1, and the downward one is for scenario 2.1 of Task 2, IPC: infection prevention and control.

**Table 2.** Results of the nonlinear fitting for Tasks 1 and 2.

| Estimated Parameter | Mean | Standard Deviation | MC_Error | Val2.5pc | Median | Val97.5pc | Start | Sample |
|---|---|---|---|---|---|---|---|---|
| λ | 1.091 | 0.336 | 0.010 | 0.510 | 1.255 | 1.388 | 6001 | 320,000 |
| α[Task 1] | 1.433 | 0.802 | 0.024 | 0.937 | 0.980 | 2.879 | 6001 | 320,000 |
| α[Task 2] | 1.176 | 0.361 | 0.014 | 0.933 | 0.977 | 1.816 | 6001 | 320,000 |
| β[Task 1] | 0.525 | 0.265 | 0.008 | 0.363 | 0.375 | 0.988 | 6001 | 320,000 |
| β[Task 2] | 0.382 | 0.045 | 0.001 | 0.351 | 0.356 | 0.462 | 6001 | 320,000 |
| ε | $8.657 \times 10^{-7}$ | $1.641 \times 10^{-6}$ | $4.859 \times 10^{-8}$ | $9.748 \times 10^{-8}$ | $2.294 \times 10^{-7}$ | $6.956 \times 10^{-6}$ | 6001 | 320,000 |

Second, this study examined the $\alpha$ values shown in Table 2, representing agents' risk attitudes toward outcomes through the VF. The $\alpha$ value (1.433) for Task 1 is higher than 1. In the context of the entrance occurrence of possibly infected stakeholders, the findings suggest that most respondents exhibit risk-averse behavior. Similarly, the estimated $\alpha$ (1.176) for Task 2 is over one but close to 1, indicating that the participants have low risk aversion under conditions in which asymptomatic stakeholders entered into facilities.

Lastly, the $\beta$ values obtained in this study are used to describe subjects' attitudes toward probabilities. A greater $\beta$ means that the risk preference of an agent is more neutral than biased. In contrast, a smaller $\beta$ suggests that agents present severely biased behaviors to enhance small probabilities and reduce higher probabilities. As shown in Table 2, $\beta$ values for Tasks 1 and 2, 0.525 and 0.382, respectively, are smaller than 1, implying that respondents' probability judgmental distortions under the circumstances of Tasks 1 and 2.

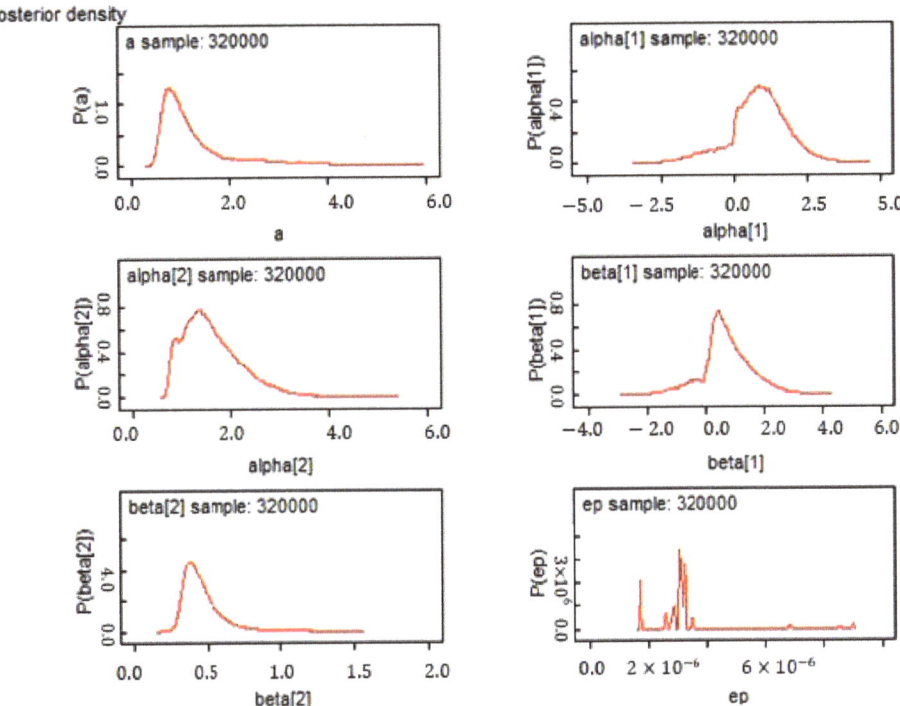

**Figure 2.** Posterior density distributions for all estimated parameters.

*4.3. Regression Results for the Effects of Individual and Organizational Factors*

Table 3 shows the regression results in which some coefficients of the factors are significantly different from 0, suggesting distortive effects of individual and organizational factors exist. Regarding VFs, the greater the α value is, the more risk-averse a participant behaves. Sociodemographic factors, including LTCF type, facility scale, and strategy type, significantly affect participants' VFs. The coefficient values of α parameter row of −0.06, 0.1, and −0.03 suggest that administrators of general nursing homes, larger facilities, and cost-leadership organizations, respectively, have cognitive value bias. Particularly, large-scale organizations with a coefficient value of 0.1 exhibit higher risk-averse behaviors.

**Table 3.** Regression results for six factors.

| Estimated Parameter | $\theta_0$ | Gender | Job Title | Funding Status | LTCF Type | Facility Scale | Strategy Type |
|---|---|---|---|---|---|---|---|
| α | 0.9 | 0.14 | −0.27 | −0.03 | −0.06 * | 0.1 * | −0.03 ** |
| β | 0.9 | 0.09 * | −0.16 ** | −0.27 * | −0.03 * | 0.05 * | 0.14 ** |

Note: * p-value < 0.1, ** p-value < 0.01. Gender: female (coded as 1 in the regression analysis) and male (coded as 2); Job title: facility (1) and healthcare (2); Funding status: public (1) and for profit (2); LTCF type: nursing homes (1), residential homes (2), and mixed LTCFs (3); Scale: less than 99 beds (1), 100~399 beds (2), and more than 400 beds (3); Strategy type: cost-leadership (1), differentiation (2), and hybrid (3).

The values of the β parameter row show factor effects on the PWFs. The results in Table 3 identified all six variables' bias effects on the perceived likelihood of an event occurrence. Given that our coding assigned values of 1 for females and 2 for males, the 0.09 coefficient of gender suggests that male executives are generally more sensitive to changes in probabilities than their female counterparts. Compared to medical administrators, facility managers with a coefficient value of −0.16 tend to distort infection risk probabilities or decision weights more. The estimated coefficient value of −0.27 suggests that public LTCF managers are more likely to enhance low probabilities and reduce high probabilities than for-profit organizations. Similar to the VFs, LTCF factors such as type, scale, and strategy, particularly in the general nursing homes, larger LTCFs, and hybrid care organizations, affect participants' PWFs, leading to biased behaviors when estimating the occurrence of infected cases.

## 5. Discussion

### 5.1. Risk Perception and Attitude

Table 2 shows that VFs of participants exhibit different risky behavior when facing varying decision tasks. The $\alpha$ value for Task 1 (1.433) is higher than that for Task 2 (1.176). The graphed results in Figure 3 show that the curves on the top left and bottom left panes are slightly concave for infection risk of possible cases (i.e., Task 1) and linear for infection risk of asymptomatic stakeholders (i.e., Task 2). Administrators tend to invest relatively large amounts in compensating for comparatively small losses resulting from possible infection cases, but they become risk-neutral or even risk-seeking when considering relatively damaging losses caused by this pandemic. In line with the previous literature [15,19,35], our results suggest that executives' diminishing sensitivity to the VFs for increasingly damaging losses thus determines how facilities engaged in healthcare preparedness and medical supply respond to COVID-19.

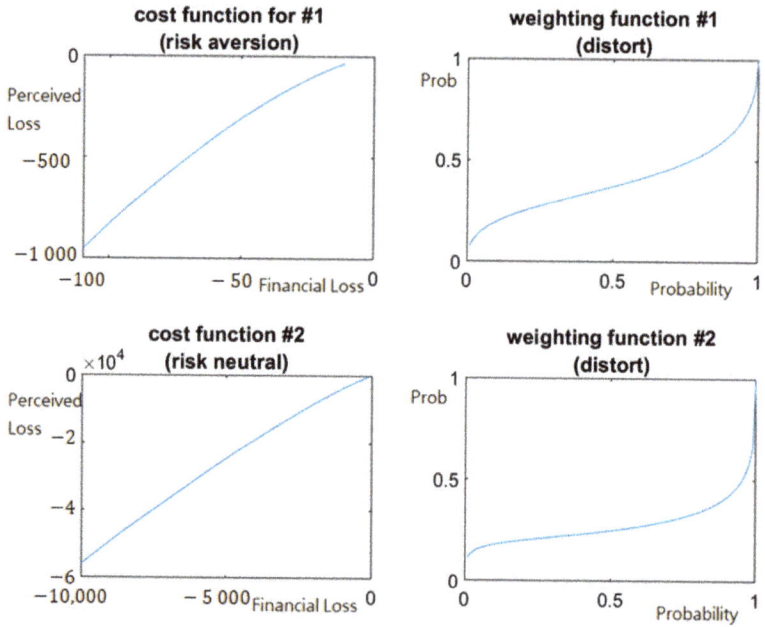

**Figure 3.** Value function $v(\cdot)$ (**left column**) and weighting function $w(\cdot)$ (**right column**) for Tasks 1 (**upward row**) and 2 (**downward row**), respectively.

Regarding PWFs, Table 2 shows that administrators underweight large probabilities and overweight small probabilities in both tasks, as predicted by CPT [19,35]. LTCF administrators show severe biased weighting behavior in which they may have inadequate awareness of emergencies such as COVID-19 and may not make optimal decisions to prevent the possible adverse effects. Task 2 has a smaller $\beta$ value (0.382) than Task 1 (0.525). The right column results of Figure 3 show that more considerable bias in probability weighting exists when managers weigh asymptomatic stakeholders' entrance occurrence

(Task 2) than that of possibly infected cases (Task 1). The findings also suggest that the PWFs vary depending on agents' attitudes toward different risk circumstances, such as the entrance occurrence of possible or asymptomatic cases. Overall, the results support that managers' risk perception and behavioral characteristics can affect decisions because of human bounded rationality in disaster response [16,25,52].

This study further considered the VF and the PWF jointly, suggesting risk attitude as a combination of attitudes toward outcomes and probabilities [19]. In Task 1 of possibly infected cases, as the PWF result of Task 1 distorts less significantly than Task 2 (see the right column of Figure 3), managers' decisions are more influenced by their risk-averse behavior response to this pandemic. By contrast, as the VF for Task 2 is close to linear, managers' risk response is entirely determined by the PWF rather than jointly by the functions $v(\cdot)$ and $w(\cdot)$. The findings highlight that decision-making can be influenced by either probability weighting or outcome sensitivity or a combination of probability and outcomes, leading to over- or under-estimation of risks and choice of inappropriate strategies. Hence, practitioners need to consider human cognitive limitations in risk preference and management. If agent bias could be counteracted, it is possible to avoid the same healthcare mistakes during the outbreak [10,12], reduce bias impacts on optimal decisions for medical resource governance [13,14], or raise awareness of inadequate contingency preparedness and risk response for healthcare operations [29]. Overall, our evidence fits the CPT elements proposed by Kahneman and Tversky [34] and Tversky and Kahneman [35], reflecting healthcare leaders' loss aversion and bias in response to the ongoing COVID-19 pandemic.

### 5.2. Biased Effects of Individual and Organizational Factors

Consistent with the findings of early studies on risk-taking behaviors [20,21,23–25], our results empirically identify subjective effects of either individual or contextual factors or both on editing and evaluating outcomes of complex choice situations. Regarding VFs, although the influence of individual variables is not significant, our findings identify the distortive effects of organizational factors, i.e., LTCF type, facility scale, and strategic orientation, on investment valuation for IPC practices [23]. In particular, large-scale organizations with a more considerable $\alpha$ coefficient value of 0.1 exhibit higher risk-averse behaviors and burden leaders to consider monetary spending to avoid relatively more minor losses. To respond to COVID-19, care organizations need to manage varying clinical and non-clinical resources and equipment supported by different sourcing systems and strategies. Thus, the findings highlight the vital roles of organizational characteristics in shifting decision-making toward a broader consideration of facilities' systems [29].

As for the results of PWFs, all six variables' biased effects are ratified. Administrators' risk perceptions that depend on a combination of individual characteristics, mental operations, and decision circumstances may impact their decisions [21,36]. Assessing is exacerbated by the contextual unpredictability and fragmented information involved in agents' subjective valuation [4,16,36] and their incomprehensive lens on impending business disruptions [11] in this evolving emergency. As shown in Table 3, a public organization, denoted by a higher coefficient value of $-0.27$, more strongly affects managers' assessments of probabilities of adverse events than other contextual determinants [10]. Accordingly, personal and organizational aspects require enhanced attention if care organizations want improvements in preparedness and responsiveness for medicine's long-term quality and security during a pandemic [14].

The regression results for the $\alpha$ parameter and $\beta$ parameter rows in Table 3 suggest that the factors of facility type, scale, and strategy simultaneously affect participants' VFs and PWFs. For considering facility type and scale, administrators of general nursing homes and larger facilities present perception bias in assessing outcomes and probabilities. Except for daily care planning, residents at general nursing homes who need skilled nursing care are at heightened risk of exposure to infection; larger LTCFs tend to enhance surveillance practices to minimize the danger of cluster infections [6,44]. In this regard, this unprecedented emergency makes decisions complicated, suggesting that managers' reference points vary considerably as their choice situations evolve. For general nursing homes and larger facilities, a participant's attitude toward risk is thus easily biased [36,41].

Specifically, the results in Table 3 show that the effect of facility strategy on the VF and the PWF is different. Cost-leadership LTCFs with a coefficient value of −0.03 exhibit biased valuation of IPC monetary spending, whereas hybrid-oriented organizations (the coefficient value of 0.14) appear biased in measuring probabilities. The literature notes that cost leaders in hospitals mainly focus on cost control and the efficiency of existing operations [46,47]. Similarly, our findings show that administrators of cost-oriented organizations think about the consequences of COVID-19 risk in a loss-averse way. Further, Kumar and Subramanian [46] and Ghiasi et al. [48] identified that hybrid organizations in the healthcare sector lack a clear focus on strategy formulation and implementation and therefore struggle to sustain their competitiveness and financial performance. Perception bias in PWFs of hybrid LTCF has managerial problems. Over- and underweighting risk probabilities may result in biased decisions, affecting IPC effectiveness and medicine supply responsiveness [4,13].

Overall, bias may occur and be exacerbated by individuals' subjective valuation of the severity of outcomes and rating of risk occurrence. Unwanted results are likely to happen in the subsequent decision-making process. If cognitive limitations on human reasoning and organizational features are addressed, risky choice problems can be evaluated and managed effectively and efficiently. The present results stress the importance of considering the effects of personal- and organization-specific variables, particularly facility type, scale, and strategy, on estimating risk probability and outcomes when making actual choices to respond to future pandemics.

## 6. Conclusions and Implications

Coronavirus disease 2019 (COVID-19) has posed severe threats to human safety and healthcare continuality and quality, particularly in residents in LTCFs at a higher risk of morbidity and mortality. This study adopted the policy Delphi technique to explore LTCF administrators' risk perceptions and attitudes, developed a CPT-based decision analysis model to understand their risky behaviors, and finally explored the roles of sociodemographic variables in influencing decisions under risk. The findings show that participants appeared risk-averse in the context of small losses and became risk-neutral when considering extensive, devastating damages. LTCF managers exhibited perception bias that led to over- and under-estimation of the occurrence of infection risk. Participants in general nursing homes, larger care organizations, and cost-leadership LTCFs demonstrated bias concerning this pandemic's outcomes. All six contextual determinants distort decision weights under risk. Public care organizations present relatively severe distortive weighting behavior. Specifically, organizational factors, including LTCF type, scale, and strategy, simultaneously affect leaders' risk perception toward consequences and probabilities. Concerning the effect of organization strategy, cost-leadership facilities behave in a loss-averse way, whereas hybrid-strategy LTCFs appear biased in measuring probabilities.

This study provides implications for academia and practice. First, this study extends CPT to risk management in the healthcare sector at an organizational level rather than the individual level, as the extant literature does [42,43]. The findings complement COVID-19 literature by exploring managers' interpretations (i.e., perception and attitude) on varying mixed gain–loss circumstances involving healthcare demand and capacity considerations that influence healthcare management and risk practices [4,15,29]. Second, this study observes participants' diminishing sensitivity to consequences and biased probability weighting behaviors. Administrators need to counteract individual subjective estimation of occurrence and outcomes, which likely avoid the human errors and systems failures that this coronavirus has revealed [10,12], make optimal decisions for supply risk governance [13], or enhance contingency preparedness for timely, adequate risk response [14]. Last, given rapidly evolving situations and inadequate information, this study suggests that administrators pay attention to their changing perception and reference points depending on the current state of COVID-19 [41,43] and the affordance and capabilities of their care organizations [27,29]. Specifically, our results suggest that proper risk management strongly depends on organizational characteristics such as LTCF type, scale, and strategy. The issues associated with organizational-level risk assessment and decision behavior should be considered when urging LTCFs to provide continuous care while implementing effective IPC practice and risk management.

Some limitations need to be addressed. First, this study primarily collected data from Taiwanese LTCFs. This obstacle may limit the generalizability of the results to other countries or healthcare organizations such as hospitals. Another limitation is the focus on infection risk, which precludes examining the impacts of other clinical and non-clinical risks and neglects intertwined relationships among other health systems' adverse events. Future research could consider more decision tasks that complement risky choice situations with other risks or unexpected events such as earthquakes. Last, the literature emphasizes competitiveness and facility intra-relationships [48,54] and complex stakeholders and relationships in the healthcare sector [13,14]. Future studies could consider other sociodemographic factors in examining decision-making under risk and influencing reorienting healthcare strategy, particularly organization-specific considerations when facing ongoing COVID-19 and future pandemics.

**Funding:** The research was founded by Ministry of Science & Technology, Taiwan. MOST 109-2511-H-344-001; MOST 110-2511-H-344-001-MY3.

**Institutional Review Board Statement:** Ethical review and approval were waived for this study, due to the following conditions issued by the Governance Framework for Human Research Ethics at National Cheng Kung University in Taiwan: (1) participants of this study are not homeless, children and adolescents, native citizens, new immigrants, pregnant women, handicappers, or psychiatric patients; (2) the likelihood of damages or discomfort derived from participating in this study is not higher than the chance of any other damages or discomfort in participants' daily life; (3) decisions to take or not to take part in this study do no influence participants' rights and benefits; (4) participants do not provide personal information; (5) the collection data is appropriately saved by researchers' institutions and used only for this study, and (6) the collection data is unrelated to any specific participant, organization, or circumstance.

**Informed Consent Statement:** This study verbally informed interviewees about information concerning the research background, aims, methods, analysis tools, and future publication of this study and asked participants to act as representatives of their facilities rather than individual anonymous interviewees. This study did not use written informed consent for survey participants. The survey questionnaires were mailed to potential organizations and received the written questionnaire by mails. This study did not know who participated in the survey because of no personal identification data.

**Conflicts of Interest:** The author declares no conflict of interest.

## Appendix A

1. Demographic data: gender, job title, the funding status of the organization, LTCF type, and facility scale.
2. Organizational strategy type: On a scale of 1 (strongly disagree) to 7 (strongly agree), please select the option that most nearly corresponds with your organizations' operations strategies.
    (1) My care organization provides innovative, differentiated, diverse, and large-scale care services/programs.
    (2) My care organization engages in a cost-efficient analysis of equipment and resources, facilities, the workforce, and care services/programs.
3. Decision tasks for investing IPC measures to minimize the damages caused by COVID-19:
    (1) Decision Task 1. If a possibly infected stakeholder (i.e., resident, staff member, or visitor) enters the facilities, he/she may be a source of infection risk that causes a facility-wide outbreak. Thus, LTCFs need additional administrative

(2) Decision Task 2. If an asymptomatic stakeholder (i.e., resident, staff member, or visitor) enters the facilities, he/she may be a source of infection risk that causes a facility-wide outbreak. Five financial loss scenarios were assumed, namely, USD 200,000, 500,000, 800,000, 1,100,000, and 1,400,000. For each loss scenario of Task 2, we assumed five probabilities of an asymptomatic case entrance occurrence, namely, 0.1% (i.e., one asymptomatic agent among 1000 agents who entered the facilities), 0.3%, 1%, 3%, and 9%. The amount of IPC investment included five choices, namely, USD 10,000, 30,000, 100,000, 300,000, and 1,000,000. Task 2 involved answering the question, "What is the acceptable amount of investment in IPC measures that your organization would choose to minimize the damages caused by COVID-19 under numerous decisions when considering various probabilities and different loss scenarios simultaneously?"

and financial resources to support IPC activities focused on the abovementioned stakeholders to prevent damage. Five financial loss scenarios were presented, namely, USD 10,000, 40,000, 70,000, 100,000, and 130,000. We assumed five probabilities of a possibly infected stakeholder's entrance occurrence for each loss scenario, namely, 1% (i.e., one possible agent among 100 agents who entered the facilities), 3%, 10%, 30%, and 90%. This study assumed that LTCFs would invest in the IPC practices suggested by the WHO and CDC to prevent infection risk. The amount of IPC investment included five choices, namely, USD 1000, 3000, 10,000, 30,000, and 100,000. Task 1 included answering the question, "What is the acceptable amount of investment in IPC measures that your organization would choose to minimize the damages caused by COVID-19 under numerous decisions when considering various probabilities and different loss scenarios simultaneously?"

## References

1. WHO. Infection Prevention and Control Guidance for Long-Term Care Facilities in the Context of COVID-19: Interim Guidance. Available online: https://apps.who.int/iris/bitstream/handle/10665/331508/WHO-2019-nCoV-IPC_long_term_care-2020.1-eng.pdf?sequence=1&isAllowed=y (accessed on 20 June 2021).
2. WHO. Strengthening the Health System Response to COVID-19. Maintaining the Delivery of Essential Health Care Services While Mobilizing the Health Workforce for the COVID-19 Response (18 April 2020). Available online: https://apps.who.int/iris/bitstream/handle/10665/332559/WHO-EURO-2020-669-40404-54161-eng.pdf?sequence=1&isAllowed=y (accessed on 20 June 2021).
3. WHO. Report Coronavirus Disease 2019 (COVID-19) Situation Report-179. Available online: https://www.who.int/docs/default-source/coronaviruse/situation-reports/20200717-covid-19-sitrep-179.pdf (accessed on 20 June 2021).
4. D'Adamo, H.; Yoshikawa, T.; Ouslander, J.G. Coronavirus disease 2019 in geriatrics and long-term care: The ABCDs of COVID-19. *J. Am. Geriatr. Soc.* **2020**, *68*, 912–917. [CrossRef] [PubMed]
5. Levitt, A.F.; Ling, S.M. COVID-19 in the Long-Term Care Setting: The CMS Perspective. *J. Am. Geriatr. Soc.* **2020**, *68*, 1366–1369. [CrossRef] [PubMed]
6. Yen, M.-Y.; Schwartz, J.; King, C.-C.; Lee, C.-M.; Hsueh, P.-R. Recommendation on protection from and mitigation of COVID-19 pandemic in long-term care facilities. *J. Microbiol. Immunol. Infect.* **2020**, *53*, 447–453. [CrossRef] [PubMed]
7. European Centre for Disease Prevention and Control. Infection Prevention and Control and Preparedness for COVID-19 in Healthcare Settings—Third Update. 13 May 2020. Available online: https://www.ecdc.europa.eu/sites/default/files/documents/Infection-prevention-control-for-the-care-of-patients-with-2019-nCoV-healthcare-settings_third-update.pdf (accessed on 20 July 2021).
8. Kamp, J.; Mathews, A.W. Coronavirus Outbreaks Spreading in Nursing Homes. Available online: https://www.wsj.com/articles/coronavirus-outbreaks-spreading-in-nursing-homes-11584628291 (accessed on 20 June 2020).
9. Carter, P.; Anderson, M.; Mossialos, E. Health system, public health, and economic implications of managing COVID-19 from a cardiovascular perspective. *Eur. Heart J.* **2020**, *41*, 2516–2518. [CrossRef]
10. Renda, A.; Castro, R. Towards stronger EU governance of health threats after the COVID-19 pandemic. *Eur. J. Risk Regul.* **2020**, *11*, 273–282. [CrossRef]
11. Sharma, P.; Leung, T.Y.; Kingshott, R.P.; Davcik, N.S.; Cardinali, S. Managing uncertainty during a global pandemic: An international business perspective. *J. Bus. Res.* **2020**, *116*, 188–192. [CrossRef]
12. McAleer, M. Prevention is better than the cure: Risk management of COVID-19. *J. Risk Financ. Manag.* **2020**, *13*, 46. [CrossRef]
13. Bhaskar, S.; Tan, J.; Bogers, M.L.; Minssen, T.; Badaruddin, H.; Israeli-Korn, S.; Chesbrough, H. At the epicenter of COVID-19–the tragic failure of the global supply chain for medical supplies. *Front. Public Health* **2020**, *8*, 821. [CrossRef]

14. Kuo, S.; Ou, H.-T.; Wang, C.J. Managing medication supply chains: Lessons learned from Taiwan during the COVID-19 pandemic and preparedness planning for the future. *J. Am. Pharm. Assoc.* **2021**, *61*, e12–e15. [CrossRef]
15. Choi, T.-M. Risk analysis in logistics systems: A research agenda during and after the COVID-19 pandemic. *Tranportation Res. Part E* **2021**, *145*, 102190. [CrossRef]
16. Liu, Y.; Fan, Z.-P.; Zhang, Y. Risk decision analysis in emergency response: A method based on cumulative prospect theory. *Comput. Oper. Res.* **2014**, *42*, 75–82. [CrossRef]
17. Bertsimas, D.; Boussioux, L.; Cory-Wright, R.; Delarue, A.; Digalakis, V.; Jacquillat, A.; Kitane, D.L.; Lukin, G.; Li, M.; Mingardi, L.; et al. From predictions to prescriptions: A data-driven response to COVID-19. *Health Care Manag. Sci.* **2021**, *24*, 253–272. [CrossRef] [PubMed]
18. Barberis, N.C. Thirty years of prospect theory in economics: A review and assessment. *J. Econ. Perspect.* **2013**, *27*, 173–195. [CrossRef]
19. Fennema, H.; Wakker, P. Original and cumulative prospect theory: A discussion of empirical differences. *J. Behav. Decis. Mak.* **1997**, *10*, 53–64. [CrossRef]
20. Cagliano, A.C.; Grimaldi, S.; Rafele, C. A systemic methodology for risk management in healthcare sector. *Saf. Sci.* **2011**, *49*, 695–708. [CrossRef]
21. Fraser-Mackenzie, P.; Sung, M.C.; Johnson, J.E. Toward an understanding of the influence of cultural background and domain experience on the effects of risk-pricing formats on risk perception. *Risk Anal.* **2014**, *34*, 1846–1869. [CrossRef]
22. Leung, T.Y.; Sharma, P.; Adithipyangkul, P.; Hosie, P. Gender equity and public health outcomes: The COVID-19 experience. *J. Bus. Res.* **2020**, *116*, 193–198. [CrossRef]
23. March, J.G.; Shapira, Z. Managerial perspectives on risk and risk taking. *Manag. Sci.* **1987**, *33*, 1404–1418. [CrossRef]
24. McNamara, G.; Bromiley, P. Decision making in an organizational setting: Cognitive and organizational influences on risk assessment in commercial lending. *Acad. Manag. J.* **1997**, *40*, 1063–1088.
25. Robinson, P.J.; Botzen, W.W. Determinants of probability neglect and risk attitudes for disaster risk: An online experimental study of flood insurance demand among homeowners. *Risk Anal.* **2019**, *39*, 2514–2527. [CrossRef]
26. Danis, K.; Fonteneau, L.; Georges, S.; Daniau, C.; Bernard-Stoecklin, S.; Domegan, L.; O'Donnell, J.; Hauge, S.H.; Dequeker, S.; Vandael, E.; et al. High impact of COVID-19 in long-term care facilities, suggestion for monitoring in the EU/EEA, May 2020. *Eurosurveillance* **2020**, *25*, 2000956.
27. Comas-Herrera, A.; Zalakaín, J. Mortality associated with COVID-19 outbreaks in care homes: Early international evidence. *Int. Long-Term Care Policy Netw.* **2020**, *12*, 1–6.
28. CDC. Infection Prevention and Control Assessment Tool for Nursing Homes Preparing for COVID-19. Available online: https://www.cdc.gov/coronavirus/2019-ncov/downloads/hcp/assessment-tool-nursing-homes.pdf (accessed on 5 July 2020).
29. Leite, H.; Lindsay, C.; Kumar, M. COVID-19 outbreak: Implications on healthcare operations. *TQM J.* **2021**, *33*, 247–256. [CrossRef]
30. De Loë, R.C.; Melnychuk, N.; Murray, D.; Plummer, R. Advancing the state of policy Delphi practice: A systematic review evaluating methodological evolution, innovation, and opportunities. *Technol. Forecast. Soc. Change* **2016**, *104*, 78–88. [CrossRef]
31. de Meyrick, J. The Delphi method and health research. *Health Educ.* **2003**, *103*, 7–16. [CrossRef]
32. Meskell, P.; Murphy, K.; Shaw, D.G.; Casey, D. Insights into the use and complexities of the Policy Delphi technique. *Nurse Res.* **2014**, *21*, 7–16. [CrossRef]
33. Paraskevas, A.; Saunders, M.N. Beyond consensus: An alternative use of Delphi enquiry in hospitality research. *Int. J. Contemp. Hosp. Manag.* **2012**, *24*, 907–924. [CrossRef]
34. Kahneman, D.; Tversky, A. Prospect theory: An analysis of decision under risk. *Econom. J. Econom. society* **1979**, *47*, 263–291. [CrossRef]
35. Tversky, A.; Kahneman, D. Advances in prospect theory: Cumulative representation of uncertainty. *J. Risk Uncertain.* **1992**, *5*, 297–323. [CrossRef]
36. Levy, J.S. An introduction to prospect theory. *Political Psychol.* **1992**, *13*, 171–186.
37. Booij, A.S.; Van de Kuilen, G. A parameter-free analysis of the utility of money for the general population under prospect theory. *J. Econ. Psychol.* **2009**, *30*, 651–666. [CrossRef]
38. Goda, K.; Hong, H. Implied preference for seismic design level and earthquake insurance. *Risk Anal. Int. J.* **2008**, *28*, 523–537. [CrossRef] [PubMed]
39. Guo, S.-M.; Wu, T.; Chen, Y.J. Over- and under-estimation of risks and counteractive adjustment for cold chain operations: A prospect theory perspective. *Int. J. Logist. Manag.* **2018**, *29*, 902–921. [CrossRef]
40. De La Maza, C.; Davis, A.; Gonzalez, C.; Azevedo, I. Understanding cumulative risk perception from judgments and choices: An application to flood risks. *Risk Anal.* **2019**, *39*, 488–504. [CrossRef] [PubMed]
41. Bern-Klug, M. Considering the CPR decision through the Lens of Prospect theory in the context of advanced chronic illness. *Gerontol.* **2017**, *57*, 61–67. [CrossRef]
42. Winter, L.; Lawton, M.P.; Ruckdeschel, K. Preferences for prolonging life: A prospect theory approach. *Int. J. Aging Hum. Dev.* **2003**, *56*, 155–170. [CrossRef]
43. Winter, L.; Parker, B. Current health and preferences for life-prolonging treatments: An application of prospect theory to end-of-life decision making. *Soc. Sci. Med.* **2007**, *65*, 1695–1707. [CrossRef]

44. ECDC. Surveillance of COVID-19 at Long-Term Care Facilities in the EU/EEA. Available online: https://www.ecdc.europa.eu/sites/default/files/documents/covid-19-long-term-care-facilities-surveillance-guidance.pdf (accessed on 20 July 2021).
45. Ghiasi, A.; Weech-Maldonado, R.; Hearld, L.; Zengul, F.; Rsulnia, M.; Hood, A.; Puro, N. The Moderating Effect of Environmental Instability on the Hospital Strategy-Financial Performance Relationship. *J. Health Care Financ.* **2019**, *Fall*, 1–18.
46. Kumar, K.; Subramanian, R. Porters Strategic Types: Differences In Internal Processes and Their Impact on Performance. *J. Appl. Bus. Res. (JABR)* **1998**, *14*, 107–124. [CrossRef]
47. Landry, A.Y.; Hernandez, S.R.; Shewchuk, R.M.; Garman, A.N. A configurational view of executive selection behaviours: A taxonomy of USA acute care hospitals. *Health Serv. Manag. Res.* **2010**, *23*, 128–138. [CrossRef]
48. Ghiasi, A.; Zengul, F.D.; Ozaydin, B.; Oner, N.; Breland, B.K. The impact of hospital competition on strategies and outcomes of hospitals: A systematic review of the US hospitals 1996-2016. *J. Health Care Financ.* **2018**, *44*, 2.
49. Topolyan, I.; Brasington, D.; Xu, X. Assessing the degree of competitiveness in the market for outpatient hospital services. *J. Econ. Bus.* **2019**, *105*, 105838. [CrossRef]
50. Turoff, M.; Linstone, H.A. *The Delphi Method-Techniques and Applications*; Addison-Wesley: Reading, MA, USA, 2002.
51. Wolf, L.A.; Delao, A.M. Establishing research priorities for the emergency severity index using a modified Delphi approach. *J. Emerg. Nurs.* **2021**, *47*, 50–57. [CrossRef] [PubMed]
52. Gonzalez, R.; Wu, G. On the shape of the probability weighting function. *Cogn. Psychol.* **1999**, *38*, 129–166. [CrossRef]
53. Wu, G.; Gonzalez, R. Curvature of the probability weighting function. *Manag. Sci.* **1996**, *42*, 1676–1690. [CrossRef]
54. Windrum, P. Third sector organizations and the co-production of health innovations. *Manag. Decis.* **2014**, *52*, 1046–1056. [CrossRef]

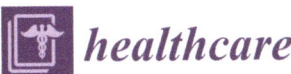

Article

# The Economic and Psychological Impacts of COVID-19 Pandemic on Indian Migrant Workers in the Kingdom of Saudi Arabia

Mohammed Arshad Khan [1,*], Md Imran Khan [2], Asheref Illiyan [2] and Maysoon Khojah [1]

1. Accounting Department, College of Administrative and Financial Sciences, Saudi Electronic University, Riyadh 11673, Saudi Arabia; m.khoja@seu.edu.sa
2. Department of Economics, Faculty of Social Sciences, Jamia Millia Islamia (A Central University), New Delhi 110025, India; imran738@gmail.com (M.I.K.); ailliyan@jmi.ac.in (A.I.)
* Correspondence: m.akhan@seu.edu.sa

**Citation:** Khan, M.A.; Khan, M.I.; Illiyan, A.; Khojah, M. The Economic and Psychological Impacts of COVID-19 Pandemic on Indian Migrant Workers in the Kingdom of Saudi Arabia. *Healthcare* **2021**, *9*, 1152. https://doi.org/10.3390/healthcare9091152

Academic Editors: Eduardo Tomé, Thomas Garavan, Ana Dias and Pedram Sendi

Received: 21 July 2021
Accepted: 27 August 2021
Published: 3 September 2021

**Publisher's Note:** MDPI stays neutral with regard to jurisdictional claims in published maps and institutional affiliations.

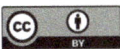

**Copyright:** © 2021 by the authors. Licensee MDPI, Basel, Switzerland. This article is an open access article distributed under the terms and conditions of the Creative Commons Attribution (CC BY) license (https://creativecommons.org/licenses/by/4.0/).

**Abstract:** The ongoing Coronavirus disease 2019 (COVID-19) pandemic has changed the working environment, occupation, and living style of billions of people around the world. The severest impact of the coronavirus is on migrant communities; hence, it is relevant to assess the economic impact and mental status of the Indian migrants. This study is quantitative in nature and based on a sample survey of 180 migrant workers. Descriptive statistics, chi-square test, dependent sample t-test, and Pearson's correlation coefficient were utilized to analyze the surveyed data. The findings of the study reveal, through the working experience of the migrants, that new international migration has reduced due to lockdown and international travel restrictions. It was also reported that the majority of the migrants worked less than the normal working hours during the lockdown, causing a reduction of salary and remittances. Chi-square test confirms that the perceptions of migrants towards the COVID-19 management by the government were significantly different in opinion by different occupation/profession. Majority of the sampled migrants reported the problem of nervousness, anxiety, and depression; however, they were also hopeful about the future. The psychological problem was severe for the migrants above the age of 40, not educated, and with a higher number of family members. Subsequently, the policy implications from the findings of the research can draw attention of the policy makers towards protective measures which need to be implemented to support migrants during the ongoing pandemic. The government should take some necessary steps, such as a financial benefit scheme, to overcome the problems in the reduction of migrant earnings and remittances. The government should not focus only on vaccination and physical fitness of the migrants but also need to find out the cure of the psychological impact arising during the pandemic.

**Keywords:** COVID-19; pandemic; migrants; sample survey; employment status; remittances; migrants' perception; economic and psychological impacts

## 1. Introduction

The dangerous ongoing pandemic, Coronavirus disease 2019 (COVID-19), reported in Wuhan city, China, in December 2019 and it is caused by a novel coronavirus called SARS coronavirus 2 (SARS-CoV-2) [1]. The director general of the World Health Organization (WHO) initially declared the spread of coronavirus as a public health emergency of international concern on 30 January 2020. Later on, the WHO declared a pandemic on 11 March 2020 [2]. The novel coronavirus is unique in nature because of high man-to-man transmission and has spread to 176 million people worldwide and caused 3.8 million deaths as of 15 June 2021 [3]. This pandemic has changed the occupation and living style of billions of people around the world and raised questions of medical facility arrangements of the different countries of the world. The government of China started imposing restrictions and the lockdown in Wuhan city began on 23 January 2020, followed by India on 24 March and Saudi Arabia on 25 March 2020 [4]. The main objective of the lockdown or curfew is to limit the spread of the virus by maintaining social distancing and creating medical facility on war footing. Lockdown; banned public gatherings; suspending religious activities; closure of business, schools, colleges, etc.; curfews; and restriction or suspension of all the travel domestically as well as internationally were followed by the majority of countries as preventative measures. The government of Saudi Arabia had suspended all its international flights on 15 March 2020 and resumes after 14 months on 17 May 2021; however, the suspension of flights will continue to 13 countries, including India due to the second wave of corona virus [5].

The COVID-19 pandemic is not only a health emergency but also a labor market and economic crisis because of its effects on the business status of millions of individuals. The Saudi health ministry took the initiative to provide free corona vaccine and also offered free corona screening and health care services to all of its citizen, including migrants workers, and made vaccine compulsory for the health care workers participating in Hajj and Umrah (Islamic pilgrimage to Mecca) initially and later on made it compulsory for all male and female private and public sector workers to attend the workplace [5–7]. COVID-19 immunization will be required to participate in any socio-cultural, commercial, economic, entertainment, or supporting affairs in Saudi Arabia from 1 August 2021 [7,8]. The government of Saudi Arabia is strict towards the enforcement of COVID-19 regulations to reduce its spread and violators are fined between Saudi Riyal (SAR) 10,000 to SAR 100,000; however, a second wave of COVID-19 hit the country in the beginning of February 2021 [9].

According to Indian Census-2011, India had 45.6 crore migrant population (38%) and, according to the recent report published by "United Nations Department of Economic and Social Affairs—2019", India continues to have the maximum of its people (17.5 million) living overseas and highest remittance receiving country (USD 78.6 billion). Saudi Arabia is the third top remittances sending country (USD 36.1 billion) in the world and ranked third (13 million) in largest number of international migrants in the world. India–Saudi Arabia shifted from the tenth (2000–2010) to seventh largest bilateral migration corridor in the world [10,11].

The COVID-19 pandemic had reduced the new international migration and increased the returnee migrants, which happens to be the first time in recent history. According to an estimate by World Bank, a total of 6,000,000 migrants were evacuated through special flights (Vande Bharat Mission) and Kerala was affected the most by 4,000,000 returnee migrants. The estimated remittances (World Bank) to India will fall by 9% in 2020 and 14% in 2021 and the flow of foreign direct investment will fall by 36% in 2020; however, India will continue to be the top remittance recipient country globally, with approximately USD 76 billion which will be 2.9% of its Gross Domestic Product (GDP). The monetary emergency accentuated by COVID-19 could be long, profound, and inescapable when seen through a relocation focal point [12]. The oil rich country and job-rich sector in Saudi Arabia was drastically affected by Corona virus because of the drop in trade, disruption of production, tourism (Hajj and umrah), and hospitality. Lockdown and travel restriction reduce the demand for oil globally, and consequently oil prices had fallen by 50% in March 2020. To recuperate the economic slowdown, the Saudi government allowed private sector companies to cut the salaries of the workers up to 40% for a period of six month and thereafter could also terminate the contract [13,14]. The majority of the migrant workers in Saudi Arabia are engaged in the construction sector, agriculture, hospitality, and domestic work, which are highly affected by the ongoing pandemic. The acutely affected migrants in the state during the pandemic are domestic workers, low skilled/low-income workers, contract terminated or completed workers, informal workers, women migrant workers, and salaried employees. In this context, the present study attempts to make a deeper analysis of economic and psychological impacts of COVID-19 pandemic on Indian migrant workers in Saudi Arabia. The paper is coordinated as follows: Section 1 is introductory, Section 2 reviews the literature, Section 3 describes the research gap, Section 4 delineates the research methodology, and Section 5 details the results and findings of the study. The last section, i.e., Section 6, concludes the paper. The limitations and future scope for work are also described in this section.

## 2. Review of Literature

The Kingdom of Saudi Arabia identified its first Corona virus positive case in Qatif (Eastern Region): a person returned from Iran through Bahrain on 2 March 2020. The Saudi government reacted accordingly by limiting domestic travel, suspending the e-visa program, closing schools and colleges, closing non-essential industries, and imposing lockdown in Qatif region on 8 March 2020, followed by a temporary ban on international flights on 15 March and domestic flights on 21 March [15]. The Saudi government issued general guidelines as preventive measures to limit the spread of virus in the early stage by ensuring social distancing, measuring temperature before entering in public places, and mandatory of wearing face mask in public places. Lack of compliance was penalized with SAR 1000 (Saudi Riyal) [16].

The undocumented immigrants (with no legal rights to reside in the country) in any country are at higher risk during the pandemic, as they are probably not getting the relief benefits provided by the local government and are living in fear of deportation. The Saudi government has decided to provide proper health care services to undocumented migrants without any legal action or deportation; however, not everybody is enjoying the legal access to health care facilities due to fear of deportation [17,18].

The COVID-19 pandemic has influenced the worldwide economy as well as Saudi Kingdom's economy. The most impacted sector, due to a ban on religious Hajj and Umrah, was the hospitality sector, especially in Makkah and Madinah. The International Air Transport Association estimates USD 7.2 billion loss of the Saudi aviation sector in 2020 due to suspension of international flights, which also affected the job status of 287 thousand people in this sector. Lockdown and suspension of international flights globally reduces the demand for oil to approximately 80 million barrel per day: consequently, the oil price was decreased by 58% in the beginning of 2020. The total decline in export of chemical and related industries due to blocked international trade were estimated to be more than SAR 10 billion in 2020 [19,20].

One study reveals that the wage cut among the gulf workers ranges between 25% to 50%, especially in education, hospitality, and other service-related industries, and income of foreign workers had substantially reduced (83% in Dubai and 35% in Jeddah) due to closure of industries as well as a drop in remittances to their respective countries by 44% during the initial wave of pandemic. Many migrants (from the Philippines, Pakistan, and Egypt) in Saudi Arabia do not want to return back to their respective countries because of the good health and emergency services in the destination country and poor medical services, high unemployment rate, and lower wage rate in their country of origin. In the same survey (N = 117), a majority of the studied migrants (89.7%) responded that they believe that gulf cities have effectively controlled the pandemic and 53% of respondents believe that locals' attitudes towards the migrant did not change, 29.9% positively changed, and 17% reported negative changes in their attitude during the pandemic [20].

The world economy is suffering from economic slowdown and an unemployment crisis due to COVID-19. One research survey by APCO worldwide (The Association of Public-Safety Communications Officials) shows that 40% of Saudi citizens spend a lesser amount on the purchases of goods and services than before COVID-19; however, the majority of the respondents (81%) believe that the Kingdom will recover from the pandemic faster than other countries in the region because of the immediate action taken by the government [21]. In order to recover the economy from the pandemic and overcome the effect on private sector, the Saudi government implemented a relief package of USD 32 billion, which will help the hospitality sector to recover. The Kingdom of Saudi Arabia also focuses on the SME (small and medium enterprises) sector by announcing a financial support of SAR 50 billion. To manage the budgetary deficit raised because of the fall in petrochemical revenue, the Saudi government chose to expand the Value Added Tax (VAT) from 5 percent to 15 percent and also attempt to help the economy by implementing technology-based solution especially for the education sector and e-businesses [22].

Another study estimates a total 21% loss of the expected earning of low skilled Indian migrant workers in Saudi Arabia and a 36% loss adding recruitment cost and total remittances could fall by USD 2 billion due to COVID-19. This estimation was done by using simple estimation model and used the data collected by KNOMAD-ILO (The Global Knowledge Partnership on Migration and Development along with International Labor Organization) in 2016-17 [23].

Psychological impact (anxiety and depression) on well-being is normal during any pandemic outbreak. Coronavirus disease had to have severe psychological effects due to the uncertainty associated with it. It is important to focus attention on physical health along with measures to balance the mental status of the people. A sample study on psychological impact on the general population in the context of Saudi Arabia was carried out at the time of COVID-19 curfew and lockdown, and revealed that stress, anxiety, and depression were majorly found in medical workers, students, females, and persons with a mental disorder, and 1/4th of the sample population experienced moderate to serious psychological effects [24,25]. Another sample study for Saudi Arabia during the first wave of Corona virus disease stated that a marginal but substantial portion of the general population had found symptoms of anxiety and depression, and a majority of them reported symptoms of psychological distress [26]. The emotional wellbeing in any society is defined by measuring distress, depression, anxiety, and behavioral control among the people. The emotional wellbeing in the general population of Saudi Arabia was found to be moderate during the COVID-19 pandemic. It was positively affected because the health authority of the Saudi government responded in a timely manner and adopted effective measures to control the spread of the virus [27]. Job status of the workers (employed or unemployed) during the pandemic has drastically changed, which also influences the mental status of the people. The symptom of depression, as evidence from South Africa suggests, was less frequent among individuals who retained paid employment during lockdown than those who lost their job [28].

The migrants in the society are more prone to have psychological distress during any outbreak because of the job insecurity and loneliness. A study assessing the psychological impact on Indian migrant-workers during COVID-19 lockdown reveals that the symptoms of anxiety and depression are severe in migrant workers. A majority of the respondents (73.5%) reported the symptom of depression, half of them were positive for anxiety, and nearly 51% of the migrant workers were found to have the symptom of both anxiety and depression [29]. Another study about the low wage migrant workers in Singapore during the pandemic revealed they are at higher risk of bearing significant health, mental, and socio-economic effects [30]. A study was carried out to understand the prevalence of anxiety, stress, and depression among repatriated Indonesian migrant workers during coronavirus pandemic. It was found that symptoms of anxiety, stress and depression were somewhat lower when contrasted with overall public and medical care in the country. The risk of anxiety and depression were found to be low in educated, young, and married people. The risk is higher among the people who had negative perceptions about the wellbeing and COVID sicknesses. Better health care services and improved quarantine facilities were found to be crucial to reduce psychological problems of repatriated migrant workers [31].

### 3. Research Gap

To date, many studies have considered the socio-economic impacts of Corona virus on the general population, ignoring the economic impacts on migrants and their perceptions of the COVID-19 management by the government. Several studies also assess the psychological or mental effect of Corona virus on the general populace of the country; however, in the current paper we also analyze the psychological impact on the migrants.

## 4. Research Methodology

The present study assesses the economic and psychological impacts on Indian migrant workers in the Kingdom of Saudi Arabia during the Corona virus pandemic. This study is quantitative in nature and depends on a sample-survey approach. Both primary and secondary information are utilized. Primary data were collected through a process of structured Google Forms questionnaire. The respondents of this study were Indian migrant workers in Saudi Arabia who were selected through non-probability snowball sampling techniques. This technique of data collection was used so that researchers could identify the Indian migrants in the Saudi Arabia due to COVID-19 related restrictions. The survey was in English language and titled as 'COVID-19 Pandemic and Indian Migrants in Saudi Arabia', and data were collected by sharing the link of the Google form through different social networking sites for literate migrants and through telephonic interview for illiterate migrants. The survey contained 29 open-ended questions, which required 4 to 6 min in total to complete. There were three segments in the overview poll. Section 1 collected the information associated with the respondent's profile (13 items) such as name, age, gender, religion, domicile, educational qualification, profession, working experience, monthly salary, remittances, number of dependent people, and other sources of family income. Section 2 of the questionnaire (8 items) includes questions on the COVID-19 pandemic disruption of daily life, job status, salary reduction, and perception of the COVID-19 management by the government. The third section includes the questions (8 items) on psychological impact (depression, anxiety, and stress) during the lockdown due to the pandemic. The sample data of 180 Indian migrants in the Kingdom of Saudi Arabia belonging to different regions (states) were collected during the months of April and May 2021. The sample data consist of 98.8% male migrants and 1.2% female migrants. The majority of the working Indian migrants in the Saudi Arabia are male. According to UNDESA-2019, in total female migrants were around 30% of the total migrants; however, the majority of them are dependent and not working [32]. This paper includes the sample of only those migrants who were working, and therefore the sample of female migrants is smaller. A five-point Likert scale was used to collect the perception towards COVID-19 management by the government and a two-point Likert scale was used to assess psychological impact on migrants during the COVID-19 pandemic. The collected data were scrutinized through the 'statistical package for social sciences' (SPSS) version 28 (IBM, Armonk, NY, USA) and descriptive statistics were used for all covariates and survey responses.

## 5. Results, Findings, and Discussion

### 5.1. Demographic Profile of the Migrants

Table 1 illustrates the demographic profile of the surveyed migrants. It is depicted that the majority of Indian migrants in the Saudi Arabia (68.3%) were aged between 30 to 50. 15% were in between 20–30 and 16.7% were above 50 years of age. Migration to Saudi Arabia for work is mostly undertaken by males: around 98.8% were male migrant-workers and only 1.2% were female workers. The maximum number of the migrants (90.5%) belong to the religion of Islam (Muslims), 7.8% were Hindus, and 1.7% were Christians. Around 56.1% of the migrants belong to Uttar Pradesh (a state in India), 26.7% were from Bihar, 4.4% were from the National Capital of Delhi and Madhya Pradesh each, 2.8% were from Kerala, and only 5.6% were from the other states of India. The majority of the respondents (35.6%) hold bachelor's degree (graduation), 26.7% hold an intermediate (senior secondary schooling) degree, 16.1% had studied until high school (10th class), 12.2% were post graduates, and only 2.2% hold a doctorate degree; however, 7.2% of the migrant workers were not educated.

**Table 1.** Demographic Profile of the Migrants.

| Variables | Levels | Data in Number | Data in % |
|---|---|---|---|
| Age | 20–30 | 27 | 15.0% |
|  | 30–40 | 58 | 32.2% |
|  | 40–50 | 65 | 36.1% |
|  | 50–60 | 30 | 16.7% |
| Gender | Male | 178 | 98.8% |
|  | Female | 2 | 1.2% |
| Domicile | Uttar Pradesh | 101 | 56.1% |
|  | Bihar | 48 | 26.7% |
|  | Delhi | 8 | 4.4% |
|  | Madhya Pradesh | 8 | 4.4% |
|  | Kerala | 5 | 2.8% |
|  | Other | 10 | 5.6% |
| Education | Doctorate | 4 | 2.2% |
|  | Post-Graduation | 22 | 12.2% |
|  | Graduation | 64 | 35.6% |
|  | Intermediate | 48 | 26.7% |
|  | High School | 29 | 16.1% |
|  | Not Educated | 13 | 7.2% |

Source: Calculated by the authors from Google-Form questionnaire.

### 5.2. Occupational Structure and Earnings of the Migrants

Table 2 presents the structure of employment, earnings, and remittances of Indian migrants in Saudi Arabia. Migration from India to Saudi Arabia consists of semi-skilled labor or unskilled labor. The majority of the surveyed respondents (24.4%) were engaged as technicians, 23.3% were sales workers, 10.6% were clerical support workers, 16.1% were plant and machine operators, and 12.2% were casual laborers (elementary activities). However, 10.6% were managers and professionals (skilled labor). Nearly half of the surveyed migrants (48.9%) earned less than SAR 2500 (Saudi Riyal) in a month and 42.8% were earning between SAR 2500 to 5000. Only 8.3% of the migrants were earning above SAR 5000; however, 91.7% were earning less than SAR 5000. The majority of the migrants (78.3%) did not have any other sources of income, however 21.7% had other sources of income from agriculture, rent, and income from businesses. India holds the highest number of international migrants and is the highest remittance receiving country in the world. The majority of the migrants (47.2%) remit less than SAR 1000, 32.8% were remitting between SAR 1000 to 3000, and 16.7% were sending between SAR 3000 to 5000; however, only 3.3% were remitting above SAR 5000 per month. The number of family members dependent on the remittances by the migrants varied: 51.6% of the migrants had 5 or more than 5 family members, 36.4% had 4 family members, and 12.3% had less than 3 family members.

### 5.3. Employment Status and Working Conditions during Lockdown (COVID-19)

Table 3 and Figure 1 describe the employment status and working hours of the surveyed migrants. The majority of the migrants (50.6%) did not work during the lockdown period of the pandemic in Saudi Arabia; however, 32.8% of the respondents worked between 5 to 8 hours in day, 2.8% worked only 1 to 3 hours a day, 8.3% were working for 3 to 5 hours, and 5.5% of them worked more than 8 hours in a day. Lockdown had reduced the working hours of the migrants; hence the majority of the migrant workers were doing activities other than work. In total, 22.2% of the respondents spent majority of their time watching TV, 13.3% using social networking sites, 6.7% in telephonic conversations, 6.7% playing games, and 18.3% on other activities. Only 32.8% of the respondents were spending their maximum time on work.

Table 2. Structure of Employment Status and Earnings.

| Variables | Levels | Data in Number | Data in % |
|---|---|---|---|
| Profession/Occupation | Professionals | 19 | 10.60% |
| | Technicians | 44 | 24.40% |
| | Clerical Support Workers | 19 | 10.60% |
| | Service & Sales Workers | 42 | 23.30% |
| | Elementary Occupation | 22 | 12.20% |
| | Plant & Machine Operator | 29 | 16.10% |
| | Others | 5 | 2.80% |
| Monthly Salary (in SAR) | Below 2500 | 88 | 48.90% |
| | 2500–5000 | 77 | 42.80% |
| | 5000–7500 | 6 | 3.30% |
| | 7500–10,000 | 4 | 2.20% |
| | Above 10,000 | 5 | 2.80% |
| Remittances (in SAR) | Below 1000 | 85 | 47.20% |
| | 1000–3000 | 59 | 32.80% |
| | 3000–5000 | 30 | 16.70% |
| | 5000–10,000 | 2 | 1.10% |
| | Above 10,000 | 4 | 2.20% |
| Number of Dependents | 2 | 3 | 1.70% |
| | 3 | 19 | 10.60% |
| | 4 | 65 | 36.10% |
| | 5 | 51 | 28.30% |
| | More than 5 | 42 | 23.30% |
| Does your family have other sources of income? | Yes | 39 | 21.70% |
| | No | 141 | 78.30% |

Source: Calculated by the authors from Google-Form questionnaire. SAR: Saudi Riyal.

Table 3. Employment Status and Working Condition during Lockdown (COVID-19).

| Statements | Levels | Frequency | Percentage |
|---|---|---|---|
| Number of daily working hour during lock down | Not Worked | 91 | 50.60% |
| | 1–3 | 5 | 2.80% |
| | 3–5 | 15 | 8.30% |
| | 5–8 | 59 | 32.80% |
| | Above 8 | 10 | 5.50% |
| Maximum time spent during lockdown | Work | 59 | 32.80% |
| | Watching TV | 40 | 22.20% |
| | Using social networking sites | 24 | 13.30% |
| | Telephonic conversation | 12 | 6.70% |
| | Playing games | 12 | 6.70% |
| | Others | 33 | 18.30% |
| For how many years you have been working in Saudi Arabia | Below 1 Year | 4 | 2.20% |
| | 2–4 Year | 62 | 34.50% |
| | 4–6 Year | 60 | 33.30% |
| | 6–8 Year | 25 | 13.90% |
| | More than 8 Year | 29 | 16.10% |
| Have you returned to India during lockdown? | Yes | 15 | 8.30% |
| | No | 165 | 91.70% |
| Average Salary loss during Corona (in SAR) | Below 500 | 110 | 61.10% |
| | 500–1000 | 47 | 26.10% |
| | 1000–2000 | 17 | 9.50% |
| | Above 2000 | 6 | 3.30% |
| Remittances during lockdown (in SAR) | Below 1000 | 105 | 58.30% |
| | 1000–3000 | 47 | 26.10% |
| | 3000–5000 | 22 | 12.20% |
| | Above 5000 | 6 | 3.40% |

Source: Calculated by the authors from Google-Form questionnaire.

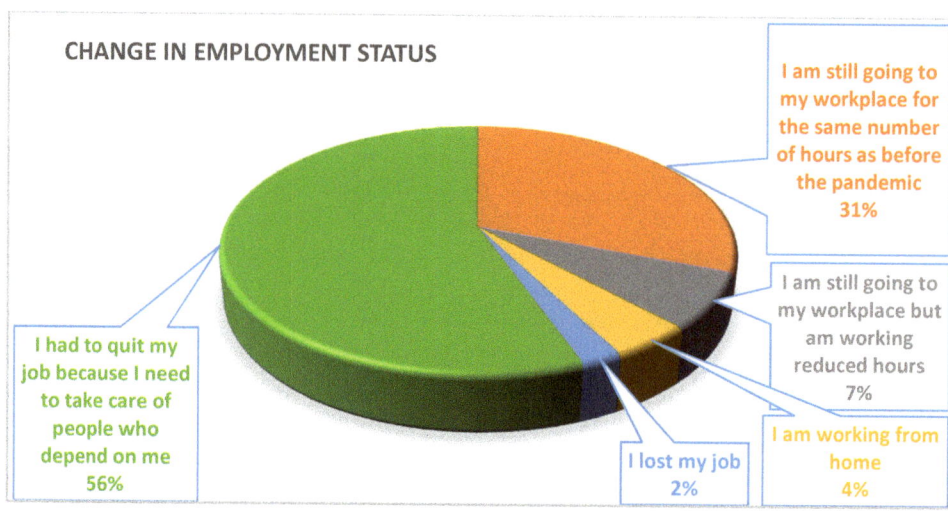

**Figure 1.** Changes in Employment Status during Corona Pandemic.

The collected data for working experience reveal the fact that the number of new migrants is low: only 2.2% of the respondents had been working in Saudi Arabia for only one year, which overlaps with the era of the pandemic. In total, 34.5% of the respondents had been working for the last 2 to 4 years, 33.3% for 4 to 6 years, 13.9% for 6 to 8 years, and only 16.1% had been working over 8 years in the Kingdom of Saudi Arabia. Lockdown and travel restrictions in India and in Saudi Arabia restrict the movement of migrants. Only 8.3% of the migrants return back to India during the pandemic and 91.7% of migrants decided to stay in the destination country. The main reason for return back to India during the pandemic is the job losses and salary cuts. This pandemic not only changed working hours but also impacted the earnings of the migrant workers. Around 26.1% of the migrants had experienced losses in their average earnings between SAR 500 to 1000, 9.5% had lost between SAR 1000 to 2000, and 3.3% had lost above SAR 2000; however, 50.6% of the migrants lost below SAR 500. Loss in earning will directly affect the remittances. The majority of the migrants (58.3%) remit below SAR 1000 during lockdown period, 26.1% were remitting between SAR 1000 to 2000, 12.2% were sending between SAR 2000 to 3000, and only 3.4% were sending above SAR 3000 to India during the lockdown period. Employment status has drastically changed during the pandemic. The majority of the respondents (55.6%) quit their job because they needed to take care of their family, 30.6% of the respondents were still going to work for the same number of hours as before the pandemic, 7.2% were working reduced hours, 4.4% were working from home, and 2.2% of the respondents lost their job in the pandemic.

*5.4. Changes in Remittances*

Figure 2 represents the changes in the distribution of remittances affected by the pandemic. The majority of the migrants were remitting below SAR 1000 before and after pandemic; however, before the pandemic, 47.2% of the migrants were remitting this amount but during the lockdown period of the pandemic that figure rose to 58.3%. This means that more migrants were remitting a lesser amount. The reduction in remittance was captured from those who were remitting either in between SAR 1000–2000 and 2000–3000 by 32.8% and 26.1%, respectively, before the pandemic, and 26.1% and 12.2% after pandemic. It was also found that remittance by higher income group tends to rise during the lockdown period of the pandemic. Before the pandemic, 3.3% of the migrants were remitting above SAR 5000 but during lockdown period the remittances in this category rose to 3.4%.

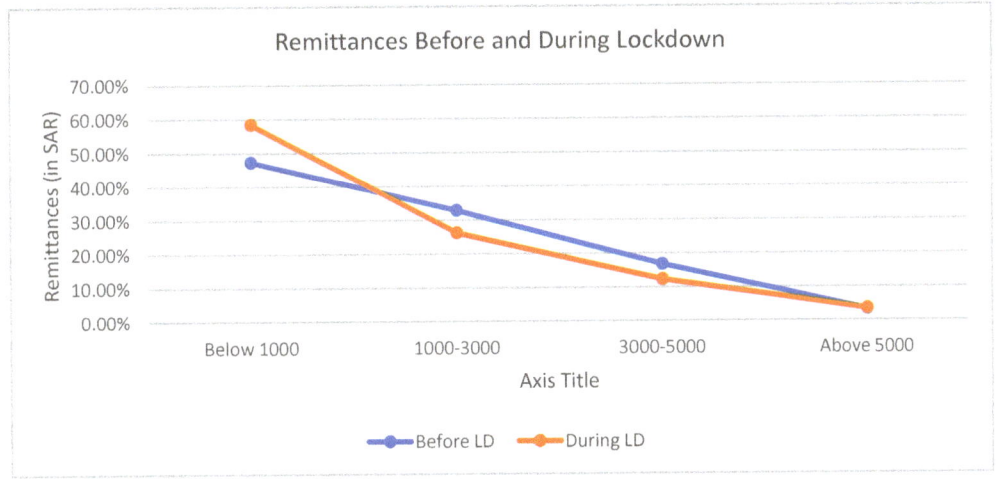

**Figure 2.** Change in remittances during the pandemic.

### 5.5. Dependent Sample t-Test

Dependent or paired sample *t*-test is used to compare the differences in the value of same sample at two different times. To test whether the comparison of remittances shown in Figure 2 is statistically significant, a *t*-test is applied. The null hypothesis was 'there is no statistical difference in remittances before and during the lockdown of the pandemic'. The mean and standard deviation of remittances before lockdown were estimated to be 1.78 and 0.917, respectively, and during lockdown the mean = 1.62 and Std. Deviation = 0.885. Table 4 describe the results of the paired *t*-test. T statistics of 3.924 with 179 degree of freedom corresponded to the *p*-value = 0.000, which is less than 0.05; therefore, we reject the null hypothesis. It means that there is statistically a difference in the remittances before and during lockdown

**Table 4.** Paired Sample *t*-Test.

| | Paired Sample *t*-Test | | | | | | | |
| --- | --- | --- | --- | --- | --- | --- | --- | --- |
| | | | | 95% Confidence Interval of the Difference | | | | |
| | Mean | Std. Deviation | Std. Error Mean | Lower | Upper | t | df | *p*-Value |
| Remittances before lockdown—Remittances during lockdown | 0.161 | 0.551 | 0.041 | 0.080 | 0.242 | 3.924 | 179 | 0.000 |

Source: Calculated by the authors from Google Form questionnaire.

### 5.6. Migrants' Perception of the COVID-19 Management by the Government of Saudi Arabia

The researchers used six questions to assess respondents' perceptions of the COVID-19 management by the government of Saudi Arabia. The responses were registered in a five-point Likert scale varying from 'very good' to 'very poor', as presented in Table 5. The migrants were found to be satisfied with the COVID protection related information provided by the government. In total, 51.1% responded 'very good', 46.1% responded as 'good', only 2.8% believed that 'average' information was provided, and none of the migrants responded 'poor' or 'very poor'. Half of the migrants reported 'very good' and 48.9% responded 'good' in regard to safety measures taken by the Saudi government. Almost the same perception was found in the case of medical facilities provided by the government: 54.4% reported as very good, 44.4% as good, and only 1.1% were average. In response to whether migrants had faced any difficulties sending money to their family during the lockdown period, 51.1% reported 'very good', 42.8% reported 'good', 3.9% reported 'average', and only 2.2% reported 'poor' facilities to send money during the lockdown period. The researchers also asked about the food and other basic facilities provided by the government: 46.7% responded 'very good' and 'good' separately; however, 6.7% responded 'average'. Furthermore, 46.1% of the respondents reported 'very good' living conditions, 49.4% responded 'good', and only 4.4% reported 'average' living condition during the lockdown period.

Table 5. Perceptions of the migrants towards COVID-19 management by Government of Saudi Arabia.

| Statement | Very Good | Good | Average | Poor | Very Poor | Total |
|---|---|---|---|---|---|---|
| COVID protection related information by Saudi Govt. | 51.1% | 46.1% | 2.8% | NIL | NIL | 100.0% |
| Safety measures taken by Saudi Government | 50.0% | 48.9% | 1.1% | NIL | NIL | 100.0% |
| Medical facility provided by Saudi Government | 54.4% | 44.4% | 1.1% | NIL | NIL | 100.0% |
| Facility to send money to India during lockdown | 51.1% | 42.8% | 3.9% | 2.2% | NIL | 100.0% |
| Food and other facilities provided by Saudi Government | 46.7% | 46.7% | 6.7% | NIL | NIL | 100.0% |
| Living conditions in Saudi Arabia during lockdown | 46.1% | 49.4% | 4.4% | NIL | NIL | 100.0% |

Source: Calculated by the authors from Google Form questionnaire.

### 5.7. Migrants' Perceptions of COVID-19 Management by Government of India

The researchers also tried to analyze the perceptions of the migrants towards the facility provided in the evacuation of migrants during the lockdown period. Two questions were asked of the respondents, and responses are presented in Table 6. The first question was related to the help provided by the embassy of India in Saudi Arabia: 33.9% of the respondents reported 'very good', 56.1% responded 'good', 7.2% responded 'poor', and 0.6% responded 'very poor'. This question was relevant because some migrants may face the problem of visa expiry, passport renewal, or issues related to working contracts. The second question was related to the evacuation of the migrants through transport facilities: 56.1% of the respondent reported 'very good', 31.7% reported 'good', 8.3% reported 'average' and 3.9% responded 'very poor'. This question was also relevant because the uncertainty which arises due to the spread of Corona virus forces migrants to return to India.

Table 6. Migrant's perceptions towards COVID management by Government of India.

| Statements | Very Good | Good | Average | Poor | Very Poor | Total |
|---|---|---|---|---|---|---|
| Help provided by Embassy of India in Saudi Arabia | 33.9% | 56.1% | 7.2% | 2.2% | 0.6% | 100.0% |
| Transport facility provided by Government of India | 56.1% | 31.7% | 8.3% | 3.9% | NIL | 100.0% |

Source: Calculated by the authors from Google Form questionnaire.

### 5.8. Combined Mean of Perceptions

Table 7 presents the combined mean of the perceptions towards COVID-19 management by the Government of India and Government of Saudi Arabia. A lower mean value indicates better perceptions. The combined mean of the perceptions towards government of Saudi Arabia is 1.54, which is less than the combined mean value 1.7 of the perception towards the government of India. This result shows that the government of Saudi Arabia managed COVID-19 better than the government of India according to migrants' perceptions. However, this perception is based on few variables and the responses of the migrants available in Saudi Arabia during lockdown period.

Table 7. Combined mean of the perceptions.

| Perceptions | N | Minimum | Maximum | Mean | Std. Deviation |
|---|---|---|---|---|---|
| Perception towards government of India | 180 | 1 | 5 | 1.7 | 0.76 |
| Perception towards government of Saudi Arabia | 180 | 1 | 4 | 1.54 | 0.58 |

Source: Calculated by the authors from Google Form questionnaire.

### 5.9. Chi-Square Test

A chi-square test was applied to discover the association between perceptions of COVID-19 management by the government across the different professions/occupations. The sample data of occupational structure were classified as Professionals, Technicians, Clerical Support Workers, Service and Sales Workers, Elementary Occupation, Plant and Machine Operator, and others. The null hypothesis was 'There is no significant difference in the opinion/perception of the migrant workers towards the COVID-19 management by the government across different occupations', and the alternative hypothesis was 'there is significant difference in the opinion/perception of the migrant workers towards the COVID-19 management by the government across different occupations. The relationship between these variables was found to be significant as calculated by chi-square value and $p$-value which is less than 0.05 (5% level of significance) as presented in the Table 8. Therefore, we reject the null hypothesis. It means that there was a significant difference in opinion of the migrant workers towards the COVID-19 management by the government of Saudi Arabia and India. Professionals, technicians, and elementary occupational workers were found to have low negative opinion towards COVID-19 management by the government, especially towards transport facilities provided by the government of India, help provided by the embassy of India, and facilities to send money from Saudi Arabia to India. However, clerical support workers, service and sales workers, and plant and machine operators had highly positive opinions concerning the COVID management by the government.

Table 8. Chi-Square Analysis of Perceptions of COVID-19 Management by Govt. Within Different Professions/Occupations.

| Perceptions | Chi Square Value | $p$-Value |
|---|---|---|
| COVID protection related information by Saudi Government | 51.36 | 0.000 |
| Safety measures taken by Saudi Government | 29.18 | 0.004 |
| Medical facility provided by Saudi government | 21.64 | 0.042 |
| Facility to send money to India during lockdown | 39.44 | 0.002 |
| Help provided by Embassy of India in Saudi Arabia | 56.37 | 0.000 |
| Transport facility provided by Government of India | 40.14 | 0.002 |
| Food & other facility provided by Saudi Government | 28.86 | 0.004 |
| Living condition in Saudi Arabia during lockdown | 36.02 | 0.000 |

Source: Calculated by the authors from Google Forms questionnaire.

### 5.10. Comparing the Perceptions of Migrants with Other Citizens

Perceptions of the citizens or migrants may differ or be the same in different countries, depending upon the infrastructure and decisions taken by the government. Several studies were carried out to investigate the perceptions of the citizens or migrants in a country. For instance, a study on the perception of health care workers during the COVID-19 pandemic in the case of Saudi Arabia was conducted, which confirmed that the majority of the respondents (93.6%) were happy and felt safe in regard to the government decision of lockdown and 94.7% supported the travel restriction imposed by the government [33]. Similarly, our study also confirms that the majority of the migrants strongly agreed or agreed with the government decision. For instance, 97.2% of the migrants agreed with the information provided by Saudi government related to the protection from Corona virus. In total, 98.8% of the respondents were happy with the safety measures taken by the Saudi government. Another study was conducted to explore the perception of the public of the government of Singapore in relation to COVID-19 related information. The results of the study confirm that majority of the respondents (99.1%) agreed or strongly agreed on the COVID-19 related information provided by the government and 97.9% believed the Singapore news agency [34]. Another study was carried out in Bangladesh to explore the public perception of government measures related to COVID-19. The result of the sample survey reveals the fact that the majority of the respondents (58%) were not satisfied by the measures taken by the government of Bangladesh. However, 40% of the respondents were found to be satisfied with government decisions [35]. Our study reveals the fact that the majority of the migrants were satisfied by the decision taken by the Saudi government. Another study for Bangladesh was conducted and revealed the fact that the majority of the respondents (62%) strongly agree that the healthcare system was not able to handle the pandemic and 68.6% believe that the government of Bangladesh needs support from the public to handle the pandemic [36]. In our study, 98.8% of the respondents were happy with the medical facilities provided by the government of Saudi Arabia, 93.8% were satisfied with the facility to send money, 90% were happy with the help provided by the embassy of India, and 87.7% were satisfy with the transport facility provided by government of India during the lockdown period.

### 5.11. Mental Health Status of the Migrants

COVID-19 had not only influenced the economic and physical health of the people but also their mental status. This pandemic had drastically changed the mental status of the Indian migrant workers in Saudi Arabia. Table 9 describes the levels of anxiety, depression, and stress among the migrant workers. The majority of the migrants feel nervous (67.8%), depressed (63.3%), and lonely (72.2%) during the pandemic. It was also reported that 70% had difficulties in concentrating and 66.7% had a hard time in sleeping; however, the majority of them (91.7%) were feeling hopeful about the future, which shows silver lining at the end of the tunnel. It was also observed that only 2.2% of the migrants were Corona positive, 1.7% of their member households were Corona positive, and most of them (78.3%) were not scared of virus.

**Table 9.** Mental health of the migrants during pandemic.

| Statements | Variables | Frequency | (%) |
|---|---|---|---|
| Have you felt nervous, anxious, or on edge? | Yes | 122 | 67.80% |
|  | No | 58 | 32.20% |
| Have you felt depressed? | Yes | 114 | 63.30% |
|  | No | 66 | 36.70% |
| Have you felt lonely? | Yes | 130 | 72.20% |
|  | No | 50 | 27.80% |
| Have you felt hopeful about the future? | Yes | 165 | 91.70% |
|  | No | 15 | 8.30% |
| I have a hard time sleeping because of the Corona | Yes | 120 | 66.70% |
|  | No | 60 | 33.30% |
| I have had difficulties concentrating because of Corona | Yes | 126 | 70.00% |
|  | No | 54 | 30.00% |
| Have you been tested Corona positive in Saudi Arabia? | Yes | 4 | 2.20% |
|  | No | 176 | 97.80% |
| Are you scared of Corona virus? | Yes | 39 | 21.70% |
|  | No | 141 | 78.30% |
| Does any of your family member infected of Corona virus? | Yes | 3 | 1.70% |
|  | No | 177 | 98.30% |

Source: Calculated by the authors from Google Forms questionnaire.

## 5.12. Comparison of Mental Health of the Migrants by Age, Domicile and Education

### 5.12.1. Felt Nervous, Anxious, or on Edge

Figure 3 describes feeling nervous, anxious, or on edge during pandemic by Indian migrants in Saudi Arabia. Around half of the young population aged between 20 to 40 felt nervous, and 78.5% of the migrants between the age of 40 to 50 and 90% of the age group above 50 felt nervous during the pandemic. The sample data reveal the fact that young migrants were less nervous than older migrants. The migrants from Bihar were found to be less nervous than Uttar Pradesh and other states of India. The nervousness of the migrants was also influenced by the levels of education of the migrants. Higher level of education implies a lower level of nervousness: 25% of doctorate, 59% of post-graduates, 64% of graduates reported nervousness during pandemic; however, 75% of intermediate, 79% of high school educated, and 61.5% of uneducated migrants reported nervousness. To investigate the relationship between nervous feeling by age, domicile, and education, correlation coefficient was applied. The result of correlation coefficient is shown in Table 10. Pearson's correlation between felt nervous and age of the migrants was found to be negative and statistically significant ($r = -0.311$, $p < 0.01$). Similarly, the relationship between felt nervous and domicile of the migrants was found to be positive and statistically significant ($r = 0.262$, $p < 0.01$). However, the relationship between felt nervous and education level of migrants was found to be positive but statistically insignificant ($r = 0.133$, $p > 0.01$).

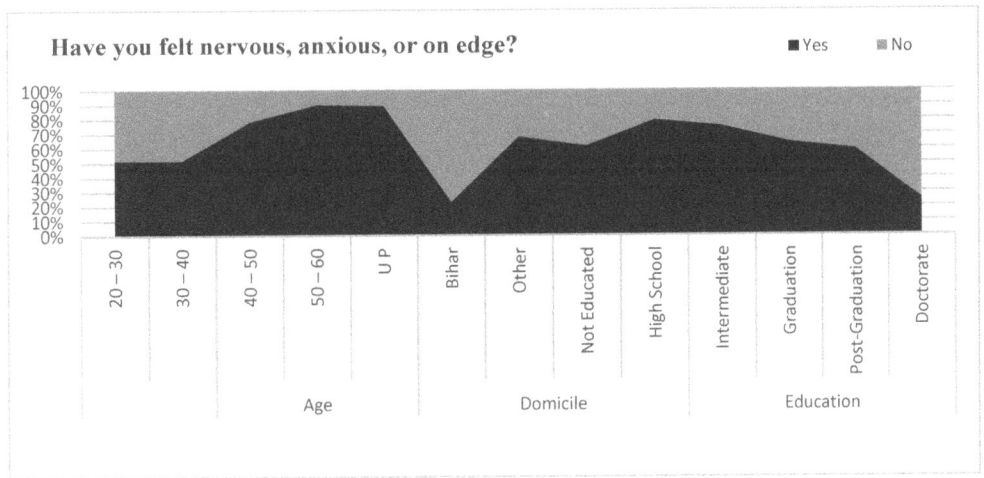

**Figure 3.** Comparison of feeling nervous.

### 5.12.2. Felt Depressed

Figure 4 represents the level of depression among the sample migrant workers during the pandemic. Less than half of the young migrants aged between 20 to 40 reported feeling depressed, however 72% of the migrants between the ages of 40 to 50 and 90% of the migrants aged above 50 reported feeling depressed during the pandemic. The sample data reveal that young aged migrants were less depressed than old age migrants. The 84.1% migrants from Uttar Pradesh reported feeling depression, however only 18.8% of the migrants from Bihar reported depression and 64.5% from other states were in depression during the pandemic. Lower levels of depression were reported by highly educated migrants (25% of doctorate, 54% of postgraduate, and 56% of graduate) and uneducated migrants (53%); however, 75% of the intermediate and high school educated migrants reported depression. To investigate the relationship between feelings of depression by age, domicile, and education, a correlation coefficient was applied. The result of the correlation coefficient is shown in Table 11. Pearson's correlation between felt depressed and age of the migrants was found to be negative and statistically significant (r = −0.368, $p < 0.01$). Similarly, the relationship between felt depressed and the domicile of the migrants was found to be positive and statistically significant (r = 0.236, $p < 0.01$). However, the relationship between felt depressed and education level of migrants was found to be positive but statistically insignificant (r = 0.140, $p > 0.01$).

**Table 10.** Pearson's correlation matrix.

| Statements | Age Pearson Correlation | p-Value |
|---|---|---|
| Felt Nervous, Anxious, or on Edge | −0.311 | 0.000 |
| Felt Depressed | −0.368 | 0.000 |
| Felt Lonely | −0.333 | 0.000 |
| Hard time sleeping | −0.372 | 0.000 |
| Difficulties in concentration | −0.315 | 0.000 |
| Hopeful about the future | −0.132 | 0.077 |
| Statements | Domicile Pearson correlation | p-Value |
| Felt Nervous, Anxious, or on Edge | 0.262 | 0.000 |
| Felt Depressed | 0.236 | 0.001 |
| Felt Lonely | 0.178 | 0.017 |
| Hard time sleeping | 0.320 | 0.000 |
| Difficulties in concentration | 0.289 | 0.000 |
| Hopeful about the future | 0.165 | 0.027 |
| Statements | Education Pearson correlation | p-Value |
| Felt Nervous, Anxious, or on Edge | 0.133 | 0.075 |
| Felt Depressed | 0.140 | 0.061 |
| Felt Lonely | 0.106 | 0.158 |
| Hard time sleeping | 0.175 | 0.019 |
| Difficulties in concentration | 0.151 | 0.044 |
| Hopeful about the future | 0.027 | 0.717 |
| Statements | Number of Family Member Pearson correlation | p-Value |
| Felt Nervous, Anxious, or on Edge | −0.403 | 0.000 |
| Felt Depressed | −0.464 | 0.000 |
| Felt Lonely | −0.382 | 0.000 |
| Hard time sleeping | −0.446 | 0.000 |
| Difficulties in concentration | −0.429 | 0.000 |
| Hopeful about the future | −0.143 | 0.055 |

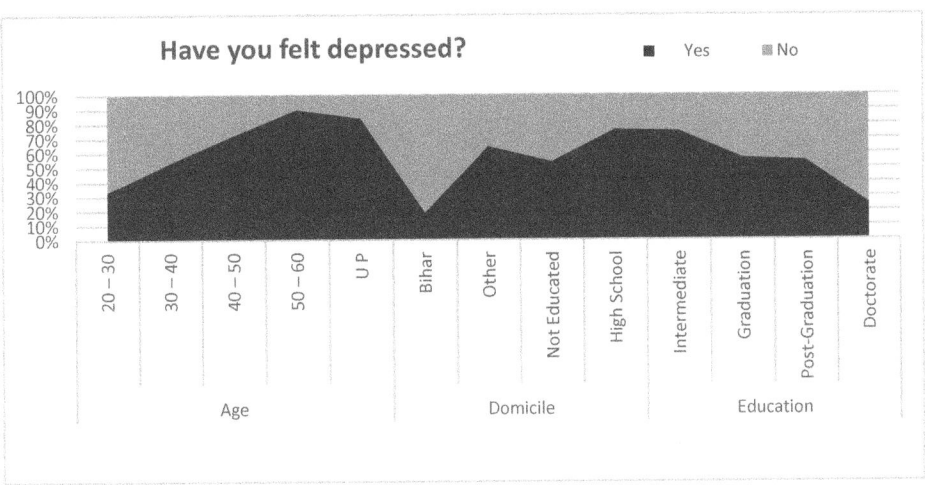

**Figure 4.** Comparison of feeling depressed.

**Table 11.** Comparison of psychological effect by number of family members.

| Statements | Levels | Number of Family Member | |
|---|---|---|---|
| | | Below 5 | 5 or More |
| Have you felt nervous, anxious, or on edge? | Yes | 50.0% | 77.5% |
| | No | 50.0% | 22.5% |
| Have you felt depressed? | Yes | 35.9% | 78.4% |
| | No | 64.1% | 21.6% |
| Have you felt lonely? | Yes | 53.1% | 82.8% |
| | No | 46.9% | 17.2% |
| Have you felt hopeful about the future? | Yes | 87.5% | 94.0% |
| | No | 12.5% | 6.0% |
| I have a hard time sleeping because of the orona | Yes | 42.1% | 80.2% |
| | No | 57.9% | 19.2% |
| I have had difficulties concentrating because of corona | Yes | 50.0% | 81.1% |
| | No | 50.0% | 18.9% |

### 5.12.3. Felt Lonely

Figure 5 shows the loneliness among the different types of the migrants. The migrants in the age group of below 40 reported less loneliness than the migrants above the age of 40. All migrants above the age of 50 reported that they felt lonely during the pandemic; however, 78.5% in the age group of 40 to 50, and around 56% of the age below 40 reported feeling loneliness during the pandemic. The migrants from Bihar were feeling less loneliness than the migrants from other states of India. The loneliness among differently educated migrants were not educated migrants (61.5%), high school (86.2%), intermediate (77.1%), graduation (67.2%), post-graduation (72.7%), and doctorate only 25%. To investigate the relationship between felt lonely by age, domicile and education, a correlation coefficient was applied. The result of the correlation coefficient is shown in Table 10. Pearson's correlation between felt lonely and age of the migrants was found to be negative and statistically significant ($r = -0.333$, $p < 0.01$). Similarly, the relationship between felt lonely and domicile of the migrants was found to be positive and statistically significant at the level of 0.05 ($r = 0.178$,

$p < 0.05$). However, the relationship between felt lonely and education level of migrants was found to be positive but statistically insignificant ($r = 0.106, p > 0.01$).

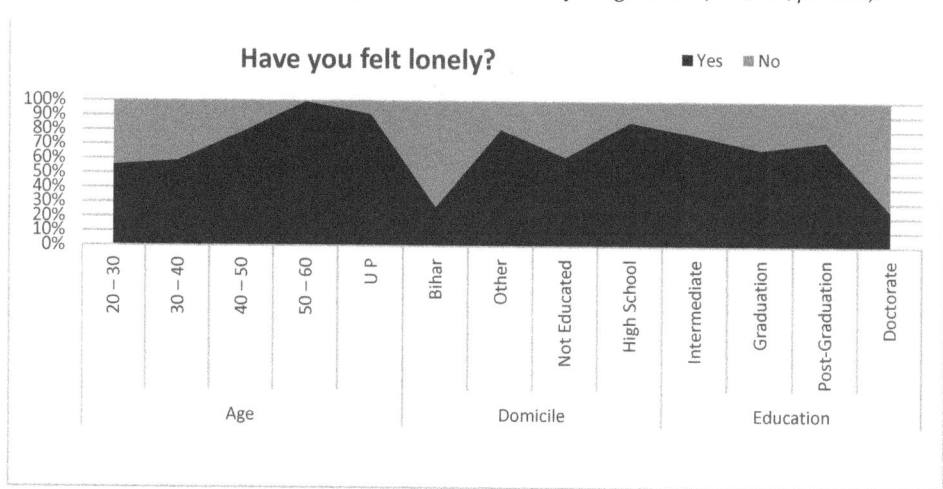

Figure 5. Comparison of feeling lonely.

5.12.4. Felt Hopeful about the Future

Figure 6 expresses the hopefulness about the future by migrant workers during the pandemic. The majority of all age groups of migrants, from all states and levels of education, reported hoping for better events to happen in the future; however, hopefulness in highly qualified migrants was reported to be less than in all other migrants. To investigate the relationship between felt hopeful about the future and age, domicile, and education, a correlation coefficient was applied. The result of correlation coefficient is shown in Table 10. Pearson's correlation between felt hopeful about the future and age of the migrants was found to be negative but statistically insignificant ($r = -0.132, p > 0.05$). Similarly, the relationship between felt hopeful about the future and domicile of the migrants was found to be positive and statistically significant at the level of 0.05 ($r = 0.165, p < 0.05$). However, the relationship between felt hopeful about the future and education level of migrants was found to be positive but statistically insignificant ($r = 0.027, p > 0.05$).

5.12.5. Difficulties in Sleeping and Concentration

Figures 7 and 8 describe the anxiety among migrant workers through sleeping problems and difficulty in concentrating. The problem of anxiety was reported as more severe in the age group of above 40 than the age group below 40. It was also seen that migrants who belongs to Bihar were found to have less of an anxiety problem than the migrants from other states. The problems of anxiety were also correlated to the level of education of the migrants. More educated migrants reported less anxiety than the lower educated migrants during the pandemic. To investigate the relationship between difficulty sleeping and difficulties in concentration by age, domicile, and education, a correlation coefficient was applied. The result of the correlation coefficient is shown in Table 10. Pearson's correlation between difficulty sleeping and age of the migrants was found to be negative and statistically significant ($r = -0.372, p < 0.01$) and difficulties in concentration and age was also found to be negative and statistically significant ($r = -0.315, p < 0.01$). Similarly, the relationship between difficulty sleeping and domicile of the migrants was found to be positive and statistically significant ($r = 0.320, p < 0.01$) and the relationship between difficulties in concentration and domicile was also found to be positive and statistically significant ($r = 0.289, p < 0.01$). The relationship between difficulty sleeping and education level of migrants was found to be positive but statistically significant at the level of 0.05. (r = 0.175, $p < 0.05$) and the relationship between difficulties in concentration and education level of the migrants was also found to be positive and statistically significant at the level of 0.05 (r = 0.151, $p < 0.05$).

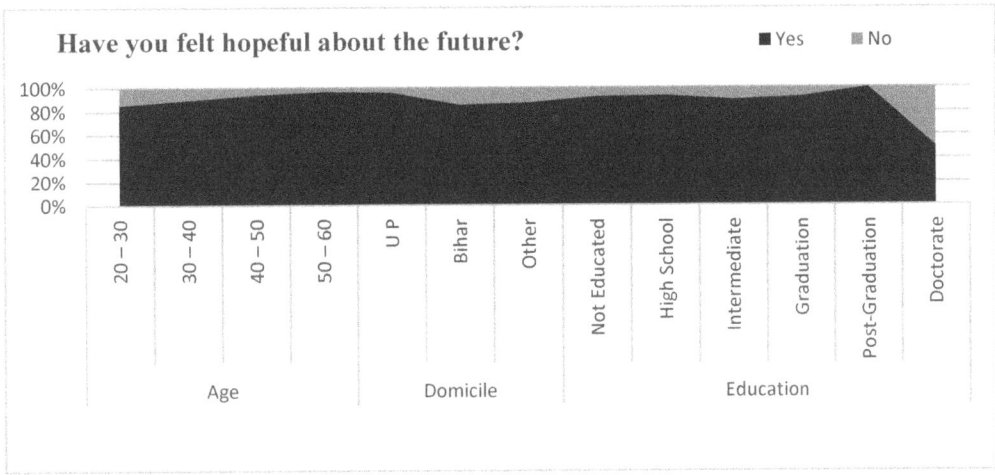

Figure 6. Comparison of feeling hopeful about future.

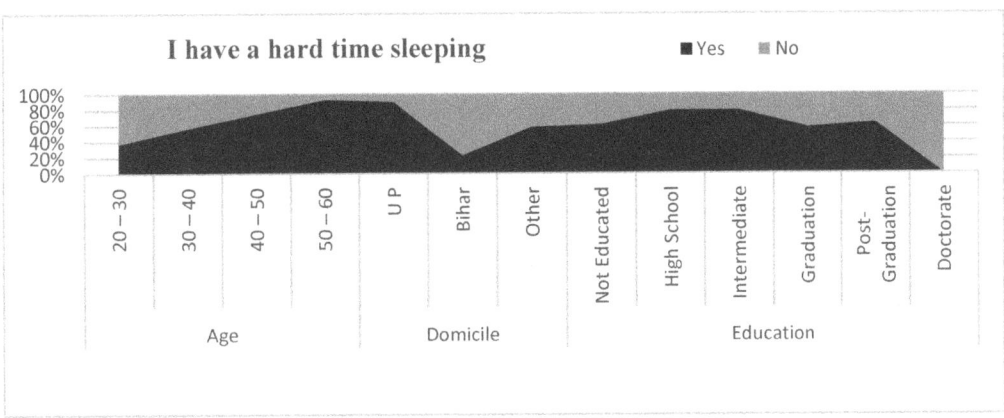

Figure 7. Comparison of hard time sleeping.

5.12.6. Comparison of Mental Health Effect by Number of Family Members

Table 11 presents the comparison of mental health impacted by number of family members of the migrants. Sample data disclose the fact that number of family members is directly related to the psychological stress on migrants. Only 50% of migrants with family members below 5 felt nervous, 35.9% depressed, 53.1% lonely, 42.1% had a hard time sleeping, and 50% had difficulties in concentrating; however, 77.5% of migrants with family members equal to 5 or above felt nervous, 78.4% depressed, 82.8% lonely, 80.2% have a hard time sleeping, and 81.1% had difficulties in concentration. The majority of the migrants (87.5% with family member below 5 and 94% with family member equal to 5 or above) felt hopeful about the future. The psychological problems are severe in the case of the migrants above the age of 40 and migrants with higher number of family members, because of social responsibility and low capabilities to face interpersonal challenges. To test the hypothesis and investigate the relationship between these statements and the number of family members, a correlation coefficient was applied. The result of correlation coefficient is shown in Table 9. Pearson's correlation between these statements and the number of family members of the migrants was found to be negative and statistically significant. However, the relationship between felt hopeful about the future and number of family member is positive but statistically insignificant ($r = -0.143, p > 0.05$).

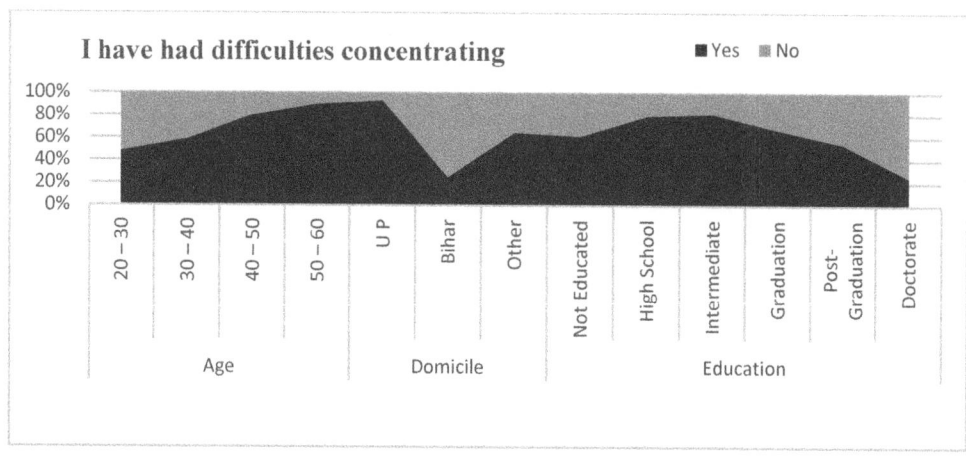

**Figure 8.** Comparison of having difficulties in concentration.

5.12.7. Comparing the Psychological Impact on Migrants before and during COVID-19

The results of the study confirm that 67.8% of the respondent migrants reported feeling nervous and 63.3% were depressed due to the COVID-19 pandemic. The level of psychological impact is much higher and severe among the migrant workers than before. One study was carried out to find out the prevalence of depression among migrant workers in AL-Qassim, Saudi Arabia, by taking a cross-sectional survey of 400 workers in 2016. The results of the study confirmed that 20% of the migrants reported the symptom of depression. It was also reported that level of depression varied by age but not by duration of stay [37]. Another similar study was conducted in 2011 to find out the prevalence of depression among migrant workers of UAE. The survey results of the 239 samples revealed that 25.1% of the migrants reported symptoms of depression. They also concluded that prevalence of depression is correlated with physical illness. In the same study, 6.3% of the respondents reported suicidal ideation and 2.5% had already attempted suicide [38]. Another study to find out the prevalence of depression among migrant workers was carried out in case of Qatar in 2016, which reported that 57.9% of the migrants had symptoms of depression [39]. Hence, it is clear that the percentage of migrants in our study which reported symptoms of depression and feeling nervous is much higher than the earlier studies; therefore, the COVID-19 pandemic had a severe psychological impact on Indian migrants working in Saudi Arabia.

## 6. Limitations

The main limitations of the study are that it focuses on the Indian male migrants in Saudi Arabia with a sample data of 180, however the sample of female migrants are very less. It also uses few tests and strategies. The current study does not emphasis the effect on migrant's family in India during pandemic. Apart from it, this study does not consider COVID-19 vaccination process, problems and its impact on migrants in Saudi Arabia. The future scope of study in this area needed to analyze the economic and psychological impacts of COVID-19 on female migrants, migrant's wife, children or family. In addition to it, the similar type of study can be done considering the female migrants.

The policy implications from the findings of the research draw attention of the policy makers towards protective measures need to be implemented to save migrants during ongoing pandemic. The government should take some necessary steps such as financial benefit scheme to overcome the problems in the reduction of migrant earnings and remittances. Employment status of the migrants had drastically changed, which also drawing attention of policy makers to create more employment opportunities to reduce unemployment and underemployment. The government should not focus only on vaccination and physical fitness of the migrants but also need to find out the cure of the psychological impact arising during the pandemic.

## 7. Conclusions

The ongoing pandemic COVID-19 has severe economic and psychological effects on the world economy. This pandemic has changed the working environment and living style of the people across the world. This study analyzed the economic impact and health status of the Indian migrants in Saudi Arabia. The study revealed that majority of the migrants do not worked during the lockdown period and 42% of the migrants worked less than 8 hours in a day. Working experience of the migrants reveals a tendency is reduction in new international migration. Only 2.2% of the migrants reported work experience below one year, 35.5% were reported between 2 to 4 year and more than 60% of the migrants reported the work experience above 4 years.

During lockdown period migrants who were not working or working for less number of hours spent his maximum time on watching TV or surfing social networking sites. Majority of the migrants (48.9%) were earning below SAR 2500 (Saudi Riyal) and remitting below SAR 1000 in a month and majority of them were either 5 members family or more than 5. Around half of the migrants do not worked during the lockdown period and 42% of the migrants worked less than 8 hours in a day. Around 61% of the migrants reported an average loss in salary of below SAR 500 and 26% reported a loss between SAR 500 to 1000, however only 12% reported a loss above SAR 1000 during lockdown period of the pandemic. It has also been observed that number of migrants who were remitting below SAR 1000 had increased and remittances by middle income group were found to be decreased during lockdown period of the pandemic. The major reason of loss in salary and reduction in remittances were change in the employment status (reduced working hours, job loss, etc.) of the migrants. The perceptions of the migrants towards COVID management by the Saudi Arabia were found to be more positive than COVID management by the government of India. Chi-square test result showed there is significant difference in opinion of the migrant workers towards the COVID-19 management by the government of Saudi Arabia and India within different professions/occupations. The majority of respondents reported of feeling nervous, depressed, lonely, hard time sleeping and difficulties in concentrating, however majority of them also hopeful about the future. The problem of anxiety and depression were found to be more in the age group of above 40 than the age below 40. It was also been observed that migrants from Bihar were feeling less nervous, depressed and lonely than the migrants from other states of India. Not educated migrants were more affected of nervousness, depression and anxiety problem than the other migrants. The psychological problems are severe in case of the migrants above the age of 40 and migrants with higher number of family member, because of social responsibility and low capabilities to face interpersonal challenges.

**Author Contributions:** Conceptualization, M.A.K., A.I. and M.K.; methodology, M.A.K., M.I.K. and A.I.; software, M.I.K. and A.I.; validation, M.A.K., M.I.K. and M.K.; formal analysis, M.A.K., M.I.K. and A.I.; investigation, M.A.K. and A.I.; resources, M.A.K. and M.K.; data curation, M.A.K., M.I.K. and A.I.; writing—original draft preparation, M.A.K. and M.I.K.; writing—review and editing, M.A.K., A.I. and M.K.; visualization, M.I.K., A.I. and M.K.; supervision, A.I. and M.K. All authors have read and agreed to the published version of the manuscript.

**Funding:** This research received no external funding.

**Institutional Review Board Statement:** Not applicable.

**Informed Consent Statement:** Not applicable.

**Data Availability Statement:** The data used to support the findings of this study are available from the corresponding author upon request.

**Conflicts of Interest:** The authors declare no conflict of interest.

## References

1. World Health Organization. Novel Coronavirus (VoCn-2019). Available online: https://www.who.int/emergencies/diseases/novel-coronavirus-2019?gclid=EAIaIQobChMIlp6V_ITf8gIVCbqWCh1hRA-HEAAYASAAEgKiKvD_BwE (accessed on 23 December 2020).
2. World Health Organization. World Health Organization Declares COVID-19 a '1Pandemic.' Here's What That Means. 2020. Available online: https://time.com/5791661/who-coronavirus-pandemic-declaration/ (accessed on 11 March 2020).
3. World Health Organization. WHO Coronavirus (COVID-19) Dashboard. 2021. Available online: https://covid19.who.int/ (accessed on 25 August 2021).
4. Koh, D. COVID-19 lockdowns throughout the world. *Occup. Med.* **2020**, *70*, 322. [CrossRef]
5. Arab News. Saudi Passengers Flock to Airports as Foreign Travel Resumes. 2020. Available online: https://www.arabnews.com/node/1860336/saudi-arabia (accessed on 18 May 2021).
6. Arab News. Saudi Health Minister: COVID-19 Vaccines Will Be Available at Pharmacies for Free. Available online: https://www.arabnews.com/node/1819076/saudi-arabia (accessed on 17 December 2020).
7. The Economic Times. Saudi Arabia to Allow Only Vaccinated Back to Workplace. 2021. Available online: https://economictimes.indiatimes.com/news/international/saudi-arabia/saudi-arabia-to-allow-only-vaccinated-back-toworkplace/articleshow/82456308.cms?utm_source=contentofinterest&utm_medium=text&utm_campaign=cppst (accessed on 7 May 2021).
8. Al Arabia News. Saudi Arabia Will Require COVID-19 Immunization during Most Events as of August. Available online: https://english.alarabiya.net/coronavirus/2021/05/18/Saudi-Arabia-will-require-COVID-19-immunization-during-most-events-as-of-August (accessed on 18 May 2021).
9. The Times of India. Saudi Arabia Includes Fines in COVID-19 Regulations. 2021. Available online: https://timesofindia.indiatimes.com/world/middle-east/saudi-arabia-includes-fines-in-covid-19-regulations/articleshow/82549798.cms (accessed on 11 May 2021).
10. Census of India. Population Classified by Place of Birth and Sex. 2011. Available online: https://censusindia.gov.in/2011census/d-series/d-1.html (accessed on 20 August 2021).
11. UNDESA. *International Migration 2019*; UNDESA: New York, NY, USA, 2019; Available online: https://www.un.org/en/development/desa/population/migration/publications/migrationreport/docs/InternationalMigration2019_Report.pdf (accessed on 26 August 2021).
12. World Bank. *Phase II: COVID-19 Crisis through a Migration Lens, Migration and Development Brief 33*; World Bank Group: Washington, DC, USA, 2020.
13. IMF. COVID-19 Pandemic and the Middle East and Central Asia: Region Facing Dual Shock. Available online: https://blogs.imf.org/2020/03/23/covid-19-pandemic-and-the-middle-east-and-central-asia-region-facing-dual-shock/ (accessed on 23 March 2020).
14. Arabian Business. COVID-19: Companies in Saudi Arabia Can Reduce Salaries by 40%. 2020. Available online: https://www.arabianbusiness.com/politics-economics/446151-covid-19-companies-in-saudi-arabia-can-reduce-salaries-by-40 (accessed on 5 May 2020).
15. Al-Tawfiq, J.A.; Memish, Z.A. COVID-19 in the Eastern Mediterranean Region and Saudi Arabia: Prevention and therapeutic strategies. *Int. J. Antimicrob. Agents* **2020**, *55*, 105968. [CrossRef]
16. Sayed, A.A. The Progressive Public Measures of Saudi Arabia to Tackle COVID-19 and Limit Its Spread. *Int. J. Environ. Res. Public Health* **2021**, *18*, 783. [CrossRef]
17. Page, K.R.; Venkataramani, M.; Beyrer, C.; Polk, S. Undocumented US immigrants and COVID-19. *N. Engl. J. Med.* **2020**, *382*, e62. [CrossRef] [PubMed]
18. Alsharif, F. Undocumented migrants in Saudi Arabia: COVID-19 and amnesty reforms. *Int. Migr.* **2021**, 1–17. [CrossRef]

19. Althaqafi, T. The Impact of Corona Virus (COVID 19) on the Economy in the Kingdom of Saudi Arabia: A Review. *IJBMR* **2020**, *8*, 34–40.
20. Konrad-Adenauer-Stiftung e. V. Migration and the COVID-19 Pandemic in the Gulf. 2020. Available online: https://www.kas.de/documents/286298/8668222/Policy+Report+No+15+Migration+and+The+COVID-19+Pandemic+in+the+Gulf.pdf/87dd88bd-ed47-41c7-be23-48c5a5eb8d7c?version=1.0&t=1603448109241 (accessed on 14 October 2020).
21. Saudi Gazette. Saudis Confident in Kingdom's Ability to Bounce Back from COVID-19: Research. Available online: https://saudigazette.com.sa/article/591686 (accessed on 9 April 2020).
22. Parveen, M. Challenges Faced by Pandemic Covid 19 Crisis: A Case Study in Saudi Arabia. *Challenge* **2020**, *63*, 349–364. [CrossRef]
23. Abella, M.I.; Sasikumar, S.K. Estimating Earnings Losses of Migrant Workers Due to COVID-19. *IJLE* **2020**, *63*, 921–939. [CrossRef] [PubMed]
24. Johns Hopkins Aramco Healthcare. COVID-19 Mental Health Tool Kit. Available online: https://medicine.umich.edu/dept/psychiatry/michigan-psychiatry-resources-covid-19/healthcare-providers/covid-19-mental-health-toolkit (accessed on 23 August 2021).
25. Alkhamees, A.A.; Alrashed, S.A.; Alzunaydi, A.A.; Almohimeed, A.S.; Aljohani, M.S. The psychological impact of COVID-19 pandemic on the general population of Saudi Arabia. *Compr. Psychiatry* **2020**, *102*, 152192. [CrossRef] [PubMed]
26. Joseph, R.; Lucca, J.M.; Alshayban, D.; Alshehry, Y.A. The immediate psychological response of the general population in Saudi Arabia during COVID-19 pandemic: A cross-sectional study. *J. Infect. Public Health* **2021**, *14*, 276–283. [CrossRef]
27. Al Mutair, A.; Alhajji, M.; Shamsan, A. Emotional Wellbeing in Saudi Arabia during the COVID-19 Pandemic: A National Survey. *Risk Manag. Healthc. Policy* **2021**, *14*, 1065. [CrossRef] [PubMed]
28. Posel, D.; Oyenubi, A.; Kollamparambil, U. Job loss and mental health during the COVID-19 lockdown: Evidence from South Africa. *PLoS ONE* **2021**, *16*, e0249352. [CrossRef] [PubMed]
29. Kumar, K.; Mehra, A.; Sahoo, S.; Nehra, R.; Grover, S. The psychological impact of COVID-19 pandemic and lockdown on the migrant workers: A cross-sectional survey. *Asian J. Psychiatry* **2020**, *53*, 102252. [CrossRef] [PubMed]
30. Yee, K.; Peh, H.P.; Tan, Y.P.; Teo, I.; Tan, E.U.; Paul, J.; Rangabashyam, M.; Ramalingam, M.B.; Chow, W.; Tan, H.K. Stressors and coping strategies of migrant workers diagnosed with COVID-19 in Singapore: A qualitative study. *BMJ* **2021**, *11*, e045949.
31. Harjana, N.P.; Januraga, P.P.; Indrayathi, P.A.; Gesesew, H.A.; Ward, P.R. Prevalence of Depression, Anxiety, and Stress Among Repatriated Indonesian Migrant Workers during the COVID-19 Pandemic. *Front. Public Health* **2021**, *9*, 630295. [CrossRef] [PubMed]
32. UNDESA. *International Migrant Stock 2019*; UNDESA: New York, NY, USA, 2019; Available online: https://www.un.org/en/development/desa/population/migration/data/estimates2/estimates19.asp (accessed on 23 August 2021).
33. Abolfotouh, M.A.; Almutairi, A.F.; Ala'a, A.B.; Hussein, M.A. Perception and attitude of healthcare workers in Saudi Arabia with regard to Covid-19 pandemic and potential associated predictors. *BMC Infect. Dis.* **2020**, *20*, 719. [CrossRef] [PubMed]
34. Lim, V.W.; Lim, R.L.; Tan, Y.R.; Soh, A.S.; Tan, M.X.; Othman, N.B.; Dickens, S.B.; Thein, T.L.; Lwin, M.O.; Ong, R.T.; et al. Government trust, perceptions of COVID-19 and behaviour change: Cohort surveys, Singapore. *Bull. WHO* **2021**, *99*, 92. [PubMed]
35. Islam, M.D.; Siddika, A. COVID-19 and Bangladesh: A Study of the Public Perception on the Measures Taken by the Government. Available online: https://doi.org/10.13140/RG.2.2.30042.49608 (accessed on 20 August 2021).
36. Bodrud-Doza, M.; Shammi, M.; Bahlman, L.; Islam, A.R.; Rahman, M. Psychosocial and socio-economic crisis in Bangladesh due to COVID-19 pandemic: A perception-based assessment. *Front. Public Health* **2020**, *8*, 341. [CrossRef] [PubMed]
37. Nadim, W.; AlOtaibi, A.; Al-Mohaimeed, A.; Ewid, M.; Sarhandi, M.; Saquib, J.; Alhumdi, K.; Alharbi, A.; Taskin, A.; Migdad, M.; et al. Depression among migrant workers in Al-Qassim, Saudi Arabia. *J. Affect. Dis.* **2016**, *206*, 103–108. [CrossRef]
38. Al-Maskari, F.; Shah, S.M.; Al-Sharhan, R.; Al-Haj, E.; Al-Kaabi, K.; Khonji, D.; Schneider, J.D.; Nagelkerke, N.J.; Bernsen, R.M. Prevalence of depression and suicidal behaviors among male migrant workers in United Arab Emirates. *J. Immigr. Minority Health* **2011**, *13*, 1027–1032. [CrossRef]
39. Khaled, S.M.; Gray, R. Depression in migrant workers and nationals of Qatar: An exploratory cross-cultural study. *Int. J. Soc. Psychiatry* **2019**, *65*, 354–367. [CrossRef] [PubMed]

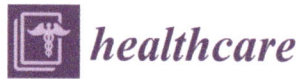 

Article

# The COVID-19 Pandemic Strain: Teleworking and Health Behavior Changes in the Portuguese Context

Teresa Forte [1], Gonçalo Santinha [2,*] and Sérgio A. Carvalho [3,4]

[1] Department of Social, Political and Territorial Sciences, University of Aveiro, 3810-193 Aveiro, Portugal; teresaforte@ua.pt
[2] GOVCOPP, Department of Social, Political and Territorial, University of Aveiro, 3810-193 Aveiro, Portugal
[3] Hei-Lab: Digital Human-Environment Interaction Lab, School of Psychology and Life Sciences, Lusófona University, 1749-024 Lisbon, Portugal
[4] Centre for Research in Neuropsychology and Cognitive and Behavioural Intervention (CINNEIC), University of Coimbra, 3000-115 Coimbra, Portugal; sergio.andcarvalho@gmail.com
* Correspondence: g.santinha@ua.pt

Citation: Forte, T.; Santinha, G.; Carvalho, S.A. The COVID-19 Pandemic Strain: Teleworking and Health Behavior Changes in the Portuguese Context. *Healthcare* **2021**, *9*, 1151. https://doi.org/10.3390/healthcare9091151

Academic Editor: Pedram Sendi

Received: 29 July 2021
Accepted: 30 August 2021
Published: 3 September 2021

**Publisher's Note:** MDPI stays neutral with regard to jurisdictional claims in published maps and institutional affiliations.

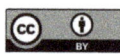

**Copyright:** © 2021 by the authors. Licensee MDPI, Basel, Switzerland. This article is an open access article distributed under the terms and conditions of the Creative Commons Attribution (CC BY) license (https://creativecommons.org/licenses/by/4.0/).

**Abstract:** The COVID-19 pandemic has forced a societal essay, based on thorough measures of individual and communitarian protection, ranging from compulsory social distancing to quarantine. Following WHO recommendations, more or less strict policies were adopted by governments worldwide in order to mitigate public health risks. In Portugal, the first state of emergency was declared on 18 March 2020 and renewed until 2 May 2020. During this time, most citizens stayed in quarantine with practical implications regarding their work and daily activities. This exploratory study, conducted within the pandemic crisis context in Portugal, intends to grasp specificities of the adaptation to the lock down and social isolation/distancing measures, concerning, specifically, teleworking conditions and physical activity practice. Data was collected from March to May 2020 through an online survey from 1148 participants of different age groups and literacy. Considering that COVID-19 features a mutual feedback loop of disease and social dynamics—governmental measures, civic adjustments, and individual coping—to know more about what was featured, the first wave may provide some cues to ensure a more efficient co-operation among social actors and, ultimately, tailor better public policies towards teleworking, online distance learning, and the promotion of healthy behaviours.

**Keywords:** COVID-19; coronavirus; SARS-Cov-2; teleworking; physical exercise; health policies

## 1. Introduction

The implementation of measures to contain and delay the spike in infection of COVID-19 has resulted in major changes in both work and social lives, allowing us to test, in a natural setting experiment, different societal iterations.

Although symptoms of COVID-19 are similar to those of other strains of coronaviruses (e.g., fever, dry cough, fatigue) asymptomatic individuals are able to spread the virus [1].The global outbreak of COVID-19 has thus prompted most countries to implement an array of measures to contain or delay the spread of the virus, from self-isolation or quarantine to public health guidance (e.g., hand washing, respiratory etiquette, social distancing) [2]. Although most countries have advised their citizens who display symptoms to self-isolate for 7–14 days, and practice social distancing to those without symptoms, the implementation of overall top-down governmental measures have differed according to each country (e.g., [3,4]). In Portugal, the first two confirmed cases of COVID-19 were reported on 2 March 2020 [5]. On the 18 March the President declared the state of emergency (President Decree no. 14-A/2020), which was consecutively renewed until 30 April with a positive impact in the number of new cases per day in this first phase, as evidenced in Figure 1.

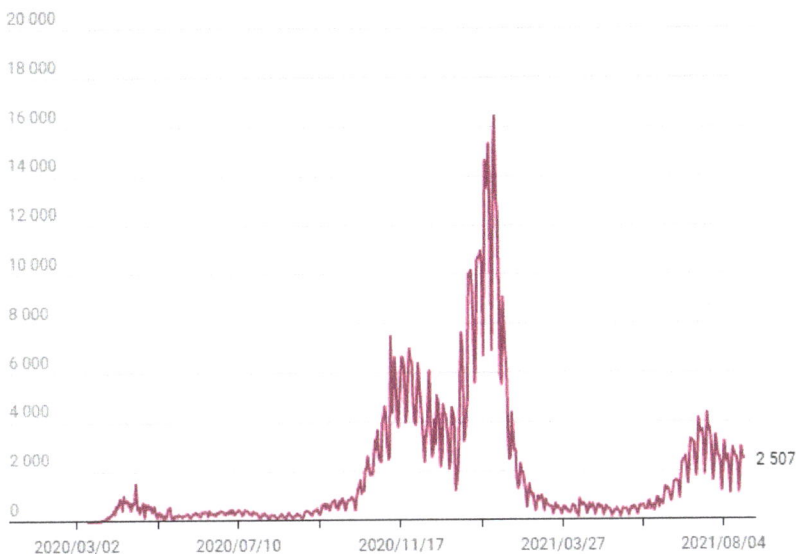

**Figure 1.** Evolution of new cases per day in Portugal. Source: https://expresso.pt/coronavirus/20-0-2021-Covid-19, accessed on 16 May 2020.

During this first period, several measures were taken which impacted work, economic, and social spheres (see [6] for an in-depth description). As the expected number of cases of an infectious disease such as COVID-19 is directly generated from contact with an infected person, social distancing is usually used as a measure to curb the spread of the disease [7]. Accordingly, one of the most poignant ideas, with unprecedented worldwide application, was the sudden adaptation and shift of the workforce into a telework format.

Epidemic models seem to project that telework is indeed critical in buffering the overall burden of COVID-19 on the population [8], and companies expect it to be an essential component in the efforts to mitigate the pandemic [9]. With the implementation of telework, allied to the quarantine measures, expectedly comes an increase in sedentary life, as well as its widely acknowledged negative health consequences [10,11].

In this article, we argue that the understanding of the ways in which teleworking will unfold and be adopted at a macro-scale level may benefit from knowledge on how individuals have adapted to it during current pandemic times with no preparation or prior training. This study, of an exploratory and descriptive nature, is thus guided by the following research question: "What featured the adaptation to tele-working and social isolation in the first lockdown?" More specifically, it sought to characterize some physical, practical, and emotional adjustments related to this shift and co-presence between home and work during the first lockdown within the Portuguese context. It also intends to explore the changes in health-related behaviours, particularly the practice of physical exercise as a way to mitigate pandemic effects.

## 2. Teleworking Background

### 2.1. Pros and Cons of Teleworking

Telework, also called telecommuting and remote working, was first outlined by [12] as an original response to urban sprawl, traffic, and scarcity of non-renewable resources. The idea gained particular momentum in the midst of a crisis of a different nature, the OPEC oil embargo and the subsequent energy scarcity and cost inflation, which added to the increasing concern over gridlocks in major urban centres. Work settings reorganization was thus seen as a measure that would promote environment sustainability in the long run.

Over the years, the appeal concerning the environmental benefits of teleworking remained, namely reducing transport-related environmental pollution, congested cities, and fostering rural development, given that people could work for city-based companies [13].

In the 1990s and 2000s, much due to technological breakthroughs that were quickly widespread, it gauged a lot of attention as a new flexible form of work organization [14] that would become a major feature of working life in western society. What is more, the claim expanded from societal and environmental benefits to how individuals and organizations could gain from this new setting [15].

Despite all, this more flexible form failed to launch at a global scale, much due to managerial and executive resistance [16]. At this level, albeit recognizing the advantages of flexible work, occupational and industry constraints, such as the fear of cultural change, inequitable outcomes and a flunk in workers' motivation kept the inertia. Accordingly, no substantial research further explored the topic up until recently within the context of pandemic compulsory measures. As a case in point, a brief search on 30 June 2021 by 'telework*' on SCimago Journal Rank (SCOPUS), the most commonly used scholar citation database in social sciences, shows a scarce interest until the 90s, a steady focus of 30 and 40 publications per year in this decade, a slight increase in the 2000s to 50 and 70, and a rise to 200 articles per year in 2020 and 2021.

Currently, teleworking is defined as the provision of service done at a distance, using online and telecommunication technologies [17], hence allowing workers to fulfil their roles and functions while keeping the connection with the employer [18]. The locale where the worker develops his activities and the use of information and communication technologies (ICT) are thus two nuclear elements of teleworking.

The economic pressure, competition, and unforeseeable changes in society and job market have challenged the traditional conception of employment, forcing organizations to adopt, up to a certain extent, flexible work practices [19]. Made possible by the advances in technology within the last decade, these practices, varying in magnitude and extent of application, are overall seen as offering a competitive edge to companies (thus being a common practice in many high-tech businesses and start-ups particularly concerned in attracting and retaining talent invested in innovation). Besides the contribution to environment-friendly and healthier cities, several advantages have been reported associated to teleworking, at an organizational and individual level [20].

An evident benefit is to reduce the costs and time spent in commuting while sparing workers from the inherent stress and tiredness with negative consequences for their physical and mental health [21]. These perks, with a clear positive impact on the daily routine, may contribute to a higher satisfaction and dedication towards work which are well known predictors of a higher productivity [18]. On the other hand, they reduce the demands of the dialectic public/private and work/family roles [22], such as schedule flexibility, reduced costs of overheads, and increase in productivity (e.g., [21,23]). It is also argued that teleworkers tend to enjoy of more free time for leisure and can easily reconcile work with family demands, being more available or, at least, more flexible to take care and give attention to children or elder family members. In addition, the employer can also be more competitive and reduce some costs, as in electricity and water, as well as those related to sick leaves and workers absenteeism.

Others have emphasized the considerable disadvantages of teleworking, such as social isolation [24], presenteeism (e.g., working longer hours, working when sick) [25], and blurred boundaries between work and home life [26], which can negatively affect psychological well-being [27] and overall family dynamics [28]. Reduced social interaction is the main problem given its potential in fostering sadness, solitude, and stress and subsequently reducing work motivation (especially for those who live alone). Mixing work and personal life can also cause entanglement and confusion [22], even more when there is an overlapping of physical spaces. In this regard, it can be substantially harder to deal with distractions at home than those that occur in a traditional workspace, thus requiring more self-discipline and time management skills to succeed in teleworking [29]. This is true in both ways, for those who get easily distracted or those who may find difficult to disconnect compromising their health and wellbeing [22].

On a different note, [18] refer that teleworking may also impair career progression because, when working remotely, workers are less on the radar for possible promotions. What is more, workers may feel less connected to the organization and miss the social contact and usual exchange with co-workers that can lead to fruitful collaborations [30]. In this regard, ref. [31] argues that personal interactions have a superior impact, particularly due to the enabled visual contact. Video calls and similar interactive devices fail to mimic this experience; hence, it is arguable that new technologies foster a particular type of distance among workers.

*2.2. Teleworking during the Pandemic*

The effective implementation of teleworking as a means to mitigate the seemingly unavoidable economic impact of the COVID-19 was especially relevant to countries such as Portugal, in which positive signs of economic growth were appearing prior to the pandemic outbreak. Through covering at least the functions compatible with working at a distance, the benefits are evident since it allows workers to keep their jobs and allows firms to continue developing their activity, reducing the economic burden [31].

However, this measure was implemented without specific regulations, only based on a general agreement on teleworking of 2002, drawn on a different stage of ICT development and EU-based policies and directives regulating work, in general, and assuming by default that the same provisions would apply. Among these, are: EU Directive 2003/88/CE, about working time schedules; EU Directive 89/391/CEE on work health and hygiene; EU directive 2019/1158 about dealing with professional and familiar life and; EU Directive 2019/1152 on transparent and predictable work conditions [32]. The highlight goes to general rights, such as the voluntary nature of the work; respect for privacy; data protection; health and safety measures.

Only in June 2020, an autonomous framework, aimed at informing a possible European-based directive on digitalization, was put forth covering four specific areas: digital competence and job security; connection and disconnection modalities; artificial intelligence and human control; respect for human dignity and vigilance. The emphasis on these areas provides cues about the main concerns of conducting work activities with such dependence on ICT. Furthermore, a few recommendations are drawn so as to protect the workers' rights on these conditions, starting with being informed about all the matters regarding equipment, working hours (normal and extraordinary), responsibilities, and costs. Other important provisions regard the costs being completely covered by the employer; the extraordinary hours reimburse; the right to sick leaves and, very importantly, an efficient and fair measurement and monitoring of working hours so as to protect workers from the risk of presenteeism.

Besides not knowing the impacts and effects on a wide array of indicators in the long-run, either related to productivity and financial aspects, the individual and social coping to the hypothetical dissemination of teleworking is also uncertain.

The literature puts forth two coping strategies: "integration" and "segmentation"/"separation" [33]; both are based on how individuals redraw cultural boundaries around "work" and "home" when these overlap, as occurs in a teleworking format. These coping strategies, although generalist, provide a conceptual lens to the practicalities of accommodating the co-presence of these two settings with the ethical and values with which they are imbued [34].

In this regard, a separatist approach features the co-presence of "work" and "home" by adhering to strict temporal regimes as expressed in fixed office hours and closed-door spaces. Thus, symbolically as well as practically, "work" and "home" are kept apart. An integrative approach, on the other hand, tends to be more flexible and is likely to follow a more laissez-faire temporal regime, integrating domestic, personal activities (as physical exercise) and professional activities in common spaces [35].

Underpinning the coping strategies lies a fundamental element regarding the gendered division of household and childcare responsibilities [36]. Domestic inequalities are still a reality, particularly in countries with lower levels of gender equality and female empowerment [37,38] and, during the pandemic, they appear to have increased, especially amongst people with children [39]. More specifically, mothers reported a decrease in working hours and an increase in domestic and house care activities, as well as supervising children's homework and didactic activities [39,40], with a negative impact on their wellbeing [36]. This is in line with the gendered expectations that remained the same and, despite the expansion of women's roles in the last decade working outside the home, they are still expected to perform most of the domestic and care work [41].

What is more, gendered roles are prescriptive and proscriptive of attitudes and behaviour, and both have been evidenced, especially in the beginning of the pandemic, with women reporting more psychological distress and anxiety, and men reporting strength, more calm, and determination [42].

This forced experience on teleworking is perceived as an opportunity to catalyse "a wider adoption of teleworking practices also after the crisis" [42]. According to the European Foundation for the Improvement of Living and Working Conditions [43], more than three quarters of EU workers prefer to work from home, at least occasionally, even without COVID restrictions. Specifically, most EU workers indicate that they had a positive experience of teleworking and, albeit not exclusively, the most favoured option is to combine teleworking and on-site work.

However, the overlapping of leisure and working time, domestic and labour routines, as well as the ICT intensive use are known to impact health and wellbeing. The negative effects are mostly psychological pressure, stress, vision problems, anxiety, headaches, fatigue, sleep disorders, and skeletal muscle functions [43].

In order to counteract the physical and mental health impact of telework, and to promote overall healthy behaviours during the pandemic, public health communication should not only focus on messaging information strictly regarding COVID-19 infection and its mitigation (e.g., prevalence, progression, death rate, mitigation measures) but also health promoting behaviours related to the management of in-door time and physical exercise. Indeed, some have advised for the maintenance of physical exercise during lockdown (e.g., [44]), and it has been argued to help reducing the negative health consequences of COVID-19 quarantine [45].

### 2.3. Occupational Health in Telework: The Importance of Physical Activity

According to the World Health Organisation [46], a healthy workforce is crucial for social and economic development. The WHO's report on occupational health states that there is a continuous two-way interaction between individuals and the physical and psychological working environment, as the latter may affect, positively or negatively, the worker's health, and productivity is, in turn, disturbed by the person's well-being. In view of this, in order to ensure occupational health in telework in the context of COVID-19, it is important to underline the health risks and benefits associated with the sudden and large-scale shift to telework, as well as the specific conditions that lead to better psychological and work outcomes [47].

Within the Portuguese context, a qualitative shift occurred in Health promotion initiatives, as evidenced in the official communication issued by The National Program for Physical Activity of the General Health Department (2020a) [42]. Aimed at counteracting the demanding restrictions, both resulting from spending more time at home collapsing routines and spaces as from being limited to enjoy public spaces, health authorities have been forceful in ensuing specific recommendations adapted to the circumstances. Very directive suggestions included: avoiding to seat or lie down for more than 30 min; reduce the time spent using technological devices; walk inside the house and conduct other physical activities; 'invest in activities of cognitive stimulation (reading, puzzles); stretch and meditate as well as play with children [48,49].

This is backed up by WHO, suggesting 30 min of intense or moderated physical activity ([49]), particularly regarding older citizens [50,51], given their higher vulnerability to health problems and COVID-19. In this regard, aerobic home exercise has been advised, due to its fairly low complexity, low risk of injury, and high popularity [52].

Also, physical activity seems to be negatively correlated to cardiovascular disease and diabetes (e.g., [53]), which is especially noteworthy in the context of COVID-19, given that these constitute risk factors associated to respective severity and mortality (e.g., [53]). Additionally, exercise has been reported to positively impact anti-inflammatory response and reduce immunologic abnormality [54,55].

It is self-evident that physical activity has been impacted by the global efforts to mitigate the progression of COVID-19 infections [56]. In this social distancing phase, the type of physical activity should prioritize interiors or secure empty public spaces. Additionally, ref. [45] puts forth that people should practice physical exercise five to seven times a week, depending on the training intensity and modality (for example, if is resistance training it should be done two to three times a week, according to [57].

However, several obstacles may hinder the engagement of at-home physical exercise, namely the unavailability of training materials and equipment for moderate to intensive physical activity (particularly from those with a lower socio-economic level with less margin to acquire them), as well as difficulties in controlling training variables, such as adequacy of training exercises.

Notwithstanding the obstacles, one may argue that the disruption of normal life and routines, allied to the sudden official Public Health communication issued by governments and reinforced by all media, led to a salience of physical activity in peoples' minds. Even though physical activity promotion and healthier lives are two common claims in western societies, the pandemic added a tone of threat and urgency to it, either as a way to reinforce the overall physical health or to mitigate the psychological impact of the quarantine measures.

In this regard, more fine-tuned research is needed to conclude the impact of the perception of public health messaging on the population´s adherence to governmental guidelines, including the appeal to physical exercise, as people tend to comply with governmental suggestions/orientations even when distrusting the government. This is particularly true in a time where information is not exclusively delivered directly by the institutions but rather mediated by both traditional and social media [58] with potential impact not only on compliance but also on mental health (e.g., [59,60]). In the context of COVID-19, studies suggest that using deontological moral advice when communicating public health advice (e.g., eliciting a sense of civic duty, ethical self-care) contributes to the engagement of behaviours that are helpful for health and wellbeing [61].

The ingrained notion of how important physical exercise is to physical and mental health found a more fertile ground because of the lack of parallel distractions.

Digital landscapes (with emphasis of YouTube and social media) played a quintessential role in this dissemination, fuelling a wide variety of online training offers, thus, expanding the outreach of gymnasium, sport clubs, and personal trainers. Recorded and live sessions, mimicking physical training, push good practices and physical activity support further, often on a daily basis [62], with the common denominator of being mainly home-based.

One may further argue that physical activity also contributes to mitigate the presenteeism and cognitive overload of connection, known to underpin physical and emotional exhaustion. In this regard, it is another aspect to take into account when drafting guidelines at EU level.

Drawing on data collected during the first locked down, the present work contributes to unveil key elements that may be considered in communication and public policies regarding teleworking and physical activity tailored to reach different segmented groups of the populations.

## 3. Materials and Methods

### 3.1. Participants and Procedure

Data was collected from 14 March 2020 to 2 of May through an online survey in google forms which was shared via institutional and personal contacts. There were 1148 participants who replied, 69.9% women ($n$ = 802) and 30.1% men ($n$= 346). The sample includes five different age groups: until 18 years old ($n$ = 8; 0.7%); 18–24 years old ($n$ = 277; 24.1%); 25–39 years old ($n$ = 261; 22.7%); 40–59 years old ($n$ = 466; 40.6%); above 60 years old ($n$ = 136; 11.2%). A substantial percentage of our sample has high education studies: nearly half is graduated at BSc level ($n$ = 563; 49%), 19.8% at Master level ($n$ = 227), and 7.1% has a PhD ($n$ = 81). 15.9% ($n$ = 182) has finished middle school and 8.3% ($n$ = 95) completed 11° grade. More than half of the participants ($n$= 722, 62.9%) has a full-time job (40 h or more per week); 18.8% ($n$ = 216) are students; 8.1% ($n$ = 93) are retired; 4.4% ($n$ = 51) work part-time jobs (16 to 30 h a week) and 44 (3.8%) are unemployed. Nearly half of the participants ($n$= 541; 47.2%) are married or living with a companion; 42.7% are single; 8.7% ($n$ = 100) are divorced, and 16 (1.4%) are widowed. More than half ($n$ = 589; 51.3%) have children. Approximately 60% of the participants indicate that their youngest child is still under age.

### 3.2. Questionnaire

The questionnaire applied was made available online and included an informed consent describing the study, the aim and topics included and informing participants about the confidentiality of their answers. Only a positive reply would allow to proceed to other items related to topics out of the scope of the present article (factual knowledge, perceptions, attitudes, and behaviours towards the virus, its transmission, and consequences), socio-demographic information, and the following sections used in the present study (Supplementary Materials):

Emotions: 5-point Likert scale items related to the emotional response felt in the last week (calm, nervous, sad, relaxed, and preoccupied).

Teleworking and physical activity: 20 items related to teleworking (physical conditions, technological dimensions, and communication) and 17 items concerning online and physical activities.

## 4. Results

### 4.1. Adaptation to Teleworking

The professional activities of most of the participants, 81.1% ($n$ = 828), are compatible with teleworking, which is exclusively conducted from home. Interestingly, 34.2% consider that their professional routine has not changed, suggesting that there were sufficient elements in this period to maintain a perception of constancy. This may result from the fact that professional activities, nowadays, rely much more on online communication and technological media than on physically grounded activities. Hence, even though the context of work differed, the work process itself, at large, did not suffer significant changes.

An aspect reported as being different was the time spent in work-related activities mediated by ICT. In this regard, 37.3% of the participants indicate spending more time online or using some ICT (e.g., computer; telephone); 26.4% indicate attending to more meetings and 34.6% to work for longer hours.

Concerning the financial practicalities of this shift, 79.4% of the participants did not receive any reimbursement for extra expenses and 74.5% were not payed for extra hours. What is more, at the time, 18.8% did not even know if they would be reimbursed.

The working hours and financial provisions appear to be at odds with the applicable European directives on this issue, regarding, in particular, the reimbursement for any extra costs related to teleworking and communications and the appropriate compensation for extraordinary working hours, particularly onerous for those participants who report working longer hours. Although these shortcomings may be understood in the light of the lack of national-based regulation on teleworking, they strengthen the need to reinforce public policy on this matter, at EU and national levels, as is currently ongoing based on the independent framework of digitalization rights (see SOC/660–EESC-2020-05278-00-00-AC-TRA (EN) 2/18).

As concerns, one of the key factors of teleworking—its physical space—among the surveyed, 72.2% (n = 594) were developing their activities in common and shared spaces, such as the living room (44.6%); the bedroom (19.6%) and the kitchen (4.5%). Only 27.8% had a specific room in the house dedicated solely to work without overlapping with other family dynamics, which is suggestive that the majority of our participants faced one of the most problematic issues in teleworking that is the physical blurred boundaries between work and home life [26]. This is even more impactful considering that 47.2% were in a relationship, 51.3% had children, of who 61% were under 18 and living at the house.

Perceived as one potential disadvantage of teleworking [22] the shortcomings of the co-presence between work and home were particularly noteworthy in the context of COVID-19, given that, due to large-scale schools closing, parents not only have to juggle work and family life, but also manage children's home schooling.

Interestingly, in line with what was found in [36], the toll was felt heavier by the women. As shown in Table 1 below, when asked about the emotions felt in the past week, men clearly reported more positive emotions than women, including feelings of calm and relaxation, and, in contrast, women differed significantly from men in showing more negative emotions, including nervousness, sadness, and preoccupation. A one-way ANOVA (data not shown) shows that there are significant differences between the groups in all the emotions assessed.

**Table 1.** Means and Standard deviation of emotions by gender.

|  |  | N | M | SD |
|---|---|---|---|---|
| Calm | Male | 346 | 3.82 | 1.01 |
|  | Female | 802 | 3.25 | 1.04 |
| Nervousness | Male | 346 | 2.25 | 1.10 |
|  | Female | 802 | 2.89 | 1.15 |
| Sadness | Male | 346 | 2.60 | 1.16 |
|  | Female | 802 | 3.12 | 1.19 |
| Relaxation | Male | 346 | 3.06 | 1.08 |
|  | Female | 802 | 2.53 | 1.04 |
| Preoccupation | Male | 346 | 3.28 | 1.11 |
|  | Female | 802 | 3.74 | 0.99 |

This strengthens the findings of [41] where women reported higher psychological distress whereas men were apparently calmer and stronger. These results may be influenced by the expected gendered display of emotions but also due to extrinsic pressures, since, in general, women were overall more burdened with more domestic and house care activities, as well as supervising children homework and didactic activities ([39,40]), with an expected negative impact on their wellbeing [36].

The analysis of the emotional reactions during this period also showed that, comparing all ages, participants above 60 years old are those that, albeit at a higher risk of pandemic-related complications and more targeted by official communication, were feeling calmer (M = 3.54; DP = 1.06), more relaxed (M = 2.77; DP = 1.12), less preoccupied (M = 3.46; DP = 1.11) and less nervous (M = 2.40; DP = 1.12) than younger individuals. Sadness was the only emotion equally felt by all groups, appropriate to the loss and disruption felt at those times.

The overall concern about older individuals' health vulnerabilities and risk of social isolation and higher emotional impact [48] is not corroborated in our sample, with younger individuals feeling more negative emotions during these times. This may be related to the work-related uncertain processes and outcomes of the pandemic impact. Interestingly, students are the ones reporting higher levels of sadness (M = 3.12; DP = 1.13) whereas workers (62.9% of our participants have a full-time job and 4.4% a part time) report more nervousness and preoccupation, particularly part-time workers, the most psychologically distressed segment. Negative emotions in workers may also be aggravated by the fact that 40% of the participants work more hours than before at their work places. This result, besides not abiding by general regulations, is at odds with the more optimist view of teleworking as allowing workers to enjoy more free time for leisure [21] and is, in turn, in line with the risk of presenteeism [25] and overall negative impacts for the psychological well-being [27].

The work spillover during leisure hours is not, however, the only problematic issue. The non-verbal overload of digital interaction is known to not only fail at mimicking a healthier personal experience as to foster tiredness and irritability [31]. This is particularly evidenced in meeting platforms, such as Zoom or Microsoft Teams, in which increasing use is also corroborated in the present study. As shown in Figure 2 below, Zoom was the more frequent new ICT platform followed by Microsoft Teams. The remaining were already commonly used for communicating with teams and co-workers, especially e-mail (99.9% of the participants), followed by WhatsApp (56.4%) and Messenger (40.8%). Other studies have reported similar results, in which the use of and dependence upon social media platforms, such as Zoom, Microsoft Teams, and WhatsApp, to stay connected for work, education, and social purposes, have seen an exponential growth in users during that time (e.g., [63,64])

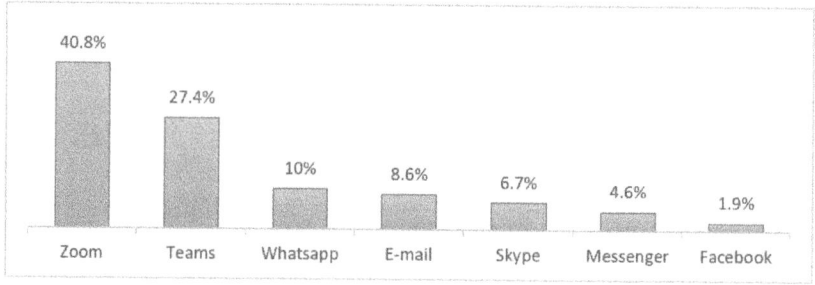

**Figure 2.** New ICT tools.

In this regard, 64.6% of our participants report not using ICT for leisure, suggesting their use as working or utilitarian tools. One of these utilitarian aims, besides work, is online shopping, with 45.8% of the participants reporting it as a common practice. For 23.1%, the frequency of on-line purchasing has increased during the pandemic that also brought a different choice of products (depicted in Table 2). Expectedly, considering the measures of social isolation and quarantine at place, there was a substantial increase in the acquisition of essential goods and foodstuffs. Gadgets and technology purchase also increased, probably due to the higher ICT use during these times for work and entertainment purposes. Interestingly, there was a fall in all of the other products, particularly clothes.

**Table 2.** Online purchases before and during the pandemic.

|  | Before | During Pandemic |
|---|---|---|
| Essential goods and foodstuffs | 26.9% | 46.8% |
| Clothes | 46.5% | 9.4% |
| Cosmetics | 5.4% | 4.7% |
| Books | 15.8% | 7.4% |
| Gadgets/Technology | 5.4% | 31.7% |

Among the 35.3% who actually use ICT for leisure, the interests and focuses are varied (see Table 3). Physical exercise classes and apps are the more frequent on-line based activities, and this interest and actual investment speaks favourably about the widespread dissemination of the importance of physical exercise. This in-home practice even surpassed the search for entertainment-based activities, as internet searches, movies and TV shows, and games.

Table 3. Categories of on-line activities for leisure.

|  | N | % |
|---|---|---|
| Physical exercise classes and apps | 107 | 27.30% |
| Internet searches (sites, YouTube) | 103 | 26.40% |
| Movies and tv shows (Netflix, HBO) | 98 | 25.10% |
| Games | 71 | 18.20% |
| Cultural activities (cinema, theater, concerts) | 50 | 12.80% |
| Social Media | 35 | 8.90% |

*4.2. Physical Activity*

The interest in being physically active is not only evidenced by searching and purchasing related physical activity apps and classes online, but also by the fact that 70.1% of the participants were already active before the pandemics, 53.1% practicing a specific sport and 46.9% recreative and leisure physical activities.

Even though 54.1% report that the physical activity decreased with the pandemic, 27.7% were still practicing up to 3 times, 19.9% once a week, and 17.3% up to seven days a week, which is not so far from the optimal practice suggested in [45,57]. These regular habits are even more important considering that 54.2% of our participants work seated at the computer with the potential sedentarism and collateral psychological pressure, stress, vision problems, anxiety, headaches, fatigue, sleep disorders, and skeletal muscle functions [57]. Furthermore, there was a substantial decrease for younger participants (52%) and for participants above 60 years old (66%), which strengthens, even more, the governmental concerns in targeting this age in particular [50].

As expected, there was a shift in the place of physical practice and whereas 91.7% of these activities were practiced outside the house with the pandemics, only 20.2% of the participants were able to keep that routine. Moreover, 79.8% of the participants report to conduct their physical activities inside the house, suggesting an adherence to the message issued by governments and reinforced by all media concerning the practice of physical activity [56]; ICTs, in particular, digital landscapes such as YouTube, social media, and sites, appear to be of nuclear importance in the adoption of this practice mimicking a real life context of physical practice and connection [62] while 39.3% of the participants report following a regular routine nowadays.

Another evidence of the compliance of governmental indications is the difference between the role of group-based activities of physical exercise before (41.6%) and during the pandemic (3.9%). There was no change, however, in the percentage of participants exercising in the company of one more person. Despite the overall frequency decrease, one may argue that what changed for most of them was the adjustment to different routines since—up to a higher or lesser degree—they have started to practice inside the house and, more often, alone (73.1% of the participants in contrast with 33.8% prior to the pandemic).

The practice of physical exercise appears to be more frequent in participants with a master degree (81%) and a PhD (79%) and the least adopted by those with a compulsory education (55.8%). These results follow the widely acknowledged association of physical exercise with health behaviour and better health in general [65] being perceived by some authors as the single most important and constant influence in health preservation [66].

On one hand, it is argued that formal education fosters knowledge and values related with seeking and comprehending health-related information as well as acting upon it. By contrast, lower educated people are at higher risk of not engaging in the desirable levels of physical activity [67], which can also be linked to more material problems (such as housing general conditions and available space) or poor health experienced by older lower educated people.

Accordingly, public health communication should emphasize beneficial and low complexity exercises (as aerobic home) assessable to all segments of the population.

## 5. Conclusions

### 5.1. Implications

The COVID-19 pandemic has embodied a major challenge, not only for the health system, but also for services, firms, workers, and employers, due to the upswing suddenly experienced by remote working technologies. The spread of teleworking and the use of technological platforms, in this context, has been considered essential to keep social distancing in workplaces and between employees and users/clients. Given the speed of change in result of political measures, services, and companies had very little time to put together a work at distance plan. Even though the COVID-19 pandemic and its mitigation methods have noticed, these past months, a gradual decrease in a number of countries concerning social distance, the extensive use of teleworking is expected to continue. As recently stated by the European Parliament Committee on Employment and Social Affairs, "the extensive use of telework poses a number of challenges and requires a re-think of the way work is performed, coordinated, and regulated" ([68], p. 14), bearing in mind its positive and negative impacts. On this, several hazards to the health of teleworkers have been highlighted in literature (see inter alia [69]), namely physical (e.g., awkward postures, repetitive movements, and long periods of continuous work, increased rate of physical inactivity, and sedentarism) and psychosocial (e.g., sleeping disorders, work-related stress, and social isolation) ones.

If COVID-19 events have transformed the working conditions and modified the employer-worker-user/client relationships, making telework unlikely to return to pre-pandemic levels, it is essential that policymakers, services, and firms realize the challenges associated with this phenomenon, building knowledge to provide the basis for change, improvement, and, accordingly, promote generative learning from research. This study, conducted within the COVID-19 crisis context in Portugal, intended to grasp specificities of the adaptation to the lock down and social distancing measures, in what concerns specifically teleworking conditions and physical activity practice.

From this study, it is possible to derive some findings with potential implications for the immediate and post-pandemic settings. First, the workload and time spent in teleworking were higher than in the physical format, i.e., before the pandemic. Besides confirming the risk of presenteeism (foreseen as disadvantage of this format) it reinforces the need to draft clear and encompassing regulations and policies protecting the workers from this probable spill over.

Our results also unveiled a problem related to the workers' personal sphere, that is, the lack of a specific space at home exclusively for work. The overlapping of spaces and blurred boundaries between work and home life is known to cause entanglement and confusion as well as be much more demanding in self-discipline and time management. Even though it is harder to tackle this issue from a public policy viewpoint, it may be mitigated at an organizational level: team-leaders and employees need to be briefed and prepared in the most co-constructive ways to conduct work in these different and heterogeneous conditions. Under a common teleworking policy, trainings, specific performance criteria and weekly check-ins to gauge their experience and address any concerns should be adopted. A people-oriented mind set would be beneficial, acknowledging and managing, as much as possible, the pressing anxiety and stress that may result from these conditions.

On the other hand, this research also suggests that women were subjected to more emotional stress and impact on psychological wellbeing. This requires a tailored approach to raise awareness about expected gendered biases while empowering women to assert and define a more balanced distribution. Given that this is a structural societal issue, it may be more effective if put forth and advocated by public or organizational policies.

The same concerns apply to the wide use of ICT, also corroborated here, known to induce a cognitive overload with a negative impact on wellbeing and physical health.

Efforts in tailoring occupational health programs and training should be put in motion and enforced by public policies. This may also include the emphasis, already noticeable, of the perks and necessity of physical activity, no longer seen as a hobby but as a complementary part of a work routine. This study indicates that, despite the difficult conditions and adverse times, there was an effort to continue to practice physical activities (also evidenced in the search for related online classes and apps), which speaks favourably of the receptivity to Health communication and individual predispositions.

In addition, the lack of reimbursement for extra work time or equipment, at par with the workers' unawareness of their rights and what they are entitled to, is indicative of the urgency in drafting regulations and legislations at the European and national level specifically covering telework. Considering the gradual shift towards flexible work practices, these regulations should be well-known by the workers.

### 5.2. Limitations of the Study and Future Research Lines

The present study has two main limitations to be taken into account and frame the results interpretation. The first concerns its exploratory and descriptive nature, reflected both in the questionnaire design and in the analyses conducted which targeted only a description of general conditions and particular behaviours and practices of the participants. The second regards the non-probabilistic sampling method through institutional and personal contacts, which resulted in an over-sampling of highly educated individuals. In this regard, the results must be considered in the light of this particular WEIRD sample and national context.

Notwithstanding, considering the increasing role teleworking is playing in society, this study highlights some patterns that may inform further research and policy design particularly in the analysed context, worth to emphasize that public policies and co-operation among social partners are crucial to ensure that new, efficient, and welfare-improving working methods emerging during the crisis are maintained and developed once physical distancing is over. To maximize productivity and welfare gains inherent in the use of more widespread telework, governments should promote investments in the physical and managerial capacity of firms and workers to telework and address potential concerns for the workers' health, well-being, and longer-term innovation related, in particular, to the excessive downscaling of workspaces.

**Supplementary Materials:** The following are available online at https://www.mdpi.com/article/10.3390/healthcare9091151/s1, Questionnaire.

**Author Contributions:** Conceptualization, T.F. and G.S.; methodology, T.F. and G.S.; formal analysis, T.F. and G.S.; writing—T.F.; G.S. and S.A.C.; proofreading—T.F.; G.S. and S.A.C. All authors have read and agreed to the published version of the manuscript.

**Funding:** This research received no external funding.

**Institutional Review Board Statement:** Ethical review and approval were waived for this study due to the absence of risk in data collection or sensible information accessed.

**Informed Consent Statement:** Informed consent was obtained from all subjects involved in the study.

**Data Availability Statement:** Not applicable.

**Acknowledgments:** This work was partly financially supported by the research unit on Governance, Competitiveness and Public Policy (UIDB/04058/2020) + (UIDP/04058/2020), funded by national funds through FCT–Fundação para a Ciência e a Tecnologia.

**Conflicts of Interest:** The authors declare no conflict of interest.

## References

1. Wang, D.; Hu, B.; Hu, C.; Zhu, F.; Liu, X.; Zhang, J. Clinical characteristics of 138 hospitalized patients with 2019 novel coronavirus-infected pneumonia in Wuhan, China. *JAMA* **2020**, *323*, 1061–1069. [CrossRef] [PubMed]
2. Bedford, J.; Enria, D.; Giesecke, J.; Heymann, D.L.; Ihekweazu, C.; Kobinger, G.; Ungchusak, K. COVID-19: Towards controlling of a pandemic. *Lancet* **2020**, *395*, 1015–1018. [CrossRef]
3. Barr, K. Coronavirus: What Is Herd Immunity and Is It a Possibility for the UK? Independent. Available online: https://www.independent.co.uk/life-style/health-and-families/coronavirus-herd-immunity-meaning-definition-what-vaccine-immune-covid-19-a9397871.html (accessed on 16 May 2020).
4. Graham-Harrison, E.; Kuo, L. China's Coronavirus Lockdown Strategy: Brutal but Effective. The Guardian. Available online: https://www.theguardian.com/world/2020/mar/19/chinas-coronavirus-lockdown-strategy-brutal-but-effective (accessed on 16 May 2020).
5. DGS. SARS-CoV-2 Situation Report. Available online: https://covid19.min-saude.pt/wp-content/uploads/2020/03/Relatório-de-Situaç~ao-1.pdf (accessed on 16 May 2020).
6. Martins, D.C. COVID-19 and Labour Law: Portugal. *Ital. Labour Law E-J.* **2020**, *13*. [CrossRef]
7. Narayanan, R.P.; Nordlund, J.; Pace, R.K.; Ratnadiwakara, D. Demographic, jurisdictional, and spatial effects on social distancing in the United States during the COVID-19 pandemic. *PLoS ONE* **2020**, *15*, e0239572. [CrossRef]
8. Di Domenico, L.; Pullano, G.; Coletti, P.; Hens, N.; Colizza, V. Expected impact of school closure and telework to mitigate COVID-19 epidemic in France. *MedRxiv* **2020**, *18*. [CrossRef]
9. Fadel, M.; Salomon, J.; Descatha, A. Coronavirus outbreak: The role of companies in preparedness and responses. *Lancet Public Health* **2020**, *5*, e193. [CrossRef]
10. Owen, N.; Healy, G.N.; Matthews, C.E.; Dunstan, D.W. Too much sitting: The population-health science of sedentary behavior. *Exerc. Sport Sci. Rev.* **2010**, *38*, 105. [CrossRef]
11. Tremblay, M.S.; Colley, R.C.; Saunders, T.J.; Healy, G.N.; Owen, N. Physiological and health implications of a sedentary lifestyle. *Appl. Physiol. Nutr. Metab.* **2010**, *35*, 725–740. [CrossRef] [PubMed]
12. Nilles, J.; Carlson, F.; Gray, P.; Hanneman, G. *The Telecommunications-Transportation Tradeoff: Options for Tomorrow*; John Wiley and Sons: New York, NY, USA, 1976.
13. Salomon, I.; Salomon, M. Telecommuting: The employee's perspective. *Technol. Forecast. Soc. Chang.* **1984**, *25*, 15–28. [CrossRef]
14. Golden, T.D. Applying technology to work: Toward a better understanding of telework. *Organ. Manag. J.* **2009**, *6*, 241–250. [CrossRef]
15. Norman, P.; Collins, S.; Conner, M.; Martin, R.; Rance, J. Attributions, cognitions, and coping styles: Teleworkers' reactions to work related problems. *J. Appl. Soc. Psychol.* **1995**, *25*, 117–128. [CrossRef]
16. Bailey, D.E.; Kurland, N.B. A review of telework research: Findings, new directions, and lessons for the study of modern work. *J. Organ. Behav.* **2002**, *23*, 383–400. [CrossRef]
17. Belzunegui-Eraso, A.; Erro-Garcés, A.; Pastor-Gosálbez, M.I. Telework as a Driver of the Third Sector and its Networks. In *Social E-Enterprise: Value Creation through ICT*; Torres-Coronas, T., Vidal-Blasco, M., Eds.; IGI Global: Hershey, PA, USA, 2013; pp. 83–95.
18. Lim, V.K.G.; Teo, T.S.H. An empirical investigation of factors affecting attitudes towards teleworking. *J. Manag. Psychol.* **2000**, *15*. [CrossRef]
19. Kowalski, K.B.; Swanson, J.A. Critical success factors in developing teleworking programs. *Benchmarking Int. J.* **2005**, *12*, 236–249. [CrossRef]
20. Montreuil, S.; Lippel, K. Telework and occupational health: A Quebec empirical study and regulatory implications. *Saf. Sci.* **2003**, *41*, 339–358. [CrossRef]
21. Sousa, A.C.T. O Meio Ambiente do Trabalho: Efeitos do Teletrabalho Regulamentado Pela Lei 13.467 de 2017. 2018. Available online: https://www.researchgate.net/profile/Angelina_Valenzuela_Rendon/publication/334001821_La_conciliacion_de_conflictos_medioambientales_relacionados_con_el_cambio_climatico/links/5d127e6c299bf1547c7f3474/La-conciliacion-de-conflictos-medioambientalesrelacionados-con-el-cambio-climatico.pdf#page=139 (accessed on 30 August 2021).
22. Tietze, S. When "Work" comes "home": Coping strategies of teleworkers and their families. *J. Bus. Ethics* **2002**, *41*, 385–396. [CrossRef]
23. Messenger, J.C.; Gschwind, L. Three generations of Telework: New ICTs and the (R)evolution from Home Office to Virtual Office. *New Technol. Work. Employ.* **2016**, *31*, 195–208. [CrossRef]
24. Golden, T.D.; Veiga, J.F.; Dino, R.N. The impact of professional isolation on teleworker job performance and turnover intentions: Does time spent teleworking, interacting face-to-face, or having access to communication-enhancing technology matter? *J. Appl. Psychol.* **2008**, *93*, 1412–1421. [CrossRef] [PubMed]
25. Biron, C.; Saksvik, P.Ø. Sickness presenteeism and attendance pressure factors: Implications for practice. In *International Handbook of Work and Health Psychology*; Cooper, C., Quick, J.C., Schabracq, M.J., Eds.; Wiley-Blackwell: Oxford, UK, 2015; pp. 77–96.
26. Ellison, N. New Perspectives on Telework. *Soc. Sci. Comput. Rev.* **1999**, *17*, 338–356. [CrossRef]
27. Mann, S.; Holdsworth, L. The psychological impact of teleworking: Stress, emotions and health. *New Technol. Work Employ* **2009**, *18*, 196–211. [CrossRef]
28. Standen, P.; Daniels, K.; Lamond, D. The home as a workplace: Work–family interaction and psychological well-being in telework. *J. Occup. Health Psychol.* **1999**, *4*, 368–381. [CrossRef] [PubMed]

29. Teo, T.S.H.; Lim, V.K.G. Factorial dimensions and differential effects of gender on perceptions of teleworking. *Women Manag. Rev.* **1998**, *8*, 253–264. [CrossRef]
30. Mann, S.; Vary, R.; Button, W. An exploration of the Emotional Impact of tele-working. *J. Manag. Psychol.* **2000**, *15*, 668–690. [CrossRef]
31. Semuels, A. Does Remote Work Actually Work? Retrieved 9 May 2020. Available online: https://eds.a.ebscohost.com/eds/pdfviewer/pdfviewer?vid=0&sid=0582bc6f-04f7-45b8b7f7-fd3d35ac37a5%40sdc-v-sessmgr01 (accessed on 30 August 2021).
32. International Labour Organization, *Teleworking during the COVID-19 Pandemic and beyond a Practical Guide*; International Labour Office: Geneva, Switzerland, 2020; Available online: https://www.ilo.org/global/publications/lang--en/index.htm (accessed on 31 August 2021)ISBN 978-92-2-032405-9.
33. Andrews, A.; Bailyn, L. Segmentation and Synergy. Two Models of Linking Work and Family'. In *Men, Work and Family*; Hood, J.C., Ed.; Sage: London, UK, 1993; pp. 262–275.
34. Campbell Clark, S. Work/Family Border Theory: A new theory of work/family balance. *Hum. Relat.* **2000**, *53*, 747–770. [CrossRef]
35. Nippert-Eng, C. Calendar and keys: The classification of home and work. *Sociol. Forum* **1996**, *11*, 563–582. [CrossRef]
36. Fisher, A.; Ryan, M. Gender inequalities during COVID-19. *Group Process. Intergroup Relat.* **2020**, *24*, 237–245. [CrossRef]
37. Fuwa, M. Macro-level gender inequality and the division of household labor in 22 countries. *Am. Sociol. Rev.* **2004**, *69*, 751–767. [CrossRef]
38. United Nations. *Gender Inequality and COVID-19 Crisis: A Human Development Perspective*; United Nations: New York, NY, USA, 2020.
39. Carlson, D.; Petts, R.; Pepin, J. Us Couples Divisions of Housework and Childcare during Covid 19 Pandemic. *SocarXiv Pap.* **2020**. [CrossRef]
40. Collins, C.; Landivar, L.; Ruppaner, L.; Scarborough, W. COVID-19 and the gender gap in work hours. *Gend. Work Organ.* **2020**, *28*, 101–112. [CrossRef]
41. Hennekam, S.; Ladge, J.; Shymko, Y. From zero to hero: An exploratory study examining sudden hero status among nonphysician health care workers during the COVID-19 pandemic. *J. Appl. Psychol.* **2020**, *105*, 1088–1100. [CrossRef]
42. OECD. *Supporting People and Companies to Deal with the COVID-19 Virus: Options for an Immediate Employment and Social-Policy Response*; OECD Briefs on the Policy Response to the COVID-19 Crisis; OECD: Paris, France, 2020; Available online: https://oecd.dam-broadcast.com/pm_7379_119_119686-962r78x4do.pdf (accessed on 30 August 2021).
43. Eurofound. *Living, Working and COVID-19 (Update April 2021): Mental Health and Trust Decline across EU as Pandemic Enters Another Year*; Publications Office of the European Union: Luxembourg, 2021.
44. Chen, P.; Mao, L.; Nassis, G.P.; Harmer, P.; Ainsworth, B.E.; Li, F. Wuhan coronavirus (2019-nCoV): The need to maintain regular physical activity while taking precautions. *J. Sport Health Sci.* **2020**, *9*, 103. [CrossRef] [PubMed]
45. Jiménez-Pavón, D.; Carbonell-Baeza, A.; Lavie, C.J. Physical exercise as therapy to fight against the mental and physical consequences of COVID-19 quara. *Prog. Cardiovasc. Dis.* **2020**, *63*, 386. [CrossRef] [PubMed]
46. World Health Organization. *The World Health Report: 2001: Mental Health: New Understanding, New Hope*; World Health Organization: Geneva, Switzerland, 2001; Available online: https://apps.who.int/iris/handle/10665/42390 (accessed on 28 July 2021).
47. Kossek, E.; Lautsch, B.; Eaton, S. "Good Teleworking": Under What Conditions Does Teleworking Enhance Employees' Well-being. In *Technology and Psychological Well-Being*; Amichai, Y., Hamburger, Y., Eds.; Cambridge University Press: Cambridge, UK, 2009. [CrossRef]
48. Ferreira, C.; Picó-Pérez, M.; Morgado, P. Covid-19 and Mental Health- What do we know so far? *Front. Psychiatry* **2020**. [CrossRef]
49. World Health Organization. Be active during COVID-19. WHO. 2020. Available online: https://www.who.int/news-room/q-a-detail/be-active-during-covid-19 (accessed on 16 May 2020).
50. World Health Organization. Global recommendations on physical activity for health. WHO. 2010. Available online: https://www.who.int/dietphysicalactivity/global-PA-recs-2010.pdf (accessed on 28 July 2021).
51. Ferreira, P.; Silva, J.; Portela, M. *IZA COVID-19 Crisis Response Monitoring*; Portigaç Iza: Bonn, Germany, 2020.
52. Hammami, A.; Harrabi, B.; Mohr, M.; Krustrup, P. Physical activity and coronavirus disease 2019 (COVID-19): Specific recommendations for home-based physical training. *Manag. Sport Leis.* **2020**, 1–6. [CrossRef]
53. Wahid, A.; Manek, N.; Nichols, M.; Kelly, P.; Foster, C.; Webster, P.; Roberts, N. Quantifying the association between physical activity and cardiovascular disease and diabetes: A systematic review and meta-analysis. *J. Am.* **2016**, *5*, e002495. [CrossRef]
54. Zhou, F.; Yu, T.; Du, R.; Fan, G.; Liu, Y.; Liu, Z.; Xiang, J.; Wang, Y.; Song, B.; Gu, X.; et al. Clinical course and risk factors for mortality of adult inpatients with COVID-19 in Wuhan, China: A retrospective cohort study. *Lancet* **2020**, *395*, 1054–1062. [CrossRef]
55. Campbell, J.P.; Turner, J.E. Debunking the myth of exercise-induced immune suppression: Redefining the impact of exercise on immunological health across the lifespan. *Front. Immunol.* **2018**, *9*, 648. [CrossRef] [PubMed]
56. Raiol, R.A. Praticar exercícios físicos é fundamental para a saúde física e mental durante a Pandemia da COVID-19. *Braz. J. health Rev.* **2020**, *2*, 2804–2813. [CrossRef]
57. Euro, L. *Staying Active during COVID-19*; EIM Blog–American College of Sport Medicine, 2020; Available online: https://www.acsm.org/read-research/newsroom/news-releases/news-detail/2020/03/16/staying-physically-active-during-covid-19-pandemic (accessed on 28 July 2021).

58. Vos, S.C.; Buckner, M.M. Social media messages in an emerging health crisis: Tweeting bird flu. *J. Health Commun.* **2016**, *21*, 301–308. [CrossRef]
59. Silver, R.C.; Holman, E.A.; Andersen, J.P.; Poulin, M.J.; Mcintosh, D.N.; Gil-Rivas, V. Mental- and physical-health effects of acute exposure to media images of the September 11 2013, 2001, attacks and the Iraq War. *Psychol. Sci.* **2013**, *24*, 1623–1634. [CrossRef]
60. Thompson, R.R.; Garfin, D.R.; Holman, E.A.; Silver, R.C. Distress, worry, and functioning following a global health crisis: A national study of Americans' responses to Ebola. *Clin. Psychol. Sci.* **2017**, *5*, 513–521. [CrossRef]
61. Everett, J.A.; Colombatto, C.; Chituc, V.; Brady, W.J.; Crockett, M. The effectiveness of moral messages on public health behavioral intentions during the COVID-19 pandemic. *PsyArXiv* **2020**. [CrossRef]
62. Liz, C.M.; Andrade, A. Análise qualitativa dos motivos de adesão e desistência da musculação em academias. *Rev. Bras. Ciênc. Esporte* **2016**, *38*, 267–274. [CrossRef]
63. Wong, A.; Ho, S.; Olusanya, O.; Antonini, M.V.; Lyness, D. The use of social media and online communications in times of pandemic COVID-19. *J. Intensive Care Soc.* **2020**. [CrossRef]
64. Affinito, A.; Botta, A.; Ventre, G. The impact of covid on network utilization: An analysis on domain popularity. In Proceedings of the 2020 IEEE 25th International Workshop on Computer Aided Modeling and Design of Communication Links and Networks (CAMAD), Pisa, Italy, 14–16 September 2020; pp. 1–6. [CrossRef]
65. Williamson, J. Awareness of Physical Activity Health Benefits can Influence Participation and Dose. *Sports Med. Rehabil. J.* **2016**, *1*, 1003.
66. Mirowsky, J.; Ross, C.E. *Education, Social Status and Health*; Aldine de Gruyter: New York, NY, USA, 2009; p. 94.
67. Droomers, M.; Schrijvers, C.T.M.; Mackenbach, J.P. Educational level and decreases in leisure time physical activity: Predictors from the longitudinal GLOBE study. *J. Epidemiol. Community Health* **2001**, *55*, 562–568. [CrossRef]
68. Samek Lodovici, M. *The Impact of Teleworking and Digital Work on Workers and Society*; Publication for the committee on Employment and Social Affairs, Policy Department for Economic, Scientific and Quality of Life Policies; European Parliament: Luxembourg, 2021.
69. Buomprisco, G.; Ricci, S.; Perri, R.; De Sio, S. Health and Telework: New Challenges after COVID-19 Pandemic. *Eur. J. Environ. Public Health* **2021**, *5*, em0073. [CrossRef]

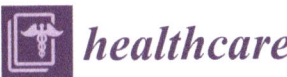 

*Article*

# Analysis of Social Effects on Employment Promotion Policies for College Graduates Based on Data Mining for Online Use Review in China during the COVID-19 Pandemic

Tinggui Chen [1,*], Jingtao Rong [1], Lijuan Peng [1], Jianjun Yang [2], Guodong Cong [3] and Jing Fang [4]

1. School of Statistics and Mathematics, Zhejiang Gongshang University, Hangzhou 310018, China; rjt323@126.com (J.R.); Cherrylijuanpeng@163.com (L.P.)
2. Department of Computer Science and Information Systems, University of North Georgia, Oakwood, GA 30566, USA; Jianjun.Yang@ung.edu
3. School of Tourism and Urban-Rural Planning, Zhejiang Gongshang University, Hangzhou 310018, China; cgd@mail.zjgsu.edu.cn
4. Department of Social Sciences, Zhejiang Gongshang University, Hangzhou 310018, China; fjhust@mail.zjgsu.edu.cn
* Correspondence: ctgsimon@mail.zjgsu.edu.cn

**Abstract:** As an important part of human resources, college graduates are the most vigorous, energetic, and creative group in society. The employment of college graduates is not only related to the vital interests of graduates themselves and the general public, but also related to the sustainable and healthy development of higher education and the country's prosperity through science and education. However, the outbreak of COVID-19 at the end of 2019 has left China's domestic labor and employment market in severe condition, which has a significant impact on the employment of college graduates. Based on the situation, the Chinese government has formulated a series of employment promotion policies for college graduates in accordance with local conditions to solve the current difficulties in employment of college graduates during the COVID-19Pandemic. Do these policies meet the expectations of the people? Is the policy implementation process reasonable? All these issues need to be tested and clarified urgently. This paper takes the employment promotion policy of college graduates under the COVID-19 as the research object, uses the PMC index model to screen the policy texts, obtains two perfect policy texts, and uses the Weibo comments to construct the evaluation model of policy measures support degree to analyze the social effects of employment promotion policies for college graduates. The results show that the public's support degree with the employment promotion policies for college graduates under COVID-19 needs to be improved. Among them, the public has a neutral attitude towards position measures and transference measures but is obviously dissatisfied with subsidy measures and channel measures. Finally, suggestions for improving policy are given to make the employment policy in line with public opinion and effectively relieve the job hunting pressure of college graduates.

**Keywords:** COVID-19; data mining; college graduates; employment policy; policy evaluation

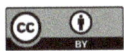

## 1. Introduction

The COVID-19 pandemic has plunged the global economy into panic and trouble [1,2]. It has caused a large-scale shutdown of work and production in the whole society, which has impacted social and economic development and the overall employment environment, and has seriously affected the employment of college graduates. As employment is the foundation of people's livelihood, steadying employment stabilizes the economy and people's expectations, livelihood, and confidence. College graduates are the main force in the job market, so promoting their stable and smooth employment is an important part of the harmonious development of the current society and the stable operation of the economy. In response to the impact of COVID-19 on the employment of college graduates, the Chinese government has launched a series of employment stabilization measures: the Ministry of Education launched a 24.365 full-day online campus employment service platform, extended the time limit for college graduates to register and settle down, expanded the enrollment scale of students in Master programs and the students upgraded from associate degree to baccalaureate, etc. In addition, if the unemployment of college graduates is not properly resolved, a waste of talents and social instability will take place. Social stability is a prerequisite for economic development, and social turbulence will inevitably affect the orderly development of the economy. For the above reasons, scientific evaluation of employment promotion policies for college graduates under the COVID-19 and corresponding suggestions are of important theoretical and practical significance.

At present, the research on the employment promotion policy of college graduates mostly focuses on the analysis of employment problems and employment-related promotion policies from a macro perspective. In particular, it mainly focuses on theoretical research and the evaluation for the effect of policy implementation. For example, Zhu and Chen [3] made comments on the development and reform of the employment-related promotion policy for college students after the reform of China's economic system and put forward suggestions for improving the employment promotion policy. Ercument and Emine [4] conducted the employment evaluation experiment of the students majoring in architecture in Hong Kong and Shanghai, and found that improving students' ability, strengthening specialization, and guiding practical ability can effectively promote the comprehensive ability of graduates in group work. However, there are few literatures from the perspective of policy-making to comprehensively evaluate different policy texts, summarize key policy content from them, and use relevant comments to analyze the social effects of the policy. In view of the inadequacy of existing research, this paper uses the Policy Modeling Consistency (PMC) index model to rate the employment promotion policy for college graduates, screens important policy content, collects Weibo comments on related topics, and constructs a support evaluation model for policy measures to respond to college graduates under the COVID-19. Further, the paper analyzes the social implementation effects of the employment promotion policy, and finally makes recommendations based on the results of the analysis.

The structure of the paper is as follows. Section 2 is a literature review. Section 3 uses the PMC index model to extract key content in the employment promotion policy for college graduates under the COVID-19. Section 4 uses the policy support degree evaluation model to analyze the impact of policy support degree evaluation model on employment promotion policy. Section 5 is the conclusions and the future work prospects.

## 2. Literature Review

The current research on employment policy mainly focuses on the following two aspects: one is the analysis of the factors affecting employment policy. The other is evaluating the effect of employment policy implementation.

Regarding the research on the factors affecting employment policies, some scholars have carried out research on individual employability, and believed that internal motivation [5], superior expectations [6] and organizational environment [7] are the main factors affecting individual employment innovation ability. The typical literature is as follows: A study conducted by Genco et al. [8] at the University of Massachusetts showed that freshmen with working experience performed better when given incentives and technical flexibility than general graduates, who have obvious differences in incentives and flexibility. Xu et al. [9] proposed that alumni feedback information systems, social evaluation systems, etc. are important resources for improving the quality of talent training in colleges and universities and for guiding and adjusting employment policies. Zhang et al. [10] and Yu [11] used questionnaire survey methods to analyze the employment area selection and graduate employment rate of college graduates in different regions. Yang and Yang [12] used regression analysis in mathematical statistics based on a large-scale sample survey of employment status of college graduates across the country, and studied the factors that affect the employment competitiveness of college graduates, including school reputation and status, employment service information, academic qualifications, academic work, and work ability, employment expectations, etc. Li and Lin [13] analyzed the factors that promoted graduates' employment and discussed their relations between each other using general system structure theory, and they constructed an employment promotion system model and its structure. Zhang [14] used a Bayesian data mining classification algorithm to explore the employment option of college graduates. Through training the existing data of the employment option of college graduates, he analyzed the feedback of graduates that were satisfied with their jobs. Furthermore, he gained the classification feature set rules and established a classification model about the employment option of college graduates. It was proved by the experiments that this model was selected user groups with high accuracy. Based on the survey data of the graduates of Jiangsu university for five consecutive years, Jie [15] adopted the method of gray relational analysis to conduct an empirical study on factors affecting the employment of college students. The results showed that there were 15 main factors affecting the employment prospects of college students. Among them, the importance of the ability of active learning was the most important one, followed by working ability. From the government, universities, enterprises, society, graduates, and other subjects, Xi and He [16] analyzed the role of a series of employment promotion and entrepreneurship guidance policies put forward by a provincial government. The results showed that the policy had not achieved the expected effect in promoting college students' independent entrepreneurship. Furthermore, the propaganda strength of the policy, the pertinence of the support object, the effectiveness of the policy, and the effectiveness of the policy supporting services for entrepreneurship need to be further improved. According to the above literature analysis, most of the research on employment policies for college graduates uses qualitative methods to explore the influencing factors of employment policies, and few policies start from the policy formulation itself to make a scientific evaluation of the social effects after the policy is implemented.

The research on the evaluation of the implementation effect of employment policies began with Edward A. Suchman's five-category evaluation, followed by Oville F. Poland's "Three E" evaluation classification framework and Wollmann's classic policy evaluation [17]. Yet most of the literature is based on empirical research, using case analysis, field questionnaire surveys, and other methods. Some examples of typical documents are as follows: Song [18] takes Guangdong Province and puts forward suggestions for optimizing policies. Hu and Chen [19] first took 1500 college students in Henan Province as the survey object and conducted a data survey on all the employment promotion policies of college students in China. If the employment policy is very practical and highly recognized by college students, it is followed by satisfaction with the employment services provided by the government. Zhao and Yao [20] jointly established the CR2 model and the corresponding projection model and constructed an evaluation index system. Using the data envelopment analysis method, they empirically analyzed the effectiveness of the public employment service policies for college students in China from 1999 to 2006. Zhang [21] believes that the historical evolution of the employment policy for college graduates has experienced three stages: the planned economic system period, the educational system reform and development period, and the social entity market economy establishment and development period. Each stage has its own different characteristics. Its characteristics are used to solve the employment problem of college graduates. The literature shows that most of the research is conducted on specific objects to test the effect of the policy after the release, and the research objects of this method are relatively one-sided and have certain timeliness. In turn, such research can neither dynamically grasp the audience's views on the policy in real time, nor make optimization suggestions for policy formulation based on the public opinion response of the people.

To sum up, the current academic circles have carried out research on employment policies that rarely combine public opinion with the evaluation and analysis of employment policies. Therefore, this paper starts from the policy text itself, ranks policy documents, digs out important policy content, trawls Weibo comments on this basis, and uses the comments to construct the employment promotion policy for college graduates under the COVID-19 to analyze the social effects of policy implementation.

## 3. Research Framework

First, this paper collected employment promotion policy documents for college graduates released by the Chinese government during the COVID-19, conducted word frequency analysis, and rated the collected policy by PMC index model to select and summarize important policy measures. Then, related topics of 4 kinds of policy measures were searched, Weibo comments were trawled, and an evaluation model of support degree of policy measures was constructed to evaluate and analyze the public support degree of policy measures, so as to study the social implementation effect of employment promotion policy for college graduates. The framework of the paper is shown in Figure 1.

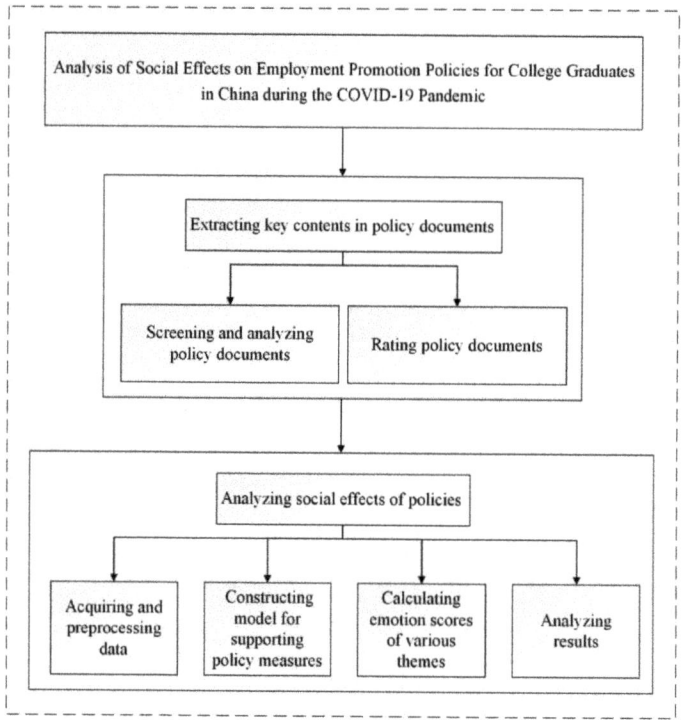

Figure 1. Research framework.

## 4. Extracting Key Contents of Employment Promotion Policy for College Graduates

### 4.1. Selecting and Analyzing Employment Promotion Policy

In order to extract the key contents of employment promotion policy for college graduates, this paper selects the related policy issued by the Chinese government from January 2020 to July 2020 during COVID-19, with reference to the graduation time of undergraduate and graduate students in previous years. In the acquisition process, following the principles of authority, rigor, completeness, and accuracy, the authors collected 16 typical policy documents that have important effects on the employment of college graduates from the websites of the Ministry of Human Resources and Social Security, People's Republic of China (PRC), the Ministry of Education, the Central People's Government, and other authority websites, as shown in Table 1.

Table 1. Documents of employment promotion policy for college graduates.

| No. | Policy Document | Issuing No. | Issuing Department | Issuing Date |
|---|---|---|---|---|
| $P_1$ | Notice on Implementing Employment Work during the Period of Epidemic Prevention and Control | Tianjin People's Office issued (2020) No. 29 | Ministry of Human Resources and Social Security of China/Ministry of Education of China/Ministry of Finance of China/Ministry of Transportation of China/National Health Commission | 2020.2.5 |
| $P_2$ | Notice on Carrying out the National Online Joint Recruitment of 2020 College Graduates-24365 Campus Recruitment Service Activities | Ministry of Education of China (2020) No. 2 | Office of the Ministry of Education of China | 2020.2.28 |
| $P_3$ | Notice on Carrying out Employment and Entrepreneurship of the 2020 National College Graduates during COVID-19 | Ministry of Education of China (2020) No. 2 | Ministry of Education of China | 2020.3.4 |
| $P_4$ | Notice on Carrying out Public Recruitment of College Graduates by Public Institutions during COVID-19 | Human Resources and Social Security of China (2020) No. 27 | General Office of the Organization Department of the CPC Central Committee of China/General Office of the Ministry of Human Resources and Social Security of China | 2020.3.11 |
| $P_5$ | Suggestions on Strengthening and Stabilizing Employment during COVID-19 | Office of the State Council of China (2020) No. 6 | Office of the State Council of China | 2020.3.18 |
| $P_6$ | Notice on Implementing Some Vocational Qualifications "First Employed then Passed the Exam" | Human Resources and Social Security of China (2020) No. 24 | Ministry of Human Resources and Social Security of China/Ministry of Education of China/Ministry of Justice of China/Ministry of Agriculture and Rural Affairs of China/Ministry of Culture and Tourism of China/National Health Commission of China/National Intellectual Property Office of China | 2020.4.21 |
| $P_7$ | Notice on Holding the 2020 National College Graduate Employment Network Alliance Recruitment Week | Ministry of Education of China (2020) No. 7 | Ministry of Education of the People's Republic of China | 2020.4.23 |
| $P_8$ | Notice on Carrying out the Pioneer base for Entrepreneurship and Employment | National Development and Reform Commission of China (2020) No. 310 | General Office of the National Development and Reform Commission of China/General Office of the State-owned Assets Supervision and Administration Commission of the Ministry of Education of China/General Office of the Ministry of Human Resources and Social Security of China | 2020.4.24 |
| $P_9$ | Notice on National SME Online Recruitment of College Graduates in 100 Days | Ministry of Industry and Information Technology of China (2020) No. 179 | Provincial Department of Industry and Information Technology of China/Provincial Department of Education of China/Provincial Department of Human Resources and Social Security of China | 2020.4.27 |
| $P_{10}$ | "Notice on Public Recruitment of Kindergarten Teachers in Primary and Secondary Schools in 2020 | Human Resources and Social Security of China (2020) No. 28 | Ministry of Human Resources and Social Security of China/Ministry of Education of China/Central Planning Office of China/Ministry of Finance of China | 2020.5.9 |

Table 1. Cont.

| No. | Policy Document | Issuing No. | Issuing Department | Issuing Date |
|---|---|---|---|---|
| $P_{11}$ | Notice on Implementation of the "Three Supports and One Support" Plan for College Graduates in 2020 | Human Resources and Social Security of China (2020) No. 57 | General Office of the Ministry of Human Resources and Social Security of China/General Office of the Ministry of Finance of China | 2020.5.19 |
| $P_{12}$ | Notice on Encouraging Scientific Research Projects to Absorb College Graduates | Ministry of Science and Technology of China (2020) No. 132 | Ministry of Science and Technology of China/Ministry of Education of China/Ministry of Human Resources and Social Security of China/Ministry of Finance of China/Chinese Academy of Sciences/Natural Science Foundation of China | 2020.5.27 |
| $P_{13}$ | Notice on Further Development of Research Assistant Positions in Colleges and Universities to Absorb Graduate Employment | Ministry of Education of China (2020) No. 23 | Office of the Ministry of Education of China | 2020.6.4 |
| $P_{14}$ | Notice on Guiding and Encouraging College Graduates to Work and Start Business in Urban and Rural Communities | Human Resources and Social Security of China (2020) No. 53 | Organization Department of the Party Committee of each city (prefecture)/Civilization Office of China/Civil Affairs Bureau of China/Education Administrative Department of China/Finance Bureau of China/Human Resources and Social Security Bureau of China/Health and Health Committee of China | 2020.6.22 |
| $P_{15}$ | Notice on Precise Assistance for Employment of College Graduates from Poor Families in 52 Poverty Counties" | Ministry of Education of China (2020) No. 21 | General Office of the Ministry of Education of China/General Office of the Ministry of Human Resources and Social Security of China/General Department of the Poverty Alleviation Office of the State Council of China | 2020.7.2 |
| $P_{16}$ | Suggestions on Allowing Medical College Graduates to Exempt from Examination to Apply for Practicing Registration of Rural Doctors | National Health Commission of China (2020) No. 11 | National Health Commission of China | 2020.7.6 |

Based on policy text, this paper uses ROST CM [22,23] software to preprocess the policy text, such as word segmentation and keyword frequency statistics, in order to extract the key content from the policy document. The specific process is as follows: first, the policy text is segmented, then the word frequency of the document after word segmentation is ranked, and finally the word segmentation results are sorted according to the word frequency from high to low. The results are shown in Table 2. In addition, the Ucient software was used to build a co-occurrence network for the documents after word segmentation, and the results are shown in Figure 2. Each node in the network represents a keyword, and if there is a line between nodes, the keywords have a symbiotic relationship. At the same time, nodes are displayed according to the keyword centrality. If the keyword has higher centrality, the keyword frequently appears together with other keywords in the network [24].

**Table 2.** Statistics of keyword frequency in employment promotion policy documents for college graduates.

| Keyword | Frequency | Keyword | Frequency |
|---|---|---|---|
| employment | 1328 | resource | 678 |
| graduate | 1322 | safeguard | 676 |
| college | 1314 | implement | 575 |
| recruitment | 1166 | society | 474 |
| service | 1130 | scientific research | 371 |
| company | 1120 | program | 271 |
| entrepreneurship | 1111 | strengthen | 168 |
| position | 890 | epidemic | 166 |
| organization | 887 | personnel | 166 |
| enterprise | 882 | policy | 164 |
| department | 781 | grassroots | 88 |

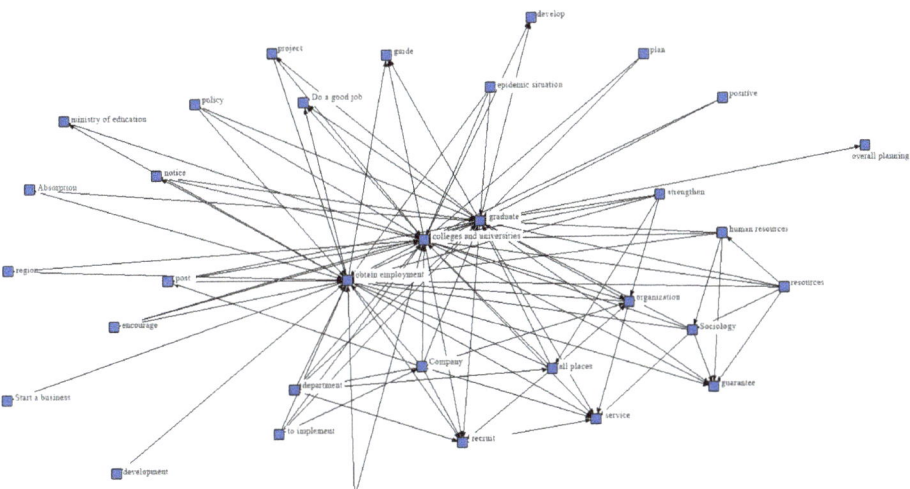

**Figure 2.** Co-citation networks of keyword in employment promotion policy documents for college graduates.

It can be seen from the keyword frequency distribution and keyword co-citation networks of the aforementioned policy documents that "employment", "service", and "position" rank first among the high-frequency words. This is different from the previous situation for college graduates. The COVID-19 has led universities and companies to cancel offline job fairs for the class of 2020, which are the main job opportunities for fresh graduates. Therefore, during COVID-19, the most important thing for the government is to mobilize all units to implement online employment services, expand employment channels and increase employment opportunities. From the two high-frequency words "entrepreneurship" and "grass-roots level", we can see that in order to increase the employment opportunities of college graduates, the government has repeatedly mentioned encouraging, supporting and guiding graduates to find jobs at the grass-roots level, stabilizing the environment for innovation and entrepreneurship, and giving full play to the important role of "mass entrepreneurship and innovation" in supporting employment.

*4.2. Evaluating Employment Promotion Policy Documents for College Graduates Based on PMC Model*

At present, the more advanced international policy text evaluation method is the PMC Index Evaluation Model established by Estrada [25]. This model believes that everything is constantly in motion and interconnected, so any relevant variable cannot be ignored. Its innovation is that it uses binarydigits 0 and 1 to balance all variables and emphasizes that the number and weight of variables should not be limited, so that the advantages and disadvantages and internal consistency of a policy can be analyzed from various dimensions [26]. Most existing policy evaluation methods have problems such as strong subjectivity and low accuracy. However, the PMC index model method can largely avoid subjectivity and improve accuracy because it obtains raw data through text mining. In addition, the effectiveness of the PMC model has been verified in the literature [25]. In the policy analysis in this paper, the PMC index model takes variables into extensive consideration, which not only can comprehensively analyze the merits and demerits of a policy, but also has the advantages of index traceability and grade identification, and scientifically quantifies the consistency level of each policy from different dimensions. Therefore, this paper introduces the PMC index model to quantitatively evaluate the employment promotion policy for college graduates under COVID-19 and obtains the key points of the policy content from the outstanding policy documents with a PMC index score of 9–10. Generally, the establishment of a PMC index model includes the following steps: (1) establishing a PMC index evaluation index system, (2) establishing a multi-input-output table, and (3) calculating twolevel variable values and PMC index.

4.2.1. Classifying the Variables and Setting Parameters of PMC Index Model

Referring to Estrada and the existing literatures [27–29] and combining with the specific characteristics of college graduates' employment promotion policy, this paper establishes 10 first-level variables and 66 s-level variables. The results are shown in Table 3.

Table 3. PMC evaluation variables of employment promotion policy for graduates.

| First-Level Variables | Second-Level Variables No. | Second-Level Variables Name | Second-Level Variables No. | Second-Level Variables Name |
|---|---|---|---|---|
| Nature of $X_1$ policy | $X_{1:1}$<br>$X_{1:3}$<br>$X_{1:5}$ | supervision<br>advisement<br>guide | $X_{1:2}$<br>$X_{1:4}$ | support<br>encourage |
| Time of $X_2$ policy | $X_{2:1}$<br>$X_{2:3}$ | transition period<br>this year | $X_{2:2}$ | short term |
| Field of $X_3$ policy | $X_{3:1}$<br>$X_{3:3}$<br>$X_{3:5}$ | economy<br>talent<br>technology | $X_{3:2}$<br>$X_{3:4}$<br>$X_{3:6}$ | public management<br>social security<br>institution |
| Function of $X_4$ policy | $X_{4:1}$<br>$X_{4:3}$<br>$X_{4:5}$ | expand demand<br>strengthen protection<br>optimize system | $X_{4:2}$<br>$X_{4:4}$ | normative guidance<br>institutional constraints |
| Objective of $X_5$ policy | $X_{5:1}$<br>$X_{5:3}$<br>$X_{5:5}$<br>$X_{5:7}$ | enterprise<br>college<br>directly subordinate agency ministries and commissions of the State Council | $X_{5:2}$<br>$X_{5:4}$<br>$X_{5:6}$ | college graduates<br>all provinces, cities, autonomous regions, and municipalities directly under the Central Government<br>key areas of the epidemic |
| Content of $X_6$ policy | $X_{6:1}$<br>$X_{6:3}$<br>$X_{6:5}$<br>$X_{6:7}$<br>$X_{6:9}$ | resumption of work and production<br>employment service<br>stable employment<br>strengthen training<br>accurate employment assistance | $X_{6:2}$<br>$X_{6:4}$<br>$X_{6:6}$<br>$X_{6:8}$ | employment subsidy<br>encourage employment and entrepreneurship<br>broaden employment channels<br>encourage grassroots work |

Table 3. Cont.

| First-Level Variables | Second-Level Variables No. | Second-Level Variables Name | Second-Level Variables No. | Second-Level Variables Name |
|---|---|---|---|---|
| Issuing agency of $X_7$ policy | $X_{7:1}$ | Ministry of Human Resources and Social Security | $X_{7:2}$ | Ministry of Education |
| | $X_{7:3}$ | Ministry of Finance | $X_{7:4}$ | Transportation Department |
| | $X_{7:5}$ | National Health Commission | $X_{7:6}$ | provinces and cities |
| | $X_{7:7}$ | Local and subordinate colleges and universities | $X_{7:8}$ | General Office of the Central Organization Department |
| | $X_{7:9}$ | Department of Justice (Bureau) | $X_{7:10}$ | Department of Agriculture and Rural Affairs (Agriculture, Animal Husbandry and Veterinary Medicine, Fishery) (Bureau, Commission) |
| | $X_{7:11}$ | Department of Culture and Tourism (Bureau) | $X_{7:12}$ | Intellectual Property Office (Intellectual Property Management Department) |
| | $X_{7:13}$ | SASAC | | |
| Incentives of $X_8$ policy | $X_{8:1}$ | employment subsidy | $X_{8:2}$ | job creation |
| | $X_{8:3}$ | tax incentives | $X_{8:4}$ | talent incentive |
| | $X_{8:5}$ | online employment | $X_{8:6}$ | multi-channel employment |
| | $X_{8:7}$ | incentives for primary services | $X_{8:8}$ | self-employed |
| | $X_{8:9}$ | skills Training | $X_{8:10}$ | employment guidance service |
| | $X_{8:11}$ | encourage teaching | $X_{8:12}$ | employment assistance |
| | $X_{8:13}$ | lower the barriers to employment | | |
| Evaluation of $X_9$ policy | $X_{9:1}$ | clear objective | $X_{9:2}$ | feasible plan |
| | $X_{9:3}$ | sufficient reference | $X_{9:4}$ | detailed planning |
| | $X_{9:5}$ | encourage employment | | |
| Publication of $X_{10}$ policy | — | | | |

The weights of the second-level variables in Table 3 are set to the same value, and all the parameter values of the second-level variables are set to binarydigits 0 and 1. If the content of the policy document involves the meaning of the second-level variables, it is assigned the value 1; otherwise, it is 0.

4.2.2. Constructing Input-Output Table

The input-output table is a data analysis framework that can store a large amount of data and use multidimensional measurement of a single variable. It is composed of numerous first-level variables and second-level variables that are not restricted by variables. The first-level variables have no fixed order and are independent of each other, and the weights of the second-level variables are equal [30], as shown in Table 4.

The second-level variables' values are assigned according to the keywords obtained in Section 4.1. When the policy text data contains the keywords corresponding to the second-level variables, the value is assigned to 1; otherwise, it is 0. Compared with the subjectivity of expert scoring, this method is more objective and scientific.

Table 4. Input-output table.

| First-Level Variables | Second-Level Variables | | | | | | |
|---|---|---|---|---|---|---|---|
| $X_1$ | $X_{1:1}$ | $X_{1:2}$ | $X_{1:3}$ | $X_{1:4}$ | $X_{1:5}$ | | |
| $X_2$ | $X_{2:1}$ | $X_{2:2}$ | $X_{2:3}$ | | | | |
| $X_3$ | $X_{3:1}$ | $X_{3:2}$ | $X_{3:3}$ | $X_{3:4}$ | $X_{3:5}$ | | |
| $X_4$ | $X_{4:1}$ | $X_{4:2}$ | $X_{4:3}$ | $X_{4:4}$ | $X_{4:5}$ | | |
| $X_5$ | $X_{5:1}$ | $X_{5:2}$ | $X_{5:3}$ | $X_{5:4}$ | $X_{5:5}$ | $X_{5:6}$ | $X_{5:7}$ |
| $X_6$ | $X_{6:1}$ | $X_{6:2}$ | $X_{6:3}$ | $X_{6:4}$ | $X_{6:5}$ | $X_{6:6}$ | $X_{6:7}$ |
| | $X_{6:8}$ | $X_{6:9}$ | | | | | |
| $X_7$ | $X_{7:1}$ | $X_{7:2}$ | $X_{7:3}$ | $X_{7:4}$ | $X_{7:5}$ | $X_{7:6}$ | $X_{7:7}$ |
| | $X_{7:8}$ | $X_{7:9}$ | $X_{7:10}$ | $X_{7:11}$ | $X_{7:12}$ | $X_{7:13}$ | |
| $X_8$ | $X_{8:1}$ | $X_{8:2}$ | $X_{8:3}$ | $X_{8:4}$ | $X_{8:5}$ | $X_{8:6}$ | $X_{8:7}$ |
| | $X_{8:8}$ | $X_{8:9}$ | $X_{8:10}$ | $X_{8:11}$ | $X_{8:12}$ | $X_{8:13}$ | |
| $X_9$ | $X_{9:1}$ | $X_{9:2}$ | $X_{9:3}$ | $X_{9:4}$ | $X_{9:5}$ | | |
| $X_{10}$ | — | | | | | | |

### 4.2.3. Calculating PMC Index

The PMC index of the policy documents in Table 1 is calculated below. The calculation method is as follows:

$$X_{i:j} \sim n, \tag{1}$$

$i$ is first-level variables; $j$ is second-level variables, $i,j = 1,2,3,4,5. \ldots \infty$.

$$X_i = \left(\sum_{j=1}^{n} \frac{X_{i:j}}{n}\right), \tag{2}$$

$n$ is the amount of second-level variables, $n = 1,2,3,4,5. \ldots \infty$.

$$\begin{aligned} PMC = &X_1\left(\sum_{a=1}^{5} \frac{X_{1:a}}{5}\right) + X_2\left(\sum_{b=1}^{3} \frac{X_{2:a}}{3}\right) + X_3\left(\sum_{c=1}^{5} \frac{X_{3:c}}{5}\right) + X_4\left(\sum_{d=1}^{5} \frac{X_{4:d}}{5}\right) \\ &+ X_5\left(\sum_{e=1}^{7} \frac{X_{5:e}}{7}\right) + X_6\left(\sum_{f=1}^{9} \frac{X_{6:f}}{5}\right) + X_7\left(\sum_{g=1}^{13} \frac{X_{7:g}}{5}\right) + X_8\left(\sum_{h=1}^{13} \frac{X_{8:h}}{5}\right) \\ &+ X_9\left(\sum_{k=1}^{5} \frac{X_{9:k}}{5}\right) + X_{10} \end{aligned} \tag{3}$$

First, determine the value of the second-level variable $X_{i:j}$ according to Formula (1), then calculate the value of each first-level variable according to Formula (2), and finally bring each first-level variable into Formula (3) to calculate the PMC index of different policies. The PMC index evaluation criteria can be obtained from the literature [21]: 9–10 points (perfect level), 7–8.99 points (excellent level), 5–6.99 points (acceptable level), 0–4.99 points (bad level). This method obtains the ranking and rating of the PMC index of the employment promotion policy for college graduates, and the results are shown in Table 5.

Table 5. PMC index of employment promotion policy documents for college graduates.

| | $X_1$ | $X_2$ | $X_3$ | $X_4$ | $X_5$ | $X_6$ | $X_7$ | $X_8$ | $X_9$ | $X_{10}$ | PMC Index | Ranking | Depression Index | Rating |
|---|---|---|---|---|---|---|---|---|---|---|---|---|---|---|
| $P_1$ | 1 | 0.33 | 0.5 | 0.4 | 0.71 | 0.56 | 0.38 | 0.23 | 0.4 | 1 | 5.51 | 5 | 4.49 | acceptable |
| $P_2$ | 0.4 | 0.67 | 0.33 | 0.4 | 0.43 | 0.22 | 0.23 | 0.08 | 1 | 1 | 4.76 | 9 | 5.24 | bad |
| $P_3$ | 1 | 0.67 | 0.67 | 1 | 0.43 | 0.78 | 0.15 | 0.69 | 1 | 1 | 7.39 | 2 | 2.61 | perfect |
| $P_4$ | 0.8 | 0.67 | 0.33 | 0.6 | 0.43 | 0.56 | 0.23 | 0.31 | 0.6 | 1 | 5.53 | 4 | 4.47 | acceptable |
| $P_5$ | 1 | 1 | 1 | 0.8 | 0.86 | 0.89 | 0.15 | 0.69 | 0.6 | 1 | 7.99 | 1 | 2.01 | perfect |
| $P_6$ | 0.4 | 0.67 | 0.5 | 0.4 | 0.29 | 0.22 | 0.54 | 0.23 | 0.8 | 1 | 5.05 | 8 | 4.95 | acceptable |
| $P_7$ | 0.2 | 0.33 | 0.33 | 0.2 | 0.43 | 0.22 | 0.15 | 0.15 | 0.6 | 1 | 3.61 | 15 | 6.39 | bad |
| $P_8$ | 0.6 | 0.33 | 0.33 | 0.8 | 0.71 | 0.44 | 0.23 | 0.46 | 0.8 | 1 | 5.7 | 3 | 4.3 | acceptable |
| $P_9$ | 0.4 | 0.33 | 0.17 | 0.4 | 0.29 | 0.33 | 0.08 | 0.08 | 1 | 1 | 4.08 | 14 | 5.92 | bad |
| $P_{10}$ | 0.4 | 0.33 | 0.5 | 0.4 | 0.29 | 0.33 | 0.31 | 0.23 | 0.8 | 1 | 4.59 | 11 | 5.41 | bad |
| $P_{11}$ | 0.8 | 0.33 | 0.5 | 0.4 | 0.29 | 0.33 | 0.23 | 0.23 | 1 | 1 | 5.11 | 7 | 4.89 | acceptable |
| $P_{12}$ | 0.6 | 0.33 | 0.33 | 0.4 | 0.29 | 0.22 | 0.31 | 0.15 | 1 | 1 | 4.63 | 10 | 5.37 | bad |
| $P_{13}$ | 0.6 | 0.33 | 0.33 | 0.4 | 0.29 | 0.22 | 0.31 | 0.15 | 0.6 | 1 | 4.23 | 12 | 5.77 | bad |
| $P_{14}$ | 0.6 | 0 | 1 | 0.8 | 0.29 | 0.22 | 0.38 | 0.38 | 0.6 | 1 | 5.27 | 6 | 4.73 | acceptable |
| $P_{15}$ | 0.4 | 0 | 0.17 | 0.4 | 0.43 | 0.44 | 0.23 | 0.23 | 0.8 | 1 | 4.1 | 13 | 5.9 | bad |
| $P_{16}$ | 0.6 | 0 | 0.17 | 0.4 | 0.43 | 0.22 | 0.08 | 0.15 | 0.2 | 1 | 3.25 | 16 | 6.75 | bad |
| average | 0.61 | 0.39 | 0.45 | 0.51 | 0.43 | 0.39 | 0.25 | 0.28 | 0.74 | 1 | | | | |

From the evaluation results in Table 5, it can be seen that among the 16 college graduate employment promotion policies, eight of the policy evaluation results are acceptablelevel or above, accounting for 50%, among which two are perfect, and the policy content contained in the perfect policy document is more comprehensive. The target audience is wider, and the steps involved in the implementation measures are more detailed. Therefore, in order to extract the key points in the policy documents, the contents of the $P_3$ and $P_5$ perfect-level policy documents are selected and summarized. Due to the diversity of the measures proposed in the policy and their different focuses, the content of the policy is divided into four areas: (1) Increase the opportunities for further education and reduce the number of fresh graduates who are in urgent need of employment. (2) Broaden employment information circulation channels, and guide universities and colleges to carry out extensive online employment. (3) Provide employment subsidies, lower employment restrictions, alleviate employment anxiety of recent graduates, and improve employment benefits of recent graduates. (4) Increase position and increase labor demand. According to the above four aspects, the employment promotion policy measures for college graduates can be divided into four categories: channel measures, transference measures, subsidy measures, and position measures.

## 5. Analyzing Social Effects on Employment Promotion Policies for College Graduates

As a reflection of public sentiment and public opinion, online public opinion not only manifests its influence on major developments, but also penetrates into the political level, becoming an important channel for the government to listen to and understand public opinion. In order to dig out the public's attitude and response to the official employment promotion policy under the COVID-19 pandemic, the corresponding topic comment information on the Weibo is crawled, and social implementation effect of employment promotion policy is analyzed based on the comments.

### 5.1. Acquiring and Preprocessing Data
#### 5.1.1. Acquiring Data

This paper searches related topics for 4 kinds of measures on Weibo and selects the 15 topics discussedmost frequently as the data crawling objects. Each topic is shown in Table 6.

**Table 6.** Related Weibo topics.

| Policy | Weibo Topic |
|---|---|
| Channel measures | 24.356 all-day online campus employment service |
| | Encourage multiple methods such as webcasting |
| | Single assistance between domestic colleges and Hubei colleges |
| Transference measures | Enrollment of postgraduate students increased by 189,000 |
| | Expand the scale of enrollment for postgraduates and undergraduates |
| | Expand the postgraduate enrollment of retired soldiers in college |
| Subsidy measures | Provide employment subsidies for college graduates in many places |
| | The highest award for innovation and entrepreneurship of Tianjin college graduates is 300,000 RMB |
| | Find a job within two years and go through the employment procedures according to the current term |
| | Graduates can keep their household registration files in the school for two years |
| Position measures | State-owned enterprises expand the enrollment of college graduates this year and next two years |
| | Expand the recruitment of primary and secondary school teachers |
| | Implement "first recruited, then passed the exam" |
| | Special post teachers plan to increase recruitment by 5000 |
| | Develop research assistant position to attract college graduates |

This paper trawls the related Weibo comments on 15 topics. The trawled content includes the publisher ID, the content of the comment, comment time, commenter ID, the number of followers, the number of subscribers, and Weibo number. This paper uses python to obtain a total of 65,487 posts, including 9596 posts for channel measures topics, 17,003 posts for transference measures topics, 7671 posts for subsidy measures topics, and 28,849 posts for position measures topics. The data format is shown in Figure 3.

| A | B | C | D | E | F | G | H | I |
|---|---|---|---|---|---|---|---|---|
| Publisher ID | Comment | Comment Time | Like | Commenter ID | Gender | Subscribers | Followers | Weibo Number |
| People's Daily | Why expand the enrollment of graduate students? Won't there be too many graduate students in the future | 2020-02-19 15:39:51 | 65 | NauYuil | female | 446 | 191 | 1395 |
| People's Daily | This policy does not solve practical problems, cure the symptoms, not the disease. | 2020-02-19 15:39:19 | 134 | Beattleship | female | 34761 | 1980 | 410 |
| People's Daily | That's great. It seems that it's easier for me to find a job. | 2020-02-19 16:28:19 | 17 | HLannnnnn | female | 4163 | 101 | 24 |
| People's Daily | I don't want the school to expand admission, because graduate students will be worthless. | 2020-02-19 15:37:20 | 19 | Guimaraes1 | male | 19913 | 459 | 3783 |
| People's Daily | Come on, speed up! | 2020-02-19 15:37:00 | 4 | Ivy_yaya | female | 11711 | 723 | 2232 |
| People's Daily | Will the Medical Specialty expand its enrollment? | 2020-02-19 15:41:06 | 2 | Breatrice-- | female | 27 | 36 | 203 |
| People's Daily | Why not expand the enrollment of graduate students in Shanxi Province? | 2020-02-19 15:39:31 | 3 | Terryw- | female | 5729 | 188 | 1070 |
| People's Daily | Will the expansion of graduate enrollment reduce the score line? | 2020-02-19 15:37:45 | 19 | caciyu1 | female | 3602593 | 351 | 3868 |
| People's Daily | The expansion of graduate enrollment is too little. | 2020-02-19 15:37:20 | 23 | Cooc-Mz | male | 171392 | 999 | 571 |
| People's Daily | Will this policy be effective next year? | 2020-02-19 15:37:10 | 2 | Y-LONG- | male | 194106 | 77 | 181 |
| People's Daily | Wow, good news! | 2020-02-19 15:42:39 | 4 | Ham10479 | male | 151 | 227 | 5299 |
| People's Daily | This is not a good phenomenon, the quality of talents is getting worse and worse. | 2020-02-19 16:57:00 | 2 | Oooccupied | female | 244 | 23 | 48 |
| People's Daily | This policy is good! | 2020-02-19 16:50:50 | 0 | Instinctus | female | 19 | 51 | 77 |
| People's Daily | It's a waste of time doing meaningless things. | 2020-02-19 16:49:41 | 0 | YHTJohn | female | 439 | 481 | 2331 |
| People's Daily | Great. I'm so happy! | 2020-02-19 16:32:44 | 4 | AKASEER | male | 458 | 348 | 556 |
| People's Daily | There are too few places for expansion admission. | 2020-02-19 15:36:55 | 2 | Uzeki | male | 204412 | 146 | 80 |

**Figure 3.** Data format.

5.1.2. Data Cleaning

Because invalid data and incorrect data inevitably appear in the trawling process, these data are rarely utilized in the analysis process or cause large errors in the results, thusthey need to be deleted. Data cleaning mainly deletes repeatedly collected data, repeated expression words, shorter sentences, meaningless, or unclear sentences. After data cleaning, a total of 61,311 valid posts were obtained.

5.1.3. Word Segmentation and Word Frequency Statistics

As the content of the comments are all in Chinese, the Jieba Chinese word segmentation package [31] is used to perform word segmentation on the Weibo comments in the Python environment and remove stop words that cannot represent text characteristics. Because the research object of this paper is the employment policy for college graduates under COVID-19 pandemic, the nouns that appear frequently in the document after word segmentation are "student, society, employment", etc., such words are more neutral and have less meaning for word frequency analysis. Therefore, this type of word is also added to the stop word dictionary. On this basis, the top 100 effective high-frequency words are sorted out as follows: "teacher", "quota", "postgraduate", "epidemic", "fresh graduate", "fractional line", "condition", "file", "previous graduate", "full-time", "employment rate", "labor force", "talent", "young people", "master", "quality", "civil servant", "part-time", "housing price", "Wuhan", "workload", "research assistant", "proportion", "normal major", "doctor", "Guangdong", "qualification", "written examination", "special post teacher", "Chongqing", "student source", "mathematics", "college promotion", "unit", "age", "college", "threshold", "preliminary examination", "junior college student", "origin", "Sichuan", "energy", "household registration", "re-examination", "unemployment rate", "poor student", "welfare", "enterprise", "area", "level", "accomplishment", "bachelor", "doctoral student", "Shandong", "Henan", "junior college", "registered residence", "treatment", "Beijing", "elementary school", "salary", "subsidy", "university", "head teacher", "interview", "tripartite agreement", "vocational school", "contract", "rural area", "preschool education", "ability", "Anhui", "township", "undergraduate", "Shanghai", "region", "city", "second degree", "whole country", "government office", "hospital", "institution", "kindergarten", "domicile", "Chinese", "art", "engineering", "nurse", "pressure", "agreement", "experience", "kindergarten teacher", "counselor", "downtown", "Tianjin", "other province", "music", "English", "news", "county town".

## 5.2. Construction of Evaluation Model for Supporting Policy Measures

An evaluation model for supporting policy measures is constructed here to evaluate and analyze the public support degree of the four types of measures summarized by the above PMC index model to study the social effects of the implementation of the employment promotion policy for college graduates.

### 5.2.1. Constructing Evaluation Dimension

The degree of support for policy measures needs to be analyzed from multiple dimensions, including the theoretical goals of the policy measures, the people's expectations of the policy measures, and the specific implementation methods of the policy measures. Most of the previous studies analyzed the policy support degree from one dimension (the theoretical objectives of the policy [32], the expectations of the masses [33,34], the policy means [35], etc.). The coverage of the policy is relatively narrow and lacks objectivity, which affects the scientific statistical results. In order to improve the credibility of the research results, this paper refers to the various evaluation dimensions adopted by the existing research and redefines the evaluation dimensions. Starting from multiple dimensions, it analyzes the degree of public support for various measures of college graduate employment promotion policies. The dimensions are shown in Table 7.

**Table 7.** Evaluation dimension.

| Evaluation Dimension | | Comments |
|---|---|---|
| Dimension | Definition | |
| Theoretical objectives | The theoretical effect to be achieved at the government level under the preset expectations of policy measures | Since the epidemic is so severe this year, it is necessary to introduce policies to ensure employment. |
| Expectations of the masses | Expected effects of policy measures at the public level | With postgraduate enrollment expansions, the graduate degree will be worthless in the future. |
| Implementation means | Specific implementation methods and processes of policy measures | The policy was issued too late, the school has already sent the files back. |
| Target groups | The main body of policy measures | Hope this policy is not just for fresh graduates. |

### 5.2.2. Constructing Comment Topic Identification System

As netizens often evaluate policy measures from different positions and perspectives, each comment may correspond to different evaluation dimensions. This paper uses the framework semantic dictionary matching method, takes the policy review subject word dictionary as the label system, and completes the identification of the corresponding dimensions by extracting and matching the evaluation words of comments. Among them, the policy review topic identification word dictionary is mainly generated based on the frequency of keyword in the comments combined with manual selection. Due to the large number of identified words, the semantic logic induction method is used to summarize and refine it. Sixteen themes are generated: "national condition", "human resource", "work treatment", "work intensity", "learning form", "school roll", "employment agreement", "employer", "position", "examination", "enrollment", "region", "education", "subject", "student type", and "applicable condition". Combining the evaluation dimension system constructed in Table 7 and the corresponding 16 themes with 4 evaluation dimensions, a comment topic identification system is obtained as shown in Table 8. This can avoid semantic confusion caused by a large number of topic words, thereby improving the data structure and clarifying the evaluation dimension to which the text belongs.

**Table 8.** Comment topic identification system.

| Dimension | Theme | Identification Word |
|---|---|---|
| Theoretical objectives | National condition | employment rate, unemployment rate, epidemic, housing price |
| | Human resource | labor force, talent, young people, quality |
| Expectations of the masses | Work treatment | salary, treatment, subsidy, welfare |
| | Work intensity | pressure, workload, energy |
| Implementation means | Learning form | full-time, part-time |
| | School roll | file, student source, registered residence, origin, household registration, domicile, |
| | Employment agreement | agreement, tripartite agreement, contract |
| | Employer | kindergarten, enterprise, university, government office, hospital, institution, vocational school, elementary school, college, unit |
| | Position | nurse, kindergarten teacher, teacher, civil servant, counselor, head teacher, research assistant, special post teacher |
| | Examination | written examination, interview, preliminary examination, reexamination |
| | Enrollment | quota, proportion |
| Target groups | Region | Shandong, Wuhan, Beijing, rural area, Chongqing, Sichuan, Guangdong, Anhui, Tianjin, area, Shanghai, Henan, whole country, other province, city, downtown, region, county town, township |
| | Education | bachelor, junior college, Doctor, Master, second degree, college promotion |
| | Subject | normal major, mathematics, music, Chinese, English, news, art, engineering, preschool education |
| | Student type | fresh graduate, poor student, doctoral student, postgraduate, undergraduate, junior college student, previous graduate |
| | Applicable condition | age, qualification, threshold, condition, experience, ability, accomplishment, fractional line, level |

The above-mentioned comment topic identification system is used to map comments to different evaluation dimensions. By identifying and matching comments, a total of 51,567 pieces of comments related to 4 evaluation dimensions were extracted. The specific results are shown in Table 9.

Table 9. Classification of comments.

| Dimension | Theme | Position Measures | Transference Measures | Channel Measures | Subsidy Measures |
|---|---|---|---|---|---|
| Theoretical objectives | National condition | 2429 | 728 | 468 | 30 |
|  | Human resource | 1106 | 871 | 573 | 41 |
| Expectations of the masses | Work treatment | 3098 | 388 | 75 | 442 |
|  | Work intensity | 443 | 435 | 90 | 35 |
| Implementation means | Learning form | 40 | 466 | 37 | 9 |
|  | School roll | 160 | 5 | 41 | 1037 |
|  | Employment agreement | 146 | 77 | 327 | 692 |
|  | Employer | 2887 | 522 | 876 | 590 |
|  | Position | 5390 | 557 | 795 | 418 |
|  | Examination | 1429 | 1521 | 43 | 48 |
|  | Enrollment | 2890 | 522 | 6 | 380 |
| Target groups | Region | 1060 | 875 | 1044 | 376 |
|  | Education | 786 | 1876 | 239 | 20 |
|  | Subject | 3179 | 712 | 23 | 73 |
|  | Student type | 2939 | 1289 | 22 | 675 |
|  | Applicable condition | 2113 | 516 | 38 | 549 |

### 5.2.3. Determining Policy Theme Weight

TF-IDF weighting method is used to assign weight to each topic here. The TF-IDF method consists of two parts: the TF method and the IDF method. The TF method is to count the keyword frequency. The basic idea is the more times a word appears in the document, the stronger the word is to summarize documents. The IDF method counts how many documents a word appears in. The basic idea is if a word appears in fewer documents, its ability to distinguish between documents is stronger. The calculation formula of the TF-IDF method in this paper is

$$\text{TF-IDF} = \frac{n_i}{\sum_k n_k} \times \log\left(\frac{|D|}{1+|D_i|}\right) \tag{4}$$

where $n_i$ refers to the number of times the topic recognition word $n_i$ under the $i$th topic appears in the review data, $\sum_k n_k$ is the total number of words in the corpus, and the result of dividing the two is the word frequency. $|D|$ refers to the number of comments in the corpus, $|D_i|$ is the number of comments containing the topic identification words under the $i$th topic, and the logarithm is the inverse document frequency. The product of the word frequency and the inverse document frequency is the TF-IDF weight of the $i$th topic. From this, the weight of each theme can be obtained as shown in Table 10.

Table 10. Weight of policy theme.

| Dimension | Theme | Position Measures | Transference Measures | Channel Measures | Subsidy Measures |
|---|---|---|---|---|---|
| Theoretical objectives | National condition | 0.0675 | 0.0633 | 0.0831 | 0.0078 |
| | Human resource | 0.0122 | 0.0612 | 0.1001 | 0.0088 |
| Expectations of the masses | Work treatment | 0.1067 | 0.0304 | 0.0143 | 0.0942 |
| | Work intensity | 0.0135 | 0.0513 | 0.0161 | 0.0034 |
| Implementation means | Learning form | 0.0013 | 0.0518 | 0.0081 | 0.0016 |
| | School roll | 0.0081 | 0.0005 | 0.0094 | 0.1889 |
| | Employment agreement | 0.0099 | 0.0024 | 0.0751 | 0.1189 |
| | Employer | 0.1073 | 0.0278 | 0.1853 | 0.1243 |
| | Position | 0.1882 | 0.0605 | 0.1767 | 0.0794 |
| | Examination | 0.0528 | 0.1512 | 0.0093 | 0.0079 |
| | Enrollment | 0.1005 | 0.0252 | 0.0017 | 0.0565 |
| Target groups | Region | 0.0352 | 0.1010 | 0.2368 | 0.0545 |
| | Education | 0.0243 | 0.1478 | 0.0594 | 0.0043 |
| | Subject | 0.1046 | 0.0667 | 0.0062 | 0.0109 |
| | Student type | 0.1061 | 0.1102 | 0.0091 | 0.1277 |
| | Applicable condition | 0.0620 | 0.0486 | 0.0093 | 0.1009 |

A theme with a weight greater than 0.1 has a significant impact on policy support degree and is called a key theme. As can be seen from the above table, there are a total of six key themes in the position measures: work treatment, employer, position, enrollment, subject, and student type. This shows that the number of new jobs were created by position measures and that the employment requirements of these new jobs have a greater impact on the public support degree of positional measures. There is a total of four key themes in the transference measures: examination, region, education, and student type. This shows that the specific arrangements for entrance examinations and the object-oriented fairness of the measures have a greater impact on the public support degree of transference measures. There are 4 key themes in the channel measures: human resource, employer, position, and region. This shows that the effectiveness of policy measures in alleviating the employment situation and the fairness of the policy in terms of geographical terms have a greater impact on the degree of support for position measures. There are 5 key themes in the subsidy measures: enrollment, employment agreement, employer, student type, and applicable condition. This shows that the implementation has a greater impact on the degree of support for subsidy measures.

### 5.3. Calculating Theme Emotion Score

Due to the use of sentence structures such as irony in Weibo, the results obtained by the traditional dictionary-based lexical weight accumulation algorithm are not ideal. Because Internet irony often uses some exaggerated rhetoric to express dissatisfaction and irony, such comments often contain strong emotional colors. In order to ensure the accuracy of the emotion score, it is very important to accurately identify and score this type of comments. Therefore, this paper identifies these sentences and revises the emotion score based on punctuation features to improve the accuracy of the results.

5.3.1. Calculation of Initial Emotion Score

The emotion score of a sentence is not only determined by the emotion evaluation word itself, but also affected by degree adverbs, negative words, and punctuation. In order to improve the accuracy of the emotion score calculation, this paper combined the comment and the Chinese grammar dictionary, selected 117 degree adverbs, and defined their respective emotion strengths. The results are shown in Table 11.

Table 11. Emotion strength of degree adverbs.

| Level | Emotion Strength | Degree Adverb | Amount |
|---|---|---|---|
| High | 2 | Very, greatly | 47 |
| Middle | 1.5 | too, more | 39 |
| Low | 0.5 | a little | 31 |

Aiming at the negative words appearing in the comments, this paper combines the original negative words in HowNet dictionary and the common phrases in Weibo to sort out a total of 27 negative words after manual screening. In addition to degree adverbs, users often use continuous punctuation (such as "!!!", "???") to reflect their own emotions. In this regard, the punctuation at the end of the comment will be identified, and the emotional intensity of various punctuation will be set, as shown in Table 12 below.

Table 12. Emotion strength of punctuation.

| Punctuation | Emotion Strength |
|---|---|
| $! \times n(n \geq 1)$ | $1.5 \times n$ |
| $? \times n(n \geq 2)$ | $1.2 \times (n-1)$ |
| $\sim \times n(n \geq 1)$ | $0.8 \times n$ |

In summary, the initial emotional score of the $i$th comment, $E_i$, is expressed as follows:

$$E_i = \sum_{j}^{n} \left[ (-1)^{N_j} W_j P_m \prod_{j}^{q} L_j \right] \quad (5)$$

where $W_j$ is the $j$th emotion score in comment, and $L_j$ is the emotion strength of degree adverbs before the $j$th emotion word. $N_j$ is the number of negative words before the $j$th emotion word. $P_m$ is the emotion strength of punctuation at the end of the comment. $q$ is the amount of degree adverbs before the $j$th emotion word.

5.3.2. Modifying Emotion Score of Irony

In the Chinese context, irony has various manifestations, and the most common form is rhetorical question. When identifying rhetorical questions, the biggest challenge lies in distinguishing interrogative sentences from rhetorical questions. The common feature of the two is the ending of the question. The difference between the two is that rhetorical questions often contain vocabulary with a certain emotional inclination, while interrogative sentences do not contain emotional inclination. Therefore, the rhetorical question processing rules are as follows:

$$E_i^* = \begin{cases} -1 \times E_i & \text{ending with the question and } E_i \neq 0 \\ E_i & \text{other} \end{cases} \quad (6)$$

5.3.3. Emotion Score of Various Themes

After the above calculation, the emotion scores of various policy themes are obtained, and the results are shown in Table 13.

Table 13. Emotion score.

| Theme | Average Emotion Score | | | |
| --- | --- | --- | --- | --- |
| | Position Measures | Transference Measures | Channel Measures | Subsidy Measures |
| National condition | 0.9016 | −0.6212 | 0.5156 | −1.5795 |
| Human resource | 0.3536 | 0.1653 | −1.4315 | 0.1411 |
| Work treatment | 0.1158 | 0.0491 | −1.1797 | 2.3995 |
| Work intensity | −1.2313 | −1.3930 | −1.025 | −1.2938 |
| Learning form | −0.7427 | −0.6341 | −0.5376 | −1.7500 |
| School roll | −0.8052 | −1.1915 | −0.8409 | −3.6528 |
| Employment agreement | 0.6784 | −0.1235 | 0.4256 | −2.5643 |
| Employer | 0.1595 | −0.5430 | −1.5411 | 0.5103 |
| Position | 0.6182 | −0.3463 | −1.0509 | 0.1168 |
| Examination | −0.4551 | 1.2514 | −0.8135 | −1.5063 |
| Enrollment | −1.1651 | −0.5399 | −0.5776 | −2.7280 |
| Region | −0.6805 | −0.6057 | −1.9725 | −0.9744 |
| Education | −0.3996 | 0.7888 | 0.4036 | −1.1675 |
| Subject | −0.2259 | −1.7181 | 0.0531 | 0.5362 |
| Student type | −0.2467 | −0.8378 | −0.8663 | −0.6121 |
| Applicable condition | 0.3725 | −0.5268 | −1.1908 | −1.9126 |

It can be seen from Table 13 that the highest emotional score among position measures is "national condition", with a score of 0.9016, indicating that the public believes that position measures can increase the employment rate of college students and reduce the impact of COVID-19 on the economy. Among position measures, the lowest emotion score is "work intensity" with a score of −1.2313, which shows that the public believes that treatments of new jobs brought about by position measures needs to be improved. Among the transference measures, the highest emotion score is the "examination" with a score of 1.2514, indicating that the public believes that the transference measures have a positive impact on the entrance examination. Among the transference measures, the lowest emotion score is the "subject" with a score of −1.7181, indicating that the public believes that the subject is not comprehensive enough. Among the channel measures, the highest emotion score is "national condition" with a score of 0.5156, indicating that the public believes that channel measures have a positive impact on increasing the employment rate and promoting the rapid employment of college graduates. Among the channel measures, the region with the lowest emotional score is the "region" with a score of −1.9725, indicating that the public believes that the geographical area targeted by the transference measures is not comprehensive enough. Among the subsidy measures, the highest emotion score is "work treatment" with a score of 2.3995, indicating that the public believes that subsidy measures can effectively improve their own work treatment. Among the subsidy measures, the lowest emotion score is "school roll", with a score of −3.6528, indicating that the public believes there are some unreasonable aspects in the means related to school roll in subsidy measures.

### 5.4. Analyzing Support Degree for Various Policy Measures

The public support degree for various employment policies is calculated based on the topic weights and emotion scores obtained above. The formula is

$$S = \sum TE^*$$

(7)

where $S$ is the public support degree for the policy measures, $T$ is the theme weight, and $E^*$ is the theme emotion score. According to the above-mentioned public support degree for various measures, the results are shown in Table 14.

Table 14. Support degree for policy measures.

| Dimension | Support Degree for Policy Measures | | | |
| --- | --- | --- | --- | --- |
| | Position Measures | Transference Measures | Channel Measures | Subsidy Measures |
| Theoretical objectives | 0.8178 | −0.2047 | −0.5484 | −0.6674 |
| Expectations of the masses | −0.6851 | −0.5797 | −1.0978 | 2.2553 |
| Implementation means | 0.0232 | 0.2851 | −0.9883 | −1.9147 |
| Target groups | −0.3252 | −0.3631 | −1.4389 | −1.0839 |
| Total score | −0.0018 | −0.1373 | −1.0557 | −1.2809 |

It can be seen from Table 14 that the support for the four types is negative, indicating that the public has a negative attitude towards the employment policy for college graduates under COVID-19. Among them, the degree of support for position measures is close to 0, indicating that the public holds a neutral attitude towards position measures. As the range of support degree for policy measures set in this paper is [−5,5], although the support degree for transference measures is negative, its value is approximately −0.1, which is still in the neutral range. The support degree of subsidy measures and channel measures is lower than −1, indicating that the public is not satisfied with these two types of policies and there is room for further improvement.

Combining Tables 10 and 13, it can be found that: (1) The emotion scores of "work-treatment", "employer", and "position" in the key themes of the position measures are positive, indicating that the public is satisfied with the treatments of newly added positions. However, the emotion score of the "enrollment" is negative and less than −1, indicating that the number of new positions is not satisfactory. In addition, the emotion scores of "subject" and "student type" are less than 0, indicating that the public is dissatisfied with the subject and academic qualifications of graduates for newly added positions. This also reduces the support for position measures, so support for position measures is relatively neutral. (2) For transference measures, under the dimension of "implementation means", "examination" has the largest proportion and positive emotional score, which makes the support of this dimension positive, indicating that the public is satisfied with the fairness of the public's specific implementation. However, note that the weight of "target groups" is 0.4743, which is close to 50%, and the support for this dimension is −0.3631, which makes the overall support degree for transference measures not high. In addition, the support degree for the "theoretical objectives" and the "expectations of the masses" is also negative. This is because the people believe that the transference measures are "a temporary solution but not a root cause" and may bring about social problems such as "depreciation of academic qualifications" after implementation. (3) The emotion scores of the four key themes in the channel measures are all negative, and all are less than −1, which is the main reason for the low final support degree of the channel measures. Many people believe that the employment information platform established by channel measures is not well known. Moreover, the policy is mainly for fresh graduates in Hubei: the coverage of the policy is not wide enough. (4) In the evaluation dimension of subsidy measures, the emotion score of "implementation means" is close to −2, and the weight reaches 0.4586. In addition, the emotion score of "target groups" is also lower than −1, which makes the overall support degree for subsidy measures poor. The public believes that the channel measures on student status are not well implemented, and the policies are only targeted at individual regions, thus many regions cannot feel the employment convenience brought by the policy.

## 6. Conclusions

This paper introduced the PMC index model to quantitatively evaluate the employment promotion policy documents of college graduates under COVID-19 pandemic at first. Then, itobtained six acceptable-level policy documents and two excellent-level policy documents, summarizedfour measures according to the key contents of policy documents, as well as constructedsupport evaluation model and analyzed the social effects of the employment promotion policy for college graduates under COVID-19 pandemic.The results showed that the public was generally not satisfied. Among them, the public had a neutral attitude towards position measures and transference measures but was obviously dissatisfied with subsidy measures and channel measures. In this regard, the government should improve and optimize the existing employment policies. Based on the analysis results, this paperput forward the following suggestions:

(1) The public expresses dissatisfaction with the geographical coverage of the four types of measures and the breadth of population coverage. In this regard, the government should optimize, adjust, and expand the subjects and student types covered by the employment policy for college graduates. At the same time, local governments should learn from the advanced experience of other regions to narrow the gap in the implementation of policies among regions, so as to ensure that policies can bring equal benefits to graduates from different regions, schools, and disciplines.

(2) In response to the shortcomings of existing position measures, the government should steadily increase the number of recruits of government agencies and institutions, and can appropriately relax restrictions on the recruitment of subjects and academic qualifications according to the work content and needs of different positions.

(3) The government first needs to pay attention to the problem that transference measures "treat the symptoms but not the root cause" proposed by the public. Second, the government needs to deal with the problem of "difficulties in obtaining employment for college graduates" from a more long-term perspective. It is necessary to foresee that college graduates transferred by transference measures will face employment pressure again in a few years. Therefore, plans should be improved. In addition, in response to the "depreciation of academic qualifications" caused by the implementation of transference measures, the government needs to realize industrial upgrading as soon as possible and create more jobs that require high-end talents to meet the growing demand for high-quality talents in society.

(4) In response to the shortcomings of channel measures, first, the government should increase the promotion of employment information platforms for college graduates and cooperate with social platforms and short video platforms commonly used by young people to increase the popularity of the platform. Second, the government should cooperate with leading companies in various industries to introduce large companies to the platform, and drive many small, medium, and micro-enterprises to settle on the platform. In addition, the government should also cooperate with various universities to guide college graduates to make better use of the platform and increase the utilization rate of the platform.

(5) In response to the shortcomings of subsidy measures, relevant government departments should strengthen supervision and ensure that relevant units and enterprises in various regions implement policies and measures, so that college graduates can truly feel the effect of subsidy measures.

However, this paper still had the following shortcomings, which need further study:

(1) The research object of this paper was the employment promotion policy for college graduates issued by the government from January to July 2020. The impact of the COVID-19 epidemic is still not finished yet, and the government will issue new employment promotion policies. Therefore, further analysis of the effects of the new policy will be carried out in the follow-up.

(2) This paper mainly analyzed the social effects of the implementation of the employment promotion policy for college graduates under the COVID-19 pandemic, so the economic effects of the policy implementation should be analyzed in the follow-up as well.

(3) Based on the data of China's Weibo [36], this paper evaluated the implementation effect of the employment policy for college graduates issued by the Chinese government. However, COVID-19 has an impact on all countries in the world; therefore,

in the future, we will collect data from all countries, conduct targeted research, and give corresponding suggestions.

**Author Contributions:** T.C. described the proposed framework and wrote the whole manuscript; J.R. implemented the simulation experiments; L.P. and J.F. collected data; J.Y. and G.C. revised the manuscript. All authors have read and agreed to the published version of the manuscript.

**Funding:** This research is supported by the National Social Science Foundation of China (Grant No. 20BTQ059), the Project of China (Hangzhou) Cross-border E-commerce College (No.2021KXYJ07), the Key Project of Zhejiang Province Education Science Planning in 2021 (Grant No. 2021SB103), the General Scientific Research Project of Professional Degree Postgraduates of Zhejiang Education Department in 2020 (Grant No. Y202045139), the Scientific Research Project of Zhejiang Education Department (Grant No. Y201737899), the Contemporary Business and Trade Research Center and Center for Collaborative Innovation Studies of Modern Business of Zhejiang Gongshang University of China (Grant No. 14SMXY05YB), as well as the Characteristic & Preponderant Discipline of Key Construction Universities in Zhejiang Province (Zhejiang Gongshang University-Statistics).

**Institutional Review Board Statement:** Not applicable.

**Informed Consent Statement:** Informed consent was obtained from all subjects involved in the study.

**Data Availability Statement:** The data used to support the findings of this study are available from the corresponding author upon request.

**Conflicts of Interest:** The authors declare no conflict of interest.

# References

1. Chen, T.; Peng, L.; Yin, X.; Jing, B.; Yang, J.; Cong, G.; Li, G. A Policy Category Analysis Model for Tourism Promotion in China during the COVID-19 Pandemic based on Data Mining and Binary Regression. *Risk Manag. Healthc. Policy* **2020**, *13*, 3211–3233. [CrossRef]
2. Fu, P.; Jing, B.; Chen, T.; Xu, C.; Yang, J.; Cong, G. Propagation Model of Panic Buying Under the Sudden Epidemic. *Front. Public Health* **2021**, *9*, 675687. [CrossRef] [PubMed]
3. Zhu, S.; Chen, C. Comment on Employment Policy of College Students in China. *Res. Contin. Educ.* **2009**, *25*, 86–89. (In Chinese)
4. Ercument, G.; Emine, G. Teaching creativity: Developing Experimental Design Studio Curricula for Pre-College and Graduate Level Students in China. *Procedia-Soc. Behav. Sci.* **2012**, *51*, 714–720.
5. Liu, Y.; Shi, J. Study on the influence process of organizational innovation climate on employee innovation behavior. *China Soft Sci.* **2010**, *22*, 133–144. (In Chinese)
6. Gu, Y.; Peng, J. The affect mechanism of creative self-efficacy on employees' creative behavior. *Sci. Res. Manag.* **2011**, *31*, 65–73.
7. Aalbers, R.; Dolfsma, W.; Koppius, O. Individual connectedness in innovation networks: On the role of individuals motivation. *Res. Policy* **2013**, *5*, 624–634. [CrossRef]
8. Genco, N.; Holtta-Otto, K.; Seepersad, C.C. An Experimental Investigation of the Innovation Capabilities of Undergraduate Engineering Students. *J. Eng. Educ.* **2012**, *20*, 725–741. [CrossRef]
9. Xu, X.; Han, M.; Li, Z. Research on the Feedback of Social Evaluation for College Graduates and Teaching Adaptation System. *Res. High. Educ. Eng.* **2008**, *54*, 92–95.
10. Zhang, N.; Ding, Z.; Peng, F. An empirical study on the influencing factors of employment region selection for innovative high-level talents: Based on the employment data of graduates from three universities in Anhui Province. *Employ. Chin. Coll. Stud.* **2020**, *21*, 34–40. (In Chinese)
11. Yu, Q. Analysis on the influencing factors of the choice of employment unit of college graduates. *Stat. Decis. Mak.* **2014**, *23*, 120–122. (In Chinese)
12. Yang, C.; Yang, L. Analysis on the Competitive Force of Employment of the College Graduates. *J. Yunnan Normal Univ. (Nat. Sci. Ed.)* **2009**, *29*, 39–45.
13. Li, Y.; Lin, Y. On the construction of college graduates' employment promotion system and the realization of its function. In Proceedings of the 2011 International Conference on Business Management and Electronic Information, Guangzhou, China, 13–15 May 2011; pp. 813–816.
14. Zhang, X. Research on the Employment Option of College Graduates Based on Bayesian Algorithm of Data Mining and Inclusion Degree. *Adv. Sci. Lett.* **2012**, *46*, 185–187.
15. Jie, L. Research on Influencing Factors of College Students' Employment Based on Grey Relational Analysis-Take Jiangsu University as an Example. *Int. J. Nonlinear Sci.* **2018**, *26*, 164–168.
16. Xi, W.; He, L. Research on influencing factors and effect of entrepreneurship policy of Chinese college students—Empirical analysis based on S province. *E3S Web Conf.* **2020**, *2*, 3–11.
17. Wollmann, H. The development of a sustainable development model framework. *Energy Policy Res.* **2007**, *31*, 69–75.

18. Song, X. A Study on the Performance of Employment Policy for College Students—Taking Guangdong Province as an Example. *J. Guangxi Univ. Financ. Econ.* **2008**, *21*, 118–121. (In Chinese)
19. Hu, Y.; Chen, Z. An Analysis of College Students' Career Orientation and Policy Cognition under Financial Crisis—Based on a Questionnaire Survey of College Students. *Hubei Soc. Sci.* **2009**, *10*, 173–176. (In Chinese)
20. Zhao, J.G.; Yao, X.M. Research on Effectiveness and Improvement of Employment Policies for University Graduates: An empirical research on the basis of DEA method. *Math. Pract. Theory* **2013**, *43*, 1–11.
21. Zhang, T. Youth employment: A new difficulty in China's employment. *Beijing Youth Work Res.* **2008**, *11*, 39–41. (In Chinese)
22. Chen, T.; Yin, X.; Peng, L.; Rong, J.; Yang, J.; Cong, G. Monitoring and Recognizing Enterprise Public Opinion from High-Risk Users Based on User Portrait and Random Forest Algorithm. *Axioms* **2021**, *10*, 106. [CrossRef]
23. Chen, T.; Peng, L.; Yang, J.; Cong, G. Analysis of User Needs on Downloading Behavior of English Vocabulary APPs Based on Data Mining for Online Comments. *Mathematics* **2021**, *9*, 1341. [CrossRef]
24. Sun, H. Key words co-occurrence network and empirical research. *Intell. Mag.* **2012**, *31*, 63–67. (In Chinese)
25. Ruiz Estrada, M.A. Policy modeling: Definition, classification and evaluation. *J. Policy Model.* **2011**, *33*, 523–536. [CrossRef]
26. Ruiz Estrada, M.A.; Yap, S.F.; Nagaraj, S. Beyond the ceteris paribus assumption: Modeling demand and supply assuming omnia mobilis. *Int. J. Econ. Res.* **2008**, *24*, 185–194.
27. Yang, Z.; Chen, Y.; Chen, Y. Research on Cross-border E-commerce Policy Evaluation Based on PMC Index Model. *Int. Bus.* **2018**, *13*, 114–126.
28. Zhang, Y.; Jin, Y.; Xue, X. Evaluation of Construction Industrialization Policy Based on PMC Index Model. In Proceedings of the International Conference on Construction and Real Estate Management 2018, Charleston, CA, USA, 9–10 August 2018; pp. 192–201.
29. Zhang, Y.; Qie, H. Quantitative Evaluation Innovation Policies of the State Council-based on the PMC-Index Model. *Sci. Technol. Progress Policy* **2017**, *34*, 127–136.
30. Wang, J.; Yang, Q.; Zhang, Y. Quantitative evaluation of civil-military integration policy based on PMC-AE index model. *Intell. Mag.* **2019**, *38*, 70–77. (In Chinese)
31. Chen, T.; Rong, J.; Yang, J.; Cong, G.; Li, G. Combining Public Opinion Dissemination with Polarization Process Considering Individual Heterogeneity. *Healthcare* **2021**, *9*, 176. [CrossRef]
32. Li, S.; Zhang, J.; Shan, L. Measuring Social Security Policy Implementation Effect Based on Multidimensional and Hierarchical Scale. *Manag. Rev.* **2015**, *27*, 24–38.
33. Agyepong, I.A.; Adjei, A.S. Public social policy development and implementation: A case study of the Ghana National Health Insurance scheme. *Health Policy Plan* **2008**, *23*, 150–160. [CrossRef] [PubMed]
34. Jones, F.J.B. The Effects of Health Insurance and Self-Insurance on Retirement Behavior. *Econometrica* **2011**, *79*, 693–732.
35. Peksen, T.D. Can states buy peace? Social welfare spending and civil conflicts. *J. Peace Res.* **2012**, *49*, 273–287.
36. Chen, T.; Wang, Y.; Yang, J.; Cong, G. Modeling multidimensional public opinion polarization process under the context of derived topics. *Int. J. Environ. Res. Public Health* **2021**, *18*, 472. [CrossRef] [PubMed]

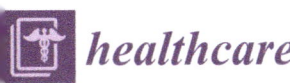

*Article*

# Assessing the Knowledge, Attitudes and Practices of COVID-19 among Quarantine Hotel Workers in China

Yi-Man Teng [1,†], Kun-Shan Wu [2,*,†], Wen-Cheng Wang [3] and Dan Xu [1]

1. College of Modern Management, Yango University, Fuzhou 350015, China; yimanteng@gmail.com (Y.-M.T.); dxu@ygu.edu.cn (D.X.)
2. Department of Business Administration, Tamkang University, Taipei 251301, Taiwan
3. College of Innovation and Entrepreneurship Education, Yango University, Fuzhou 350015, China; wcwang@go.hwh.edu.tw
* Correspondence: kunshan@mail.tku.edu.tw
† Equal first authorship.

**Abstract:** During the pandemic, quarantine hotel workers face a higher risk of infection while they host quarantine guests from overseas. This study's aim is to gain an understanding of the knowledge, attitudes, and practices (KAP) of quarantine hotel workers in China. A total of 170 participants took part in a cross-sectional survey to assess the KAP of quarantine hotel workers in China, during the COVID-19 pandemic. The chi-square test, independent $t$-test, one-way analysis of variance (ANOVA), descriptive analysis, and binary logistic regression were used to examine the sociodemographic factors associated with KAP levels during the COVID-19 pandemic. The results show that 62.41% have good knowledge, 94.7% have a positive attitude towards COVID-19, but only 78.2% have good practices. Most quarantine hotel workers (95.3%) are confident that COVID-19 will be successfully controlled and that China is handling the COVID-19 crisis well (98.8%). Most quarantine hotel workers are also taking personal precautions, such as avoiding crowds (80.6%) and wearing facemasks (97.6%). The results evidence that quarantine hotel workers in China have acquired the necessary knowledge, positive attitudes and proactive practices in response to the COVID-19 pandemic. The results of this study can provide a reference for quarantine hotel workers and their targeted education and intervention.

**Keywords:** COVID-19; quarantine hotel workers; knowledge; attitudes; practices

**Citation:** Teng, Y.-M.; Wu, K.-S.; Wang, W.-C.; Xu, D. Assessing the Knowledge, Attitudes and Practices of COVID-19 among Quarantine Hotel Workers in China. *Healthcare* **2021**, *9*, 772. https://doi.org/10.3390/healthcare9060772

Academic Editors: Thomas Garavan, Eduardo Tomé and Ana Dias

Received: 26 May 2021
Accepted: 17 June 2021
Published: 21 June 2021

**Publisher's Note:** MDPI stays neutral with regard to jurisdictional claims in published maps and institutional affiliations.

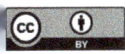

**Copyright:** © 2021 by the authors. Licensee MDPI, Basel, Switzerland. This article is an open access article distributed under the terms and conditions of the Creative Commons Attribution (CC BY) license (https://creativecommons.org/licenses/by/4.0/).

## 1. Background

The COVID-19 pandemic has made a significant impact on the health and safety of each country's population, as well as ongoing effects to their economies and societies. The World Health Organization has declared the pandemic a public health emergency of global concern [1]. As positive cases of COVID-19 escalate, hospitals face problems with overcrowding and insufficient isolation space [2]. Australia enforces home-isolation for confirmed cases with mild symptoms and suspected cases; however, this ultimately increases the risk of infection to other household members [3]. To prevent this interaction, they propose that COVID-19 patients with mild symptoms isolate themselves by staying in a hotel. In addition, due to increasing concerns regarding transmitting the virus to their families, healthcare workers [4] need temporary quarantine accommodation.

To mitigate the pandemic, countries around the world have implemented safety measures such as lockdown, social distancing, and mandatory 14-day quarantine periods for citizens and foreign visitors arriving from abroad [5]. The latter resulted in a demand for designated quarantine hotels, as this is where the majority of incoming residents and visitors will stay. As a result, many governments have expropriated hotels to be used as temporary quarantine accommodation: the 'quarantine hotel.' Quarantine hotels are a community-based public health intervention designed to mitigate the spread of COVID-19 within the community [6]. The use of quarantine hotels to isolate tourists and returning residents for medical observation over a 14-day period is the hotel industry's contribution to the control of COVID-19 [7]. Some scholars also argue that quarantine hotels reframe the taken-for-granted business model and goes beyond basic cleaning and hygiene standards to devote greater attention to the protection and safety of the quarantine guests' physical and psychosocial needs, and better fulfill stakeholder demands [8].

Currently, in China, the COVID-19 epidemic is well-controlled; however, confirmed cases from overseas continue to increase [9]. During the pandemic, while hosting quarantine guests from overseas, quarantine hotel workers face a much higher risk of infection [6] as COVID-19's main route of transmission is through respiratory droplets and direct contact with confirmed cases. Additionally, the quarantine hotel workload includes following an operation guide, complying with high-standard anti-epidemic and disinfection measures, and implementing quarantine services. The challenge for quarantine hotel workers is not only the increasing workload created by the quarantine hotel operation, but also high psychological stress associated with job insecurity, risk of exposure, and contagion for themselves, their friends, and families.

Public health education was evidenced to be the significant measure to mitigate the spread of the epidemic during the SARS, MERS, and COVID-19 pandemics [10,11]. Previous literature proposes webinars (web-based seminars) as a public health educational tool, and provide a viable method of instruction and education for school personnel who are interested in strategies for improving a school's wellness environment [12]. Recently, some scholars have also evidenced that webinars offer clear and actionable information to school staff about disease characteristics, adoptable preventive measures, and early detection and control of COVID-19 in primary schools [13]. Public health education may improve the effectiveness of preventive measures in terms of transmission of COVID-19 and other viruses.

To effectively curb the COVID-19 crisis, countries worldwide are continuously promoting different unprecedented preventive measures, including appropriate personal hygiene and public health measures [14]. Incorrect knowledge toward the diseases affects people's incorrect attitude and practices directly raise the risk of infection. Knowledge, attitudes, and practices (KAP) is a significant educational tool for public health and plays an integral role in determining a society's readiness to accept behavioral change measures from health authorities [15]. Referring to the articles, people's KAP towards COVID-19 largely affected adherence to control measures in accordance with KAP theory [16–18]. According to the previous studies, assessing the KAP toward COVID-19 would assist in providing better insight to address poor knowledge of COVID-19. This also offers the development of preventive strategies and health promotion programs [11,19]. Previous studies have evidenced the relation of a higher level of knowledge and the practice of preventive measures, as well as the positive relation of attitudes and preventive behaviors [20–22]. In the latest articles of KAP regarding COVID-19, they all demonstrated collecting KAP information has long been useful for informing prevention, control, and mitigation measures during the epidemic outbreaks [23].

Prior research provides evidence that the level of KAP possessed by inhabitants dictates the success of the adopted measures [15,18,24–26]. Recently, there are some studies investigated KAP towards COVID-19 in different group, such as general residents [19,26–36], healthcare workers [24,37–41], students [9,42–48], patients [49], hospital visitors [50] and slums [51,52], during the COVID-19 pandemic. Most of KAP studies regarding COVID-19 discuss the group of general residents. The results from these studies found that residents with a high level of knowledge about COVID-19 and positive attitudes toward it tended to have better preventive behaviors and behavioral compliance [19,26]. Furthermore, there are fewer articles that discuss KAP toward the COVID-19 system review and future direction [53,54].

Now, the increased trend in confirmed cases in China indicates they are coming from overseas. There is an urgent need to grasp quarantine hotel staff awareness of COVID-19 at this critical time, as they are providing service to host overseas quarantine guests. To the best of our knowledge, there is no published research concentrated on the KAP of quarantine hotel workers. The literature lacks an examination of quarantine hotel workers' KAP toward COVID-19 from this perspective and has rarely discussed targeted education and intervention for quarantine hotel workers in order to comply with pandemic control measures. If the quarantine hotel workers' KAPs are concerned about the virus and factors that affect their attitude and behavior, then this information can inform relevant training and policies during their work and guide them in prioritizing protection and avoiding occupational exposure. To date, peer-reviewed COVID-19 KAP surveys have comprised of a brief online survey among ordinary residents, healthcare workers, adults, students, patients, hospital visitors, and slums, and these surveys are not relevant in hospitality industry settings.

To facilitate the management of the COVID-19 pandemic in the hospitality industry, there is an imperative need to grasp the quarantine hotel workers' awareness of COVID-19 at this critical time. This study aims to assess quarantine hotel workers' KAP towards COVID-19 through an online questionnaire survey in China. The implication of this study is to anticipate to guide quarantine hoteliers to develop the key skills in the hotel industries for medical education, as well as anti-epidemic and disinfection standards for their staff during and post-pandemic.

## 2. Materials and Methods

### 2.1. Study Design

This cross-sectional study applied convenience sampling to collect samples from the quarantine hotel employees in Xiamen, Fujian Province, China, during the COVID-19 pandemics, from 20 May to 10 June 2020. There are approximately 50 quarantine hotels in Xiamen, as it is the only city in the Fujian Province with airports receiving international flights. The participating staff came from seven hotels. We called the HR manager of the quarantine hotel and asked them whether they would join the survey. Finally, the HR managers of seven hotels agreed to post the one-page recruitment poster on their WeChat (similar to WhatsApp) employee group chat and invited employees to participate in the survey. The advertisement included a brief introduction, background information, purpose, procedures, declarations of anonymity and confidentiality, and the voluntary nature of taking part. The quarantine hotel workers who understood the content of the survey and agreed to participate in the study were instructed to complete the questionnaire via clicking on the link or scanning the QR code.

### 2.2. Study Instrument

The questionnaire consisted of four sections: (1) demographics—this surveyed participants' sociodemographic information, including gender, age, education, and monthly income; (2) knowledge about COVID-19; (3) attitude toward COVID-19; and (4) practices relevant to COVID-19.

To measure COVID-19 knowledge, 12 items were adapted from Zhong et al. [26]. There were four items regarding clinical presentations (K1–K4), three regarding transmission routes (K5–K7), and five regarding prevention and control (K8–K12). 'True,' 'false,' or 'I don't know' responses were offered for these items. Correct answers scored '1' and incorrect/unknown answers scored '0.' The score total range for knowledge items was 0–12, with higher scores indicating better knowledge about COVID-19. Bloom's cut-off of 80% ($\geq 9.6$) was used to determine a better knowledge [55].

Attitudes were measured with a two-item scale developed by Zhong et al. [26]. Participants were asked to state their level of agreement on the successful control of COVID-19 (1 = agree; 0 = No/I don't know), and confidence in winning the battle against the virus (1 = yes; 0 = No). An 'I don't know' response was considered as a lack of agreement and thus, 'No' and 'I don't know' were coupled, as per previous studies [14,40]. In addition, the combinations of responses were considered for each participant. The attitude of the participants who agreed that COVID-19 could be successfully controlled and were confident that China could overcome the pandemic scored '1' and were labeled as 'optimistic attitude' [26]. 'No' or 'I don't know' responses scored '0' and were labeled 'negative attitude' [14].

Practice toward COVID-19 was measured with a two-item scale that was developed by Zhong et al. [26]. Participants were asked to state their current behaviors, e.g., going to a crowded place and/or wearing a mask when going out (yes = 1; No = 0). Participants who agreed they had not been to any crowded places and wore a mask when leaving their home scored '1' and were labeled as 'good practice' toward COVID-19. The responses that disagreed scored '0' and were labeled as 'poor practice' [14].

### 2.3. Statistical Analysis

The data were organized and analyzed using IBM SPSS Statistics (Statistical Package for the Social Sciences) 22.0 software (IBM, Armonk, NY, USA). The chi-squared test, independent $t$-test, and ANOVA with multiple comparisons between each two categories were done by post hoc analysis. Least significant difference (LSD) was applied to find the differences in KAP between groups for selected demographic variables. To identify related factors, the response binary logistic regression analysis was applied and expressed as odds ratio (OR) and 95% confidence interval (CI), with a significance level of 0.05 (two-tailed). For the final model, the Hosmer–Lemeshow test [56], which measures goodness of fit ($p$-value > 0.05), was considered an appropriate logistic regression model. $p < 0.05$ was considered to indicate significance in all tests. Internal consistency of the questionnaire's knowledge section revealed Cronbach's alpha as 0.69, which confirms acceptable internal consistency.

### 2.4. Ethical Consideration

According to the relevant laws and regulations of China and the guidelines of Yango University, an ethics approval was not required for this non-interventional study (e.g., surveys). Nevertheless, after quarantine hotel managers agreed to participate in this study, and ethical approval clearance and informed consent clearance were approved by the Luo, Zhong You, Executive principle of Yango University; hence, an ethical approval was expected. After expressing the principles of Helsinki Declaration, the participants were informed of the purpose of the research and expressed their informed consent. Participants were made clear that their participation is voluntary. The study was harmless to the participants, as no names were used and all data were analyzed anonymously in order to maintain anonymity.

## 3. Results

### 3.1. Respondent Characteristics

In terms of demographics among 170 participants, there were slightly more female respondents in this study ($n$ = 99, 58.2%) than there were male (41.8%). In terms of ages, 90 participants were Millennials (53.0%) and 32 participants were Generation Z (18.8%). In total, 103 participants (50.6%) had a junior college and above degree. In terms of departments, 28.8% participants were frontline employees (including front desk and housekeeping departments) and 71.2% participants were logistics support employees (including food & beverage, administration, and security departments). One-hundred twenty-eight participants (75.3%) indicated that their individual monthly income was 6000 RMB or below.

### 3.2. Assessment of COVID-19 Knowledge

Results of the knowledge assessment of quarantine hotel workers regarding clinical presentations, transmission routes, and prevention and control of COVID-19 are shown in Table 1. The mean COVID-19 knowledge score for quarantine hotel workers was 9.78 (Standard deviation: 1.61, range: 0–12). The rate of overall correct answer to COVID-19 knowledge was 81.5% (9.78/12 × 100). The rate of overall correct answer for all quarantine hotel workers ranged between 23.5% and 98.2%. Most workers of the quarantine hotel

(98.2%) recognize that human beings who had contact with confirmed cases should be isolated immediately for 14 days. Even so, people are obviously confused about the spread of virus. When asked if eating and contacting wild animals would cause infection, only 23.5% answered correctly (Table 1).

Table 1. Responses to the questionnaire on COVID-19 KAP.

| Items | Correct Answer Rate (n; %) | Incorrect Answer and 'I Don't Know' Rate (n; %) |
|---|---|---|
| K1. The main clinical symptoms of COVID-19 are fever, fatigue, dry cough, and myalgia. | 159 (93.5) | 11 (6.5) |
| K2. Unlike the common cold, nasal congestion, runny nose, and sneezing are less common among people infected with COVID-19 virus. | 113 (66.5) | 57 (33.5) |
| K3. At present, there is no effective treatment in COVID-19, but early symptomatic treatment can help most patients recover from infection. | 152 (89.4) | 18 (10.6) |
| K4. Not all persons with COVID-19 will develop into severe cases. Only those who are elderly, have chronic illnesses, and are obese are more likely to be severe cases. | 113 (66.5) | 57 (33.5) |
| K5. Eating or contacting wild animals would result in the infection by the COVID-19 virus. | 40 (23.5) | 130 (76.5) |
| K6. Persons with COVID-19 cannot pass the virus to others when a fever is not present. | 130 (76.5) | 23.5 (4.0) |
| K7. The COVID-19 virus spreads via respiratory droplets from infected individuals. | 162 (95.3) | 8 (4.7) |
| K8. Ordinary residents can wear general medical masks to prevent infection from the COVID-19 virus. | 162 (95.3) | 8 (4.7) |
| K9. It is not necessary for children and young adults to take measures to prevent infection from the COVID-19 virus. | 156 (91.8) | 14 (8.2) |
| K10. To prevent infection by COVID-19, individuals should avoid going to crowded places such as train stations and avoid taking public transportation. | 150 (88.2) | 20 (11.8) |
| K11. Isolation and treatment of people who are infected with the COVID-19 virus are effective ways to reduce the spread of the virus. | 159 (93.5) | 11 (6.5) |
| K12. People who have contact with someone infected with the COVID-19 virus should be immediately isolated in a proper place. In general, the observation period is 14 days. | 167 (98.2) | 3 (1.8) |
| Attitudes | Answer yes rate (n; %) | Answer no rate (n; %) |
| A1. Do you agree that COVID-19 will finally be successfully controlled? | 162 (95.3) | 8 (4.7) |
| A2. Do you have confidence that China can win the battle against the COVID-19 virus? | 168 (98.8) | 2 (1.2) |
| Practice | Answer yes rate (n; %) | Answer no rate (n; %) |
| P1. Have you been to any crowded places in recent days? | 33 (19.4) | 137 (80.6) |
| P2. Do you wear a mask when you go out in recent days? | 166 (97.6) | 4 (2.4) |

The independent $t$-test and one-way ANOVA analysis were used to assess the differences in knowledge scores among different demographic characteristics. The results showed that there were no significant differences in knowledge scores for all demographic variables (gender, age, education, department, and monthly income) ($p > 0.05$, Table 2).

**Table 2.** Relationship between socio-demographic characteristics of the participants and their knowledge scores about COVID-19 ($n = 170$).

| Characteristics | Category | | Number of Participants (%) | Knowledge Score (Mean ± SD) | t/F | p-Value |
|---|---|---|---|---|---|---|
| Gender | Male | a | 71 (41.8) | 9.54 ± 1.52 | −1.707 | 0.090 |
|  | Female | b | 99 (51.2) | 9.96 ± 1.65 |  |  |
| Age | Generation Z | a | 32 (18.8) | 9.22 ± 2.15 | 2.529 | 0.083 |
|  | Millennials | b | 90 (52.9) | 9.88 ± 1.51 |  |  |
|  | Generation X | c | 48 (28.2) | 9.98 ± 1.28 |  |  |
| Education | MSB | a | 20 (11.8) | 9.75 ± 1.07 | 0.431 | 0.731 |
|  | SHSVS | b | 47 (27.6) | 9.85 ± 1.43 |  |  |
|  | JC | c | 57 (33.5) | 9.91 ± 1.84 |  |  |
|  | UA | d | 46 (27.1) | 9.57 ± 1.70 |  |  |
| Department | Frontline | a | 49 (28.8) | 9.86 ± 1.37 | 0.385 | 0.701 |
|  | Logistics support | b | 121 (71.2) | 9.75 ± 1.70 |  |  |
| Income per month RMB [#] | 6000 and below | a | 128 (81.5) | 9.85 ± 1.53 | −0.254 | 0.800 |
|  | 6001 and above | b | 29 (18.5) | 9.93 ± 1.46 |  |  |

Note: (1) Generation Z = Born 1996+; Millennials = Born 1977–1995; Generation X = Born 1965–1976. (2) MSB = Middle school and below; SHSVS = Senior high school/vocational school; JC = Junior college; UA = Undergraduate and above. (3) [#] Exclude 'I don't want to talk about it' participants. (4) t = Student's t test, F = analysis of variance (ANOVA) test. (5) Multiple comparisons between each two categories are done by post hoc analysis (Least Significant Difference, LSD).

Initially, most (8/12) knowledge questions about COVID-19 had a high accuracy rate (80% or more) (Table 1). As a result, a cut off knowledge score of ≤9 was set for poor knowledge and ≥10 for good (adequate) knowledge (Table 3). The study found that 62.41% of quarantine hotel workers have good (adequate) knowledge, which implies that a significant proportion of quarantine hotel workers have poor knowledge about COVID-19. Further, binary logistic regression analysis found that female quarantine hotel workers had higher odds of having good (adequate) knowledge at 10% significance level (Table 4).

**Table 3.** Difference in quarantine hotel workers' KAP toward COVID-19 by demographics ($N = 170$).

| Characteristics | Knowledge | | | Attitude | | | Practice | | |
|---|---|---|---|---|---|---|---|---|---|
|  | Poor (n; %) | Good (n; %) | $\chi^2$ or t (p-Value) | Negative (n; %) | Optimistic (n; %) | $\chi^2$ or t (p-Value) | Poor (n; %) | Good (n; %) | $\chi^2$ or t (p-Value) |
| Overall | 64 (37.6) | 106 (62.41) |  | 9 (5.3) | 161 (94.7) |  | 37 (21.8) | 133 (78.2) |  |
| Gender |  |  | 5.446 (0.020) |  |  | 0.278 (0.598) |  |  | 0.043 (0.837) |
| Male | 34 (47.9) | 37 (52.1) |  | 3 (4.2) | 68 (95.8) |  | 16 (22.5) | 55 (77.5) |  |
| Female | 30 (30.3) | 69 (69.7) |  | 6 (6.1) | 93 (93.9) |  | 21 (21.2) | 78 (78.5) |  |
| Age |  |  | 1.555 (0.460) |  |  | 0.400 (0.819) |  |  | 2.112 (0.348) |
| Gen Z | 15 (46.9) | 17 (53.1) |  | 1 (3.1) | 31 (96.9) |  | 10 (31.2) | 22 (68.8) |  |
| Millennials | 31 (34.4) | 59 (65.6) |  | 5 (5.6) | 85 (94.4) |  | 18 (20.0) | 72 (80.0) |  |
| Gen X | 18 (37.5) | 30 (62.5) |  | 3 (6.3) | 45 (93.8) |  | 9 (18.8) | 39 (81.3) |  |
| Education level |  |  | 1.775 (0.620) |  |  | 7.045 (0.070) |  |  | 2.892 (0.409) |
| Middle school and below | 7 (35.0) | 13 (65.0) |  | 3 (15.0) | 17 (85.0) |  | 4 (20.0) | 16 (80.0) |  |
| Senior high school/vocational school | 19 (40.4) | 28 (59.6) |  | 4 (8.5) | 43 (91.5) |  | 8 (17.0) | 39 (83.0) |  |
| Junior college | 18 (31.6) | 39 (68.4) |  | 1 (1.8) | 56 (98.2) |  | 11 (19.3) | 46 (80.7) |  |
| Undergraduate and above | 20 (43.5) | 26 (56.5) |  | 1 (2.2) | 45 (97.8) |  | 14 (30.4) | 32 (69.6) |  |

Table 3. Cont.

| Characteristics | Knowledge | | | Attitude | | | Practice | | |
|---|---|---|---|---|---|---|---|---|---|
| | Poor (n; %) | Good (n; %) | $\chi^2$ or t (p-Value) | Negative (n; %) | Optimistic (n; %) | $\chi^2$ or t (p-Value) | Poor (n; %) | Good (n; %) | $\chi^2$ or t (p-Value) |
| Department | | | 0.024 (0.876) | | | 0.094 (0.759) | | | 1.873 (0.171) |
| Frontline | 18 (36.7) | 31 (63.3) | | 3 (6.1) | 46 (93.9) | | 14 (28.6) | 35 (71.4) | |
| Logistics support | 46 (38.0) | 75 (62.0) | | 6 (5.0) | 115 (95.0) | | 23 (19.0) | 98 (81.0) | |
| Income per month RMB [#] | | | 1.300 (0.254) | | | 0.496 (0.481) | | | 1.138 (0.286) |
| 6000 and below | 43 (33.6) | 85 (66.4) | | 5 (3.9) | 123 (96.1) | | 24 (18.8) | 104 (81.2) | |
| 6001 and above | 13 (44.8) | 16 (55.2) | | 2 (6.9) | 27 (93.1) | | 8 (27.6) | 21 (72.4) | |
| Knowledge score | 8.25 ± 1.53 | 10.71 ± 0.68 | −14.375 (0.000) | 9.33 ± 1.80 | 9.81 ± 1.60 | −0.860 (0.391) | 9.78 ± 1.57 | 9.78 ± 1.63 | 0.006 (0.995) |

Note: (1) Knowledge section total scores range from 0–12, with a cut off level of ≤9 set for poor knowledge and ≥10 for good knowledge. (2) The attitude of the participants who agreed that COVID-19 could be successfully controlled and were confident about China winning against the pandemic scored '1' and was labeled as 'optimistic attitude' toward COVID-19. Any other combinations of responses scored '0' and were labeled as 'negative attitude' toward COVID-19. (3) The practice of the participants who agreed they had not gone to any crowded places and wore a mask when leaving home in recent days scored '1' and was labeled as 'good practice' regarding COVID-19. Any other combinations of responses scored '0' and were labeled as 'poor practice' regarding COVID-19. (4) [#] Exclude 'I don't want to talk about it' participants.

Table 4. Logistic regression analysis for factors associated with good knowledge and optimistic attitude regarding COVID-19 (N = 170).

| Characteristics | Knowledge | | Attitude | |
|---|---|---|---|---|
| | OR (95% CI) | p-Value | OR (95% CI) | p-Value |
| **Gender (Reference: Male)** | | | | |
| Female | 1.881 (0.922, 3.837) | 0.082 | 0.522 (0.087, 3.139) | 0.269 |
| **Age (Reference: Generation Z)** | | | | |
| Millennials | 1.679 (0.605, 4.657) | 0.319 | 9.066 (0.349, 235.311) | 0.185 |
| Generation X | 1.517 (0.461, 4.989) | 0.493 | 9.656 (0.288, 323.420) | 0.206 |
| **Education (Reference: Middle school and below)** | | | | |
| Senior high school/ vocational school | 1.292 (0.355, 4.702) | 0.697 | 0.020 (0.001, 0.682) | 0.030 * |
| Junior college | 1.272 (0.469, 3.452) | 0.636 | 0.151 (0.009, 2.462) | 0.184 |
| Undergraduate and above | 1.964 (0.797, 4.839) | 0.142 | 1.001 (0.058, 17.420) | 0.999 |
| **Department (Reference: logistics support department)** | | | | |
| Frontline | 0.723 (0.333, 1.572) | 0.413 | 0.516 (0.079, 3.372) | 0.490 |
| **Income per month RMB (Reference: 6000 and below) [#]** | | | | |
| 6001 and above | 0.460 (0.177, 1.197) | 0.112 | 0.062 (0.003, 1.137) | 0.061 |
| Hosmer–Lemeshow goodness of fit statistic | 8.277 | 0.309 | 2.050 | 0.979 |

Note: (1) [#] Exclude 'I don't want to talk about it' participants; (2) * Statistically significant at $p < 0.05$.

### 3.3. Assessment of COVID-19 Attitudes

To assess the attitudes toward COVID-19, two questions were used. One asked whether the COVID-19 epidemic would be successfully controlled, which the majority of the quarantine hotel workers agreed with (95.3%). Another asked whether they trusted China to be able to win its battle against the virus, which again, the majority of the quarantine hotel workers agreed with (98.8%). Overall, 94.7% of quarantine hotel workers had an optimistic (positive) attitude toward COVID-19, while 5.3% had a negative attitude (Table 3). In addition, attitudes toward COVID-19 were significantly associated with education level (Table 3). Quarantine hotel workers who had a senior high school/vocational school (vs. middle school and below, OR: 0.020, 95% CI = 0.001–0.682, $p = 0.030$) were more unlikely to have optimistic attitude toward COVID-19 (Table 4).

### 3.4. Assessment of COVID-19 Practices

Quarantine hotel workers were asked two questions in assessment of practices relevant to COVID-19. The first question asked whether or not they agreed that they were avoiding crowded places in recent days; the second was whether or not they agreed that they were wearing face masks when outside the home in recent days. For the first question, 80.6% of quarantine hotel workers reported that they had been avoiding crowded places, whereas the remaining 19.4% had not been. Furthermore, 97.6% of quarantine hotel workers reported wearing a face mask when going out in public in recent days, whereas 2.4% indicated they did not. In addition, 78.2% of quarantine hotel workers had 'good practice' relevant to COVID-19. The remaining participants (21.8%) recorded 'poor practice' (Table 3). The practice relevant to COVID-19 was not significantly associated with all demographic characteristics (Table 3).

## 4. Discussion

The outbreak of COVID-19 has sent the hotel industry into an unprecedented recession. In this context, the different management policies undertaken by hotel managers are determining the industry's survival. Quarantine hotel workers' adherence to control measures is essential, and is largely affected by their KAP towards COVID-19, in accordance with KAP theory. The understanding of quarantine hotel workers' KAP toward the pandemic is helpful for hoteliers when addressing and implementing effective decision-making frameworks to ensure rapid response to unexpected events that challenge the solvency of their business. Assessing KAP related to COVID-19 provides greater insight, helping to address poor knowledge about the virus and assist with the development of preventive strategies and health promotion programs. KAP studies provide baseline information to determine the type of intervention that may be required to change misconceptions about the virus [14,15,24]. To date, there has been limited published data on quarantine hotel workers' KAP toward COVID-19. Therefore, it is tremendously important to investigate the KAP of quarantine hotel workers to help guide these efforts.

In China, the overall COVID-19 'correct' knowledge rate among quarantine hotel workers is 81.5%, with an average score of moderate (9.78 ± 1.61). This knowledge score is higher than that of US residents (80%) [34] and the Palestinian population (79%) [57], but lower than the Chinese general population (90%) [26] and Tanzanian residents (84.4%) [11]. This study found that 62.41% of quarantine hotel workers in China have good (adequate) knowledge of COVID-19, which means there is a considerable proportion of quarantine hotel workers who have poor knowledge. Recently, the research results provide evidence that the level of knowledge regarding COVID-19 was proportional to age and years of education [58]. However, this empirical result reveals that there were no significant differences in knowledge toward COVID-19 scores for the demographic variables (age, education, department, and monthly income). That result is not consistent with other studies conducted worldwide, which shows knowledge was significantly differed across age, education level, and income [26,27]. Our study demonstrated the female quarantine hotel workers were more likely to have good (adequate) knowledge compared to men, which is consistent with the contentions of Zhong et al. [26] and Banik et al. [28], and is similar to a cross-cultural KAP study by Ali et al. [59]. This result may be explained by gender difference in related activities, and can also be attributed to the fact that women will experience higher family pressure in their role of caring for families.

As a considerable amount of quarantine hotel workers in China have poor knowledge of COVID-19, quarantine hoteliers should provide extra medical education to identify microbiological characteristics and perform diagnosis, disinfection, and self-protection technology. Recently, some articles have advocated that hoteliers should improve the service of hygiene and cleaning, disinfection, and hygiene activities as the main contents response to the hotel industries development of post-COVID 19 [60–62]. Following the scholars, appropriate training in operation guides, complying with anti-epidemic and disinfection standards, and implementing quarantine services is also essential.

This study also found that a large majority of quarantine hotel workers have optimistic attitudes about controlling and overcoming COVID-19 (94.7%). Roughly 95.3% of quarantine hotel workers concurred that COVID-19 will be controlled and 98.8% of respondents believe China can win the battle against the virus. The participants' high confidence and optimistic attitudes toward the control of COVID-19 will be attributed to the severe measures taken by the government to slow down the epidemic. The staff of quarantine hotels hold a highly optimistic (positive) attitude towards COVID-19, which is consistent with recent studies, in which most participants believe that their country will fight against it, and this epidemic will be treated in Bangladesh [28], Egypt [27], Malaysia [19], and Saudi Arabia [63]. Attitudes toward COVID-19 play efficacy beliefs among the public, significantly impacting on promoting preventive behaviors [64]. This optimism attitude may be the result of strict disease control measures taken by China government, which have strengthened people's confidence in their approach.

According to the results, most quarantine hotel workers are taking precautions, such as avoiding crowded places (80.6%) and wearing face masks (97.6%) during the COVID-19 pandemic, which indicates a general willingness for quarantine hotel workers to make behavioral changes to prevent COVID-19 infections. This finding is similar to previous KAP studies regarding COVID-19 [65,66], but contradictory to a study conducted among Malaysian people, which found only 51.2% of participants reported wearing a face mask when going out in public [25]. These practices could be because of the restriction on actions imposed by the government that promote the practice of effective measure to combat the spread of COVID-19 [67].

This study focused on grasping the quarantine hotel workers' KAP towards COVID-19 at this critical time; however, we are aware of some limits of the study. First, this was a rapid survey whereby participants were recruited by the quarantine hotels' human resources managers posting a one-page advertisement on their staff group chat in WeChat (similar to WhatsApp) inviting workers to participate. We are not able to verify whether this recruitment method was affected by social desirability bias. Second, the participants were only from quarantine hotels in Xiamen city, which may not reflect the actual situation of the workers in Chinese quarantine hotels as a whole. Third, one of the main shortcomings of KAP surveys is that it is difficult to get a standard reference (cut-off point) to classify the study subjects' knowledge and practice levels. Lastly, due to the lack of infection data in this dataset, it was not possible to document the infection rates among quarantine hotel workers or the patients remaining in their care and, thus, this research could not determine causality between the variables. These problems require further study and resolution.

## 5. Conclusions

At present, the trend in confirmed cases in China indicates that they are coming from overseas. There is an imperative need to grasp quarantine hotel staff awareness of COVID-19 at this critical time, as they are the first to host overseas quarantine guests. The purpose of this study is to explore the characteristics and levels of quarantine hotel workers' knowledge about COVID-19. To the best of our knowledge, there is a gap in the literature regarding applying the theories of KAP to the hotel industry. This is the first contribution to the assessment of the quarantine hotel workers' awareness about COVID-19 risks. To enable further progress in this field, a deeper understanding of how KAP theory research in hospitality is required. The findings suggest that most quarantine hotel workers in China have adequate knowledge on COVID-19 and are generally optimistic (positive) in their outlook on overcoming the pandemic.

The survey results provide a general outline of quarantine hotel workers' COVID-19 prevention practices, which can better prepare quarantine hoteliers when addressing future health crises. The results also highlight future targeted education and intervention for quarantine hotel workers in order to comply with pandemic control measures, such as providing staff with training in anti-epidemic and disinfection standards and implementing quarantine services.

It is anticipated that in the post-pandemic future, the key skills in the hotel industry's competitive workforce will be medical education and anti-epidemic and disinfection standards. Currently and moving forward, hoteliers will focus their attention on hygiene and cleanliness and promote this message via social media, e.g., 'We have high standards of cleanliness and hygiene,' to ensure customers trust the hotel and feel comfortable and safe during their stay.

**Author Contributions:** Conceptualization, Y.-M.T. and K.-S.W.; methodology, Y.-M.T. and K.-S.W.; formal analysis, Y.-M.T. and K.-S.W.; software, Y.-M.T. and K.-S.W.; visualization, W.-C.W.; data curation, Y.-M.T. and D.X.; writing—original draft, Y.-M.T., K.-S.W., W.-C.W. and D.X.; writing—review and editing, Y.-M.T. and K.-S.W. All authors have read and agreed to the published version of the manuscript.

**Funding:** This research received no external funding.

**Institutional Review Board Statement:** Not applicable since the study is not involving humans or animals.

**Informed Consent Statement:** Not applicable since the study is not involving humans.

**Data Availability Statement:** Data sharing not applicable.

**Conflicts of Interest:** The authors declare no conflict of interest.

## References

1. World Health Organization. Mental Health and Psychosocial Considerations during the COVID-19 Outbreak. WHO. 2020. Available online: https://www.who.int/docs/default-source/coronaviruse/mental-health-considerations.pdf (accessed on 25 June 2020).
2. Feng, E.; Cheng, A. In Quarantined Wuhan, Hospital Beds for Coronavirus Patients are Scarce. National Public Radio (NPR). 2020. Available online: https://www.npr.org/goatsandsoda/2020/02/05/802896668/in-quarantined-wuhanhospital-beds-for-coronavirus-patients-are-scarce (accessed on 25 June 2020).
3. Mahmoudi, N.; Melia, A.; Lee, D.; Dalton, C.; Paolucci, F. Cost-Effectiveness Analysis of COVID-19 Case Isolation. 2020. Available online: https://ssrn.com/abstract=3603711 (accessed on 6 July 2020).
4. Rosemberg, M.A. Health and safety considerations for hotel cleaners during Covid-19. *Occup. Med.* **2020**, *70*, 382–383. [CrossRef]
5. Lin, C.Y. Social reaction toward the 2019 novel coronavirus (COVID-19). *Soc. Health Behav.* **2020**, *3*, 1–2. [CrossRef]
6. Teng, Y.M.; Wu, K.S.; Lin, K.L.; Xu, D. Mental health impact of COVID-19 on quarantine hotel employees in China. *Risk Manag. Healthc. Policy* **2020**, *13*, 2743–2751. [CrossRef] [PubMed]
7. Wong, I.A.; Yang, F.X. A quarantined lodging stay: The buffering effect of service quality. *Int. J. Hosp. Manag.* **2020**, *91*, 102655. [CrossRef] [PubMed]
8. Jiang, Y.; Wen, J. Effects of COVID-19 on hotel marketing and management: A perspective article. *Int. J. Contemp. Hosp. Manag.* **2020**, *32*, 2563–2573. [CrossRef]
9. Wen, F.; Meng, Y.; Cao, H.; Xia, J.; Li, H.; Qi, H.; Meng, K.; Zhang, L. Knowledge, attitudes, practices of primary and middle school students at the outbreak of COVID-19 in Beijing: A cross-sectional online study. *medRxiv* **2020**. [CrossRef]
10. Deng, J.F.; Olowokure, B.; Kaydos-Daniels, S.C.; Chang, H.J.; Barwick, R.S.; Lee, M.L.; Deng, C.-Y.; Factor, S.H.; Chiang, C.E.; Maloney, S.A.; et al. Severe acute respiratory syndrome (SARS): Knowledge, attitudes, practices and sources of information among physicians answering a SARS fever hotline service. *Public Health* **2006**, *120*, 15–19. [CrossRef] [PubMed]
11. Rugarabamu, S.; Byanaku, A.; Ibrahim, M. Knowledge, attitudes, and practices (KAP) towards COVID-19: A quick online cross-sectional survey among Tanzanian residents. *MedRxiv* **2020**. [CrossRef]
12. Hoke, A.M.; Francis, E.B.; Hivner, E.A.; Simpson, A.J.L.; Hogentogler, R.E.; Kraschnewski, J.L. Investigating the effectiveness of webinars in the adoption of proven school wellness strategies. *Health Educ. J.* **2018**, *77*, 249–257. [CrossRef]
13. Paduano, S.; Marchesi, I.; Frezza, G.; Turchi, S.; Bargellini, A. COVID-19 in school settings: Webinar aimed at both teachers and educators. *Ann Ig.* **2021**. [CrossRef]
14. Imtiaz, R.D.; Tripathy, S.; Kar, S.K.; Sharma, N.; Verma, S.K.; Kaushal, V. Study of knowledge, attitude, anxiety & perceived mental healthcare need in Indian population during COVID-19 pandemic. *Asian. J. Psychiatr.* **2020**, *51*, 102083. [CrossRef]
15. Ajilore, K.; Atakiti, I.; Onyenankeya, K. College students' knowledge, attitudes and adherence to public service announcements on Ebola in Nigeria: Suggestions for improving future Ebola prevention education programmers. *Health Educ. J.* **2020**, *76*, 648–660. [CrossRef]
16. Hussain, A.; Garima, T.; Singh, B.M.; Ram, R.; Tripti, R. Knowledge, attitudes, and practices towards COVID-19 among Nepalese residents: A quick online crosssectional survey. *Asian J. Med. Sci.* **2020**, *11*, 6–11. [CrossRef]
17. Tomar, B.S.; Singh, P.; Nathiya, D.; Tripathi, S.; Chauhan, D.S. Indian community knowledge, attitude & practice towards COVID-19. *medRxiv* **2020**. [CrossRef]

18. Tariq, S.; Tariq, S.; Baig, M.; Saeed, M. Knowledge, awareness and practices regarding novel coronavirus among a sample of Pakistani population, a crosssectional study. *Disaster Med. Public Health Prep.* **2020**, 1–20. [CrossRef]
19. Azlan, A.A.; Hamzah, M.R.; Sern, T.J.; Ayub, S.H.; Mohamad, E. Public knowledge, attitudes and practices towards COVID-19: A cross-sectional study in Malaysia. *PLoS ONE* **2020**, *15*, e0233668. [CrossRef] [PubMed]
20. Papagiannis, D.; Malli, F.; Raptis, D.G.; Papathanasiou, I.V.; Fradelos, E.C.; Daniil, Z.; Rachiotis, G.; Gourgoulianis, K.I. Assessment of knowledge, attitudes, and practices towards new coronavirus (SARS-CoV-2) of health care professionals in Greece before the outbreak period. *Int. J. Environ. Res. Public Health* **2020**, *17*, 4925. [CrossRef] [PubMed]
21. Afzal, M.S.; Khan, A.; Qureshi, U.U.R.; Saleem, S.; Saqib, M.A.N.; Shabbir, R.M.K.; Naveed, M.; Jabbar, M.; Zahoor, S.; Ahmed, H. Community-based assessment of knowledge, attitude, practices and risk factors regarding COVID-19 among Pakistanis residents during a recent outbreak: A cross-sectional survey. *J. Community Health* **2020**, 1–11. [CrossRef] [PubMed]
22. Alrubaiee, G.G.; Al-Qalah, T.A.H.; Al-Aawar, M.S.A. Knowledge, attitudes, anxiety, and preventive behaviours towards COVID-19 among health care providers in Yemen: An online cross-sectional survey. *BMC Public Health* **2020**, *20*, 1541. [CrossRef]
23. Austrian, K.; Pinchoff, J.; Tidwell, J.B.; White, C.; Abuya, T.; Kangwana, B.; Ochako, R.; Wanyungu, J.; Muluve, E.; Mbushi, M.; et al. COVID-19 related knowledge, attitudes, practices and needs of households in informal settlements in Nairobi, Kenya. *Bull. World Health Organ* **2020**. [CrossRef]
24. Shi, Y.; Wang, J.; Yang, Y.; Wang, Z.; Wang, G.; Hashimoto, K.; Zhang, K.; Liu, H. Knowledge and attitudes of medical staff in Chinese psychiatric hospitals regarding COVID-19. *Brain Behav. Immun.* **2020**, *4*, 100064. [CrossRef]
25. Tachfouti, N.; Slama, K.; Berraho, M.; Nejjari, C. The impact of knowledge and attitudes on adherence to tuberculosis treatment: A case-control study in a Moroccan region. *Pan. Afr. Med. J.* **2012**, *12*, 52. Available online: http://www.panafrican-med-journal.com/content/article/12/52/full/ (accessed on 6 July 2020). [PubMed]
26. Zhong, B.L.; Luo, W.; Li, H.M.; Zhang, Q.Q.; Liu, X.G.; Li, W.T.; Li, Y. Knowledge, attitudes, and practices towards COVID-19 among Chinese residents during the rapid rise period of the COVID-19 outbreak: A quick online cross-sectional survey. *Int. J. Biol. Sci.* **2020**, *16*, 1745–1752. [CrossRef] [PubMed]
27. Abdelhafiz, A.S.; Mohammed, Z.; Ibrahim, M.E.; Ziady, H.H.; Alorabi, M.; Ayyad, M.; Sultan, A.E. Knowledge, perceptions, and attitude of Egyptians towards the Novel Coronavirus Disease (COVID-19). *J. Community Health* **2020**, 1–10. [CrossRef] [PubMed]
28. Banik, R.; Rahman, M.; Sikder, T.; Rahman, Q.R.; Pranta, M.R. Investigating knowledge, attitudes, and practices related to COVID-19 outbreak among Bangladeshi young adults: A web based cross-sectional analysis. *Res. Sq.* **2020**. [CrossRef]
29. Caviglia-Harris, J.; Hall, S.; Mulllan, K.; Macintyre, C.; Bauch, S.C.; Harris, D.; Sillis, E.; Roberts, D.; Toomey, R.; Cha, H. Improving Household Surveys Through Computer-Assisted Data Collection: Use of Touch-Screen Laptops in Challenging Environments. *Field Methods* **2012**, *24*, 74–94. [CrossRef]
30. Geldsetzer, P. Knowledge and perceptions of COVID-19 among the general public in the United States and the United Kingdom: A Cross-sectional online survey. *Ann. Intern. Med.* **2020**. [CrossRef]
31. Hossain, M.A.; Hossain, K.M.A.; Walton, L.M.; Uddin, Z.; Haque, O.; Kabir, F.; Arafat, S.M.Y.; Sakel, M.; Faruqui, R.; Hossain, Z. Knowledge, attitudes, and fear of COVID-19 during the rapid rise period in Bangladesh. *PLoS ONE* **2020**. [CrossRef]
32. Lau, L.L.; Hung, N.; Go, D.J.; Ferma, J.; Choi, M.; Dodd, W.; Wei, X. Knowledge, attitudes and practices of COVID-19 among income-poor households in the Philippines: A cross-sectional study. *J. Glob. Health* **2020**, *10*, 011007. [CrossRef]
33. McFadden, S.M.; Malik, A.A.; Aguolu, O.G.; Willebrand, K.S.; Omer, S.B. Perceptions of the adult US population regarding the novel coronavirus outbreak. *PLoS ONE* **2020**, *15*, e0231808. [CrossRef] [PubMed]
34. Wolf, M.S.; Serper, M.; Opsasnick, L.; O'Conor, R.M.; Curtis, L.M.; Benavente, J.Y.; Wismer, G.; Baito, S.; Eifler, M.; Zheng, P.; et al. Awareness, attitudes, and actions related to COVID-19 among adults with chronic conditions at the onset of the U.S. outbreak: A cross-sectional survey. *Ann. Intern. Med.* **2020**. [CrossRef] [PubMed]
35. Yue, S.; Zhang, J.; Cao, M.; Chen, B. Knowledge, attitudes and practices of COVID-19 among urban and rural residents in China: A cross-sectional study. *J. Community Health* **2020**, 1–6. [CrossRef]
36. Masoud, A.T.; Zaazouee, M.S.; Elsayed, S.M.; Ragab, K.M.; Kamal, E.M.; Alnasser, Y.T.; Assar, A.; Nourelden, A.Z.; Istatiah, L.J.; Abd-Elgawad, M.M.; et al. KAP-COVIDGLOBAL: A multinational survey of the levels and determinants of public knowledge, attitudes and practices towards COVID-19. *BMJ Open* **2021**, *11*, e043971. [CrossRef]
37. Kamate, S.K.; Sharma, S.; Thakar, S.; Srivastava, D.; Sengupta, K.; Hadi, A.J.; Chaudhary, A.; Joshi, R.; Dhanker, K. Assessing knowledge, attitudes and practices of dental practitioners regarding the COVID-19 pandemic: A multinational study. *Dent. Med. Probl.* **2020**, *57*, 11–17. [CrossRef] [PubMed]
38. Khader, Y.; Al Nsour, M.; Al-Batayneh, O.B.; Saadeh, R.; Bashier, H.; Alfaqih, M. Dentists' awareness, perception, and attitude regarding COVID-19 and infection control: Cross-sectional study among Jordanian dentists. *JMIR Public Health Surveill.* **2020**, *6*, e18798. [CrossRef] [PubMed]
39. Saqlain, M.; Munir, M.M.; Rehman, S.; Gulzar, A.; Naz, S.; Ahmed, Z.; Tahir, A.H.; Mashhood, M. Knowledge, attitude, practice and perceived barriers among healthcare professionals regarding COVID-19: A cross-sectional survey from Pakistan. *J. Hosp. Infect.* **2020**, *105*, 419–423. [CrossRef] [PubMed]

40. Zhou, M.; Tang, F.; Wang, Y.; Nie, H.; Zhang, L.; You, G.; Zhang, M. Knowledge, attitude and practice regarding COVID-19 among health care workers in Henan, China. *J. Hosp. Infect.* **2020**, *105*, 183–187. [CrossRef]
41. Hossain, M.A.; Rashid, M.U.B.; Khan, M.A.S.; Sayeed, S.; Kader, M.A.; Hawlader, M.D.H. Healthcare Workers' knowledge, attitude, and practice regarding personal protective equipment for the prevention of COVID-19. *J. Multidiscip. Healthc.* **2021**, *14*, 229–238. [CrossRef] [PubMed]
42. Peng, Y.; Pei, C.; Zheng, Y.; Wang, J.; Zhang, K.; Zheng, Z.; Zhu, P. A cross-sectional survey of knowledge, attitude and practice associated with COVID-19 among undergraduate students in China. *BMC Public Health* **2020**, *20*, 1–8. [CrossRef]
43. Wu, X.L.; Munthali, G.N.C. Knowledge, attitudes, and preventive practices (KAPs) towards COVID-19 among international students in China. *Dovepress* **2021**, *14*, 507–518. [CrossRef]
44. Dilucca, M.; Souli, D. Knowledge, attitude and practice of secondary school students toward COVID-19 epidemic in Italy: A cross selectional study. *bioRxiv* **2020**. [CrossRef]
45. Taghrir, M.H.; Borazjani, R.; Shiraly, R. COVID-19 and Iranian medical students; A survey on their related-knowledge, preventive behaviors and risk perception. *Arch. Iran Med.* **2020**, *23*, 249–254. [CrossRef] [PubMed]
46. Duong, M.C.; Nguyen, H.T.; Duong, B.T. A Cross-Sectional Study of Knowledge, Attitude, and Practice Towards Face Mask Use Amid the COVID-19 Pandemic Amongst University Students in Vietnam. *J. Community Health* **2021**, 1–7. [CrossRef]
47. Jia, Y.; Qi, Y.; Bai, L.; Han, Y.; Xie, Z.; Ge, J. Knowledge–attitude–practice and psychological status of college students during the early stage of COVID-19 outbreak in China: A cross-sectional study. *BMJ J.* **2021**, *11*, e045034. [CrossRef]
48. Addis, S.G.; Nega, A.D.; Miretu, D.G. Knowledge, attitude and practice of patients with chronic diseases towards COVID-19 pandemic in Dessie town hospitals, Northeast Ethiopia. *Diabetes Metab. Syndr. Clin. Res. Rev.* **2021**, *5*, 847–856. [CrossRef] [PubMed]
49. De Lima Filho, B.F.; Bessa, N.P.O.S.; Fernandes, A.C.T.; da Silva Patrício, Í.F.; de Oliveira Alves, N.; da Costa Cavalcanti, F.A. Knowledge levels among elderly people with Diabetes Mellitus concerning COVID-19: An educational intervention via a teleservice. *Acta Diabetol.* **2020**, *4*, 1–6. [CrossRef] [PubMed]
50. Gebretsadik, G.; Ahmed, N.; Kebede, E.; Gebremicheal, S.; Belete, M.A.; Adane, M. Knowledge, attitude, practice towards COVID-19 pandemic and its prevalence among hospital visitors at Ataye district hospital, Northeast Ethiopia. *PLoS ONE* **2021**, *16*, e0246154. [CrossRef]
51. Islam, M.S.; Emran, G.I.; Rahman, E.; Banik, R.; Sikder, T.; Smith, L.; Hossain, S. Knowledge, attitudes and practices associated with the COVID-19 among slum dwellers resided in Dhaka City: A Bangladeshi interview-based survey. *J. Public Health* **2021**, *43*, 13–25. [CrossRef]
52. Abuya, T.; Austrian, K.; Isaac, A.; Kangwana, B.; Mbushi, F.; Muluve, E.; Mwanga, D.; Ngo, T.; Nzioki, M.; Ochako, R.; et al. *COVID-19-Related Knowledge, Attitudes, and Practices in Urban Slums in Nairobi, Kenya*; Population Council: Nairobi, Kenya; Ideas Evidence Impact: New York, NY, USA, 2020.
53. Sarria-Guzmán, Y.; Fusaro, C.; Bernal, J.E.; Mosso-González, C.; González-Jiménez, F.E.; Serrano-Silva, N. Knowledge, Attitude and Practices (KAP) towards COVID-19 pandemic in America: A preliminary systematic review. *J. Infect. Dev. Ctries* **2021**, *15*, 9–21. [CrossRef]
54. Gupta, P.K.; Kumar, A.; Joshi, S. A review of knowledge, attitude and practice towards COVID-19 with future directions and open challenges. *J. Public Aff.* **2020**, e2555. [CrossRef]
55. Kaliyaperumal, K. Guideline for conducting a knowledge, attitude and practice(KAP) study. *AECS Illum.* **2004**, *4*, 7–9.
56. Hosmer, D.W.; Lemeshow, S. Goodness-of-fit tests for the multiple logistic regression model. *Comm. Stat, A.* **1980**, *9*, 1043–1069. [CrossRef]
57. Qutob, N.; Awartani, F. Knowledge, attitudes and practices (KAP) towards COVID-19namong Palestinians during the COVID-19 outbreak: A cross-sectional survey. *PLoS ONE* **2021**, *16*, e0244925. [CrossRef] [PubMed]
58. Gallè, F.; Veshi, A.; Sabella, E.A.; Çitozi, M.; Da Molin, G.; Ferracuti, S.; Liguori, G.; Orsi, G.B.; Napoli, C.; Napoli, C. Awareness and Behaviors Regarding COVID-19 among Albanian Undergraduates. *Behav. Sci.* **2021**, *11*, 45. [CrossRef] [PubMed]
59. Ali, M.; Uddin, Z.; Banik, P.C.; Hegazy, F.A.; Zaman, S. Knowledge, attitude, practice and fear of COVID-19: A cross-cultural study. *medRxiv* **2020**, *26*, 20113233. [CrossRef]
60. Awan, M.I.; Shamim, A.; Ahn, J. Implementing cleanliness is half of faith in re-designing tourists, experiences and salvaging the hotel industry in Malaysia during COVID-19 pandemic. *J. Islamic Mark.* **2020**. [CrossRef]
61. Nuskiya, M.H.F.; Mubarak, K.; Mufeeth, M. COVID-19 Crisis and recovery of hotel industry: A strategic focus on Tourism sector in Srilanka. *J. Tour. Econ. Appl. Res.* **2020**, *4*. [CrossRef]
62. Teng, X.; Teng, Y.M.; Wu, K.S.; Chang, B.G. Corporate Social Responsibility in Public Health During the COVID-19 Pandemic: Quarantine Hotel in China. *Front Public Health* **2021**, *9*, 620930. [CrossRef]
63. Al-Hanawi, M.K.; Angawi, K.; Alshareef, N.; Qattan, A.M.N.; Helmy, H.Z.; Abudawood, Y. Knowledge, attitude and practice toward COVID-19 among the public in the Kingdom of Saudi Arabia: A cross-sectional study. *Front. Public Health* **2020**, *8*, 217–227. [CrossRef]
64. Lee, M.; Kang, B.A.; You, M. Knowledge, attitudes, and practices (KAP) toward COVID-19: A cross-sectional study in South Korea. *BMC Public Health* **2021**, *21*, 1–10. [CrossRef]

55. Erfani, A.; Shahriarira, R.; Ranjbar, K.; Mirahmadizadeh, A.; Moghadami, M. Knowledge, attitude and practice toward the Novel Coronavirus (COVID-19) Outbreak: A population-based survey in Iran. *Bull. World Health Organ.* **2020**. [CrossRef]
56. Rahman, A.; Sathi, N.J. Knowledge, attitude and preventive practices toward Covid-19 among Bangladeshi internet users. *Electron. J. Gen. Med.* **2020**, *17*, em245. [CrossRef]
57. Tang, K.H.D. Movement control as an effective measure against Covid-19 spread in Malaysia: An overview. *Z. Gesundh. Wiss.* **2020**, 1–4. [CrossRef] [PubMed]

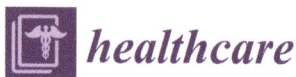 

Article

# An Examination of COVID-19 Mitigation Efficiency among 23 Countries

Emily Chia-Yu Su [1,2], Cheng-Hsing Hsiao [3], Yi-Tui Chen [3,*] and Shih-Heng Yu [4,*]

1. Graduate Institute of Biomedical Informatics, College of Medical Science and Technology, Taipei Medical University, Taipei 11031, Taiwan; emilysu@tmu.edu.tw
2. Clinical Big Data Research Center, Taipei Medical University Hospital, Taipei 11031, Taiwan
3. Department of Health Care Management, College of Health Technology, National Taipei University of Nursing and Health Sciences, Taipei 11219, Taiwan; alvul4@hotmail.com
4. Department of Business Management, National United University, Miaoli 36003, Taiwan
* Correspondence: yitui@ntunhs.edu.tw (Y.-T.C.); shihhengyu@gmail.com (S.-H.Y.); Tel.: +886-2-2822-7101 (ext. 6120) (Y.-T.C.); +886-3-7381-616 (S.-H.Y.)

**Abstract:** The purpose of this paper was to compare the relative efficiency of COVID-19 transmission mitigation among 23 selected countries, including 19 countries in the G20, two heavily infected countries (Iran and Spain), and two highly populous countries (Pakistan and Nigeria). The mitigation efficiency for each country was evaluated at each stage by using data envelopment analysis (DEA) tools and changes in mitigation efficiency were analyzed across stages. Pearson correlation tests were conducted between each change to examine the impact of efficiency ranks in the previous stage on subsequent stages. An indicator was developed to judge epidemic stability and was applied to practical cases involving lifting travel restrictions and restarting the economy in some countries. The results showed that Korea and Australia performed with the highest efficiency in preventing the diffusion of COVID-19 for the whole period covering 105 days since the first confirmed case, while the USA ranked at the bottom. China, Japan, Korea, and Australia were judged to have recovered from the attack of COVID-19 due to higher epidemic stability.

**Keywords:** COVID-19; stay-at-home order; mitigation efficiency; epidemic stability

Citation: Su, E.C.-Y.; Hsiao, C.-H.; Chen, Y.-T.; Yu, S.-H. An Examination of COVID-19 Mitigation Efficiency among 23 Countries. *Healthcare* **2021**, 9, 755. https://doi.org/10.3390/healthcare9060755

Academic Editor: Daniele Giansanti

Received: 18 April 2021
Accepted: 10 June 2021
Published: 18 June 2021

**Publisher's Note:** MDPI stays neutral with regard to jurisdictional claims in published maps and institutional affiliations.

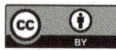

**Copyright:** © 2021 by the authors. Licensee MDPI, Basel, Switzerland. This article is an open access article distributed under the terms and conditions of the Creative Commons Attribution (CC BY) license (https://creativecommons.org/licenses/by/4.0/).

## 1. Introduction

The COVID-19 pandemic has been raging across the world since the beginning of 2020, resulting in a substantial death toll. As of 30 May 2021, the World Health Organization (WHO) indicated that more than 216 countries, areas, and territories were found to have more than 169 million confirmed cases associated with 3.53 million deaths [1]. When the epidemic broke out, the governments of most countries in the world adopted various response strategies including viral tests to identify infected persons, wearing masks and practicing social distancing to prevent infection, and closing schools and businesses, etc., to slow the spread of the epidemic. After a period of hard work, the epidemic situation in some countries significantly improved, while in others, it was still deteriorating. The number of daily new confirmed cases in some countries has fallen to single or double digits, but in some other countries, it has not reached its peak and continues to increase. This shows that the response strategies adopted in each country may have different effects on the mitigation of COVID-19 transmission.

How different response strategies affect the mitigation of new confirmed cases was analyzed by several studies. For example, Ding and Li [2] discussed the performances of various response strategies in fighting against COVID-19. Patrikar et al. [3] presented a mathematical model to predict the peak of the epidemic based on different levels of response strategies such as social distancing. Chen et al. [4] examined the effectiveness of transmission mitigation in association with the response strategies. However, very few studies focus on the analysis of the epidemic mitigation efficiency.

In this paper, we attempt to measure the relative efficiency in preventing the spread of COVID-19 using the data envelopment analysis (DEA) technique. In practice, the DEA technique has been widely used in various applications, including health industries [5,6], energy sectors [7–9], cement industries [10], agricultural production [11,12], and manufacturing sectors [13], and it has proven to be an effective approach in identifying the best practice frontiers.

In the field of medical services, DEA was also widely used to measure the efficiency of hospitals in association with patient visits, surgeries, and discharges. For example, Khushalani and Ozcan [14] employed a dynamic network DEA to examine the efficiency of production quality in hospitals and found that urban and teaching hospitals were less likely to improve quality production efficiency. Deily and McKay [15] used efficiency scores obtained from a DEA analysis as explanatory variables to determine hospital efficiency. In other fields, Oggioni et al. [10] employed DEA to analyze efficiency by using energy as an input and one desired output accompanied by undesired outputs ($CO_2$ emissions). Mousavi-Avval et al. [11] and Mohammadi et al. [12] applied the DEA technique to measure the efficiency of agricultural production to identify wasteful energy. Vazhayil and Balasubramanian [9] showed that the weight-restricted stochastic DEA method was appropriate to optimize power sector strategies.

To compare the mitigation efficiency among countries on a fair basis, the time period for each stage was calculated from the date of the first confirmed case in each country. The whole period covers 105 days from the first confirmed case and was divided into six stages. In addition to the measurement of overall efficiency covering 105 days, the efficiency at each stage was also evaluated. Firstly, the purpose of this article was to compare the relative efficiency of each country in mitigating the spread of the COVID-19 epidemic. Secondly, the trends of efficiency rank across stages for each country were analyzed. Eventually, an indicator for epidemic stability was developed to judge the status of epidemic stability for each country.

## 2. Research Methods

To compare the relative efficiency in preventing and reducing the spread of COVID-19, a total of 23 countries were selected, including 19 countries in the G20 and four other representative countries, as listed in Table 1. The reason for the selection of Iran and Spain was due to their high levels of confirmed cases and deaths. Pakistan and Nigeria were chosen due to their large populations, which reached 220.9 million and 206.1 million, respectively, at the end of 2020 [16].

Table 1. The starting and ending dates of each stage for each country.

| Country | Stage 1 | Stage 2 | Stage 3 | Stage 4 | Stage 5 | Stage 6 |
|---|---|---|---|---|---|---|
| China | 2019/12/31–2020/1/30 | 2020/1/31–02/14 | 02/15–02/29 | 02/30–03/15 | 03/16–03/30 | 03/31–04/14 |
| Japan | 01/15–02/14 | 02/15–02/29 | 03/01–03/15 | 03/16–03/30 | 03/31–04/14 | 04/15–04/29 |
| Korea | 01/20–02/19 | 02/20–03/05 | 03/06–03/20 | 03/21–04/04 | 04/05–04/19 | 04/20–05/04 |
| USA | 01/23–02/22 | 02/23–03/08 | 03/09–03/23 | 03/24–04/07 | 04/08–04/22 | 04/23–05/07 |
| Australia, France | 01/25–02/24 | 02/25–03/10 | 03/11–03/25 | 03/26–04/09 | 04/10–04/24 | 04/25–05/09 |
| Canada | 01/27–02/26 | 02/27–03/12 | 03/13–03/27 | 03/28–04/11 | 04/12–04/26 | 04/27–05/11 |
| Germany | 01/28–02/27 | 02/28–03/13 | 03/14–03/28 | 03/29–04/12 | 04/13–04/27 | 04/28–05/12 |
| India | 01/30–02/29 | 03/01–03/15 | 03/16–03/30 | 03/31–04/14 | 04/15–04/29 | 04/30–05/14 |
| Italy | 01/31–03/01 | 03/02–03/16 | 03/17–03/31 | 04/01–04/15 | 04/16–04/30 | 05/01–05/15 |
| Russia, Spain, UK | 02/01–03/02 | 03/03–03/17 | 03/18–04/01 | 04/02–04/16 | 04/17–05/01 | 05/02–05/16 |
| Iran | 02/20–03/21 | 03/22–04/05 | 04/06–04/20 | 04/21–05/05 | 05/06–05/20 | 05/21–06/04 |
| Brazil, Pakistan | 02/27–03/28 | 03/29–04/12 | 04/13–04/27 | 04/28–05/12 | 05/13–05/27 | 05/28–06/11 |
| Nigeria | 02/28–03/29 | 03/30–04/13 | 04/14–04/28 | 04/29–05/13 | 05/14–05/28 | 05/29–06/12 |
| Mexico | 02/29–03/30 | 03/31–04/14 | 04/15–04/29 | 04/30–05/14 | 05/15–05/29 | 05/30–06/13 |
| Indonesia | 03/02–04/01 | 04/02/04/16 | 04/17–05/01 | 05/02–05/16 | 05/17–05/31 | 06/01–06/15 |
| Saudi Arabia | 03/03–04/02 | 04/03–04/17 | 04/18–05/02 | 05/03–05/17 | 05/18–06/01 | 06/02–06/16 |
| Argentina | 03/04–04/03 | 04/04–04/18 | 04/19–05/03 | 05/04–05/18 | 05/19–06/02 | 06/03–06/17 |
| South Africa | 03/06–04/05 | 04/06–04/20 | 04/21–05/05 | 05/06–05/20 | 05/21–06/04 | 06/05–06/19 |
| Turkey | 03/12–04/11 | 04/12–04/26 | 04/27–05/11 | 05/12–05/26 | 05/27–06/10 | 06/11–06/25 |

The WHO [1] divided the stages of transmission into (1) no cases reported or observed (Stage 0); (2) imported cases (Stage 1); (3) localized community transmission (Stage 2); and (4) large-scale community transmission (Stage 3). As the date of the first confirmed case varied across countries, the period of each stage was not based on the same date among these countries but was calculated instead from the date of the first confirmed case in each country. The date of the first confirmed case was identified based on the daily situation report released by the WHO [1] starting on 21 January 2020. Among the 23 counties selected, China, Japan, and Korea reported having confirmed cases of COVID-19 before 21 January 2020. The information released from the WHO [1] demonstrated that some cases of pneumonia of unknown etiology were detected in Wuhan City, Hubei Province, China, on 31 December 2019. On 7 January 2020, a new type of coronavirus was isolated and identified. Thus, the first case in China may be considered to have occurred at the end of 2019. According to the WHO [1], the first confirmed cases of COVID-19 in Japan and Korea were reported on 15 and 20 January 2020, respectively.

The overall efficiency was compared based on the whole period covering 105 days since the first confirmed case for each country. The development process of COVID-19 spread was separated into 6 stages. As the number of new confirmed cases reported in earlier days is much lower, Stage 1 covers the first 30 days after the first confirmed case in each country. Each stage from Stage 2 to Stage 6 covered 15 days. The starting and ending dates of each stage for each country are listed in Table 1.

### 2.1. The DEA Model

In this paper, the DEA model was employed to measure the mitigation efficiency regarding the spread of COVID-19 at each stage for each country. The DEA model, proposed by Charnes et al. [17] based on the frontier production function defined by Farrell [18], is a nonparametric technique for measuring the relative efficiency of each decision-making unit (DMU) [19]. The mitigation of COVID-19 transmission in each country was executed by a technology whereby $N$ countries in terms of DMUs transform a non-negative vector of multiple inputs, denoted $x = (x_1, \ldots, x_m) \in \Re_+^m$, into a non-negative vector of multiple outputs, denote $y = (y_1, \ldots, y_s) \in \Re_+^s$. This paper employed the basic DEA model of Charnes, Coopers, and Rhodes (CCR) to calculate the efficiency of COVID-19 transmission mitigation. The CCR model, under the hypothesis of constant returns to scale, is expressed as follows:

$$\text{Min} \quad \theta$$
$$\text{s.t.} \quad \theta x_0 - X\lambda \geq 0$$
$$Y\lambda \geq y_0 \quad (1)$$
$$\lambda \geq 0$$

where $y_0$ is the output, $x_0$ is the input, $X$ and $Y$ are the datasets in the matrices, $\lambda$ is a semipositive vector, and $\theta$ represents the technical efficiency.

After the efficiency at each stage was obtained, Pearson correlation tests were conducted between the different stages at a $p$-value $< 0.01$ to examine the variation in efficiency ranks across stages. The correlation tests were used to explain the impact of the efficiency ranks at previous stages on subsequent stages.

In this paper, epidemic stability (ES) is defined as the recovery status from the epidemic, and the indicator ES is presented by measuring the average increase in the proportion of confirmed cases to population (PCCP) during the period of the last day of Stage 6 and a day designated to restart the economy, expressed as follows:

$$ES = \frac{S_f - S_0}{\Delta t} \quad (2)$$

where $S_f$ and $S_0$ denote the PCCP on the last day of Stage 6 and the designated day, respectively, and $\Delta t$ represents the period between the two dates.

### 2.2. The Variables

Efficiency, described as the relative performance regarding the reduction in COVID-19 transmission, was measured in this paper using the DEA method and is stated in the form of an output/input ratio. The objective of the authority administration was to minimize the total confirmed cases that occurred in each stage with a given amount of resources used. Cooper et al. [19] suggested that the DEA technique can be easily applied to a multiple input–output framework to compare the relative efficiency among various DMUs. The information produced from the DEA is valuable for identifying specific efficient units for future learning [20].

Neiderud [21] suggested that the rise of megacities may yield potential risks for new epidemics and become a threat in the world. The high human population density and close human-to-human contact are major sources for the rapid spread of respiratory diseases or avian flu. The growth and density of the human population may work as an incubator for infectious diseases, and urbanization as a driver of disease may have a negative effect on public health [22,23]. Thus, variables including (1) newly confirmed cases $n$, (2) population density $d$, and (3) urbanization degree $u$ for each country were employed to measure the relative efficiency. As more confirmed cases represent less efficiency, newly confirmed cases $n$ was treated as an input variable in Equation (1) to measure mitigation efficiency. In essence, the higher the population density and urbanization of a country are, the greater the chance of infection is. Thus, population density $d$ and urbanization degree $u$ were treated as output variables in Equation (1) for the measurement of mitigation efficiency.

*2.3. Data Collection*

The data for accumulated confirmed cases were extracted from the daily situation reports from the WHO [1], and the total confirmed cases in each stage were calculated by the difference in the accumulated confirmed cases on the last day of each stage and the previous stage. The population density data for each country were provided by Worldometer [24], and the urbanization degree data were extracted from the World Bank [16]. The descriptive statistics for the total accumulated confirmed cases across the 6 stages (i.e., 105 days since the first confirmed case), population density and urbanization degree are presented in Table 2. By the end of Stage 6 (i.e., 105 days since the first confirmed case), the USA had 1,193,452 confirmed cases, ranking at the top of the 23 countries, while Australia had the lowest number (6914) of confirmed cases. Korea had the highest population density at 527.30 persons per km$^2$, while Australia had a much lower population density at 3.32 persons per km$^2$. Argentina had the largest urbanization degree at 92% and ranked at the top. In contrast, the urbanization degree of India was much lower than the average of 71.48% based on the other countries and was only 34%.

Table 2. Descriptive statistics of study variables.

| Statistics | Total Confirmed Cases $n$ | Population Density $d$ (Person Per km$^2$) | Urbanization Degree $u$ (%) |
| --- | --- | --- | --- |
| Max. | 1,193,452 | 527.30 | 92.00 |
| Min. | 6914 | 3.32 | 34.00 |
| Average | 190,093 | 151.40 | 71.48 |
| Standard deviation | 260,495 | 146.28 | 15.45 |

The efficiency score was calculated through the assistance of the software DEA solver 13.

## 3. Results

The efficiency of COVID-19 mitigation covering the first 105 days after a confirmed case for each of the countries is depicted in Figure 1. Australia and Korea rank at the top in terms of mitigation efficiency. In contrast, the USA ranks at the bottom, followed by Brazil and Russia. The major cause affecting the efficiency rank may be attributed to the number of total confirmed cases occurring over the whole period. The total confirmed cases in Australia and Korea in the whole period (covering 105 days since the first confirmed case) were only 6667 cases and 10,801 cases, respectively, while the USA, Brazil, and Russia had 1,193,452; 739,503, and 272,043 cases, respectively.

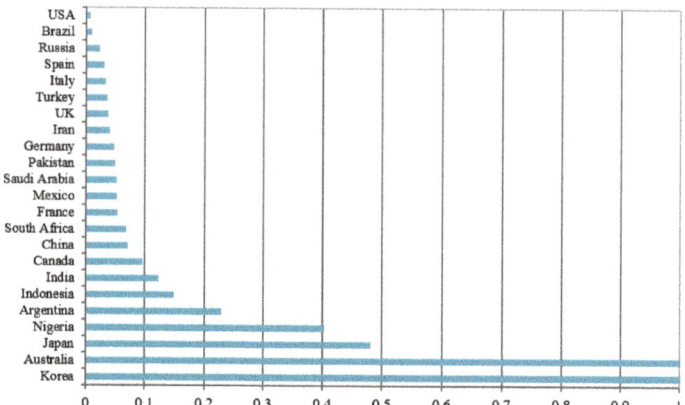

**Figure 1.** Mitigation efficiency scores among the 23 countries.

The efficiency scores and ranks at each stage for each country were also calculated according to Equation (1). Based on the shape of the efficiency ranking trend, these countries were classified into five types, as depicted in Figure 2.

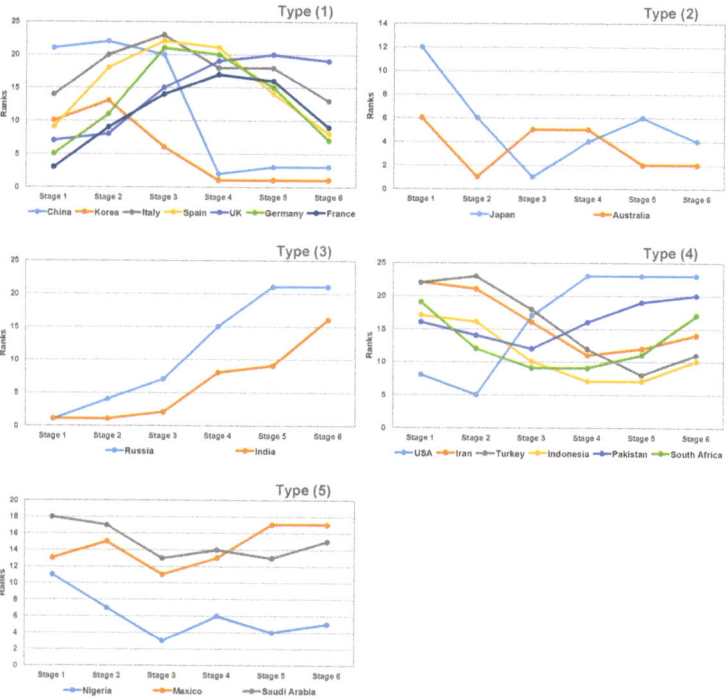

**Figure 2.** The trends in efficiency rank for countries of Types (1)–(5).

### 3.1. Type (1): An Inverted U-Shaped Pattern Including Korea, China, Italy, Spain, UK, Germany, and France

This pattern in the efficiency rank trends was characterized by a continual decline in mitigation efficiency from Stage 1, which, after reaching the lowest point in the efficiency ranks, continued to improve until the last stage (Stage 6). Efforts to mitigate newly confirmed cases through the implementation of response strategies may have eventually achieved a certain effect. In essence, the mitigation efficiency in Type (1) gradually deteriorated in the middle stages. Passing through the peak of daily new confirmed cases, the COVID-19 transmission was then reduced, and the efficiency started to improve through the last stage. For example, Italy ranked 14th in Stage 1 and then dropped to 20th in Stage 2. Italy then reached a peak of daily confirmed cases, amounting to 6557 cases on 22 March 2020, which occurred in Stage 3. After Stage 3, the COVID-19 transmission in Italy improved, and the efficiency rank rose to 13th place in Stage 6. The efficiency ranks for China after Stage 3 and for Korea after Stage 2 showed great improvement and attained a relatively more stable state. China ranked 21st place and 22nd place at Stage 1 and Stage 2, respectively, but the efficiency rank was improved to 2nd place at Stage 4 and 3rd place at Stages 5 and 6 through a great number of emergency response strategies. Similar to China, Korea ranked in 10th place and 13th place for mitigation efficiency at Stages 1 and 2, respectively, and the efficiency improved to 6th place at Stage 3 and first place at Stage 4, which was subsequently maintained until the final stage. The other countries showed similar processes, but the degree of efficiency improvement was different.

### 3.2. Type (2): An Inverted N-Shaped Pattern Including Japan and Australia

In this type, the efficiency rank fluctuated across stages, with initial improvements followed by deterioration in the middle stages, but eventually, the efficiency rank improved in the final stages. For example, the efficiency rank for Japan improved continuously from 12th place in Stage 1 to 6th place in Stage 2 to first place in Stage 3, then dropped to 4th place in Stage 4 and 6th place in Stage 5, and eventually improved to 4th place again.

### 3.3. Type (3): Continual Decreases in Efficiency Rank Including Russia and India

The trend pattern in efficiency rank for Type (3) countries is characterized by the gradual deterioration in mitigation efficiency. The efficiency ranks are not bad in the earlier stages, but they worsen progressively. For example, Russia performed at the highest level regarding mitigation efficiency in Stage 1 and was ranked in first place. Unfortunately, Russia did not maintain this advantage, and its rank continued to deteriorate to 4th place in Stage 2 and, finally, to 21st place in Stage 6.

### 3.4. Type (4): U-Shaped Pattern Including the USA, Iran, Turkey, Indonesia, Pakistan, South Africa, Argentina, and Brazil

This trend in the efficiency ranks is characterized by some improvements in mitigation efficiency in the middle stages that eventually rebound back to a worse state. For example, the response in the USA to avoid COVID-19 transmission was not bad in Stages 1 and 2, as it ranked in 8th place and 5th place, respectively. However, its efficiency continually and dramatically dropped after Stage 2 and fell to 23rd place (the bottom of the ranking) in Stages 5 and 6. The efficiency improvement from Stage 1 to Stage 2 in the USA may be attributed to its prompt travel restrictions on China from 2 February 2020 and additional travel restrictions on Iran, Italy, and Korea on 29 February [25]. The gradual deterioration in efficiency ranking in the later stages in the USA implies that its response strategies may be ineffective for avoiding the epidemic.

The trend pattern in the efficiency ranking for Brazil provides a different story. From Stage 1 to Stage 6, the efficiency ranks for Brazil were not good. On 25 June 2020 (the final observation point in Stage 6) in Brazil, newly confirmed cases remained at a high level, amounting to 39,436 cases. This implies that the response strategies adopted by Brazil contained flaws.

### 3.5. Type (5): N-Shaped and W-Shaped Patterns Including Mexico, Nigeria, and Saudi Arabia

An N-shaped pattern for Mexico and W-shaped patterns for Nigeria and Saudi Arabia were identified. At the middle stages, the efficiency ranks for these Type (5) countries fluctuated very much. For example, Mexico ranked 13th place at Stage 1 and then dropped and rose in the middle stages, eventually dropping again to 17th place at Stage 6. As the efficiency for these two patterns drops again in the last stages, this implies that the mitigation efficiency is not stable and that the future trends for these countries are not optimistic.

To examine the impact of the efficiency rank at the previous stage on the subsequent stage, a Pearson correlation test of efficiency scores between different stages was conducted. The results are listed in Table 3. The correlation coefficient between Stage 1 and Stages 4–6 was very low, ranging from 0 to $-0.1433$. In contrast, the correlation coefficient was 0.788 between Stage 4 and Stage 5, 0.760 between Stage 4 and Stage 6, and 0.983 between Stage 5 and Stage 6. Table 3 also shows that the greater the distance is between any two stages, the lower the correlation coefficient is.

**Table 3.** Correlations of mitigation efficiency between different stages.

|         | Stage 1    | Stage 2    | Stage 3   | Stage 4    | Stage 5    | Stage 6 |
|---------|------------|------------|-----------|------------|------------|---------|
| Stage 1 | 1          |            |           |            |            |         |
| Stage 2 | 0.6739 *** | 1          |           |            |            |         |
| Stage 3 | 0.4048 **  | 0.5666 *** | 1         |            |            |         |
| Stage 4 | −0.1433    | 0.0210     | 0.4297 ** | 1          |            |         |
| Stage 5 | −0.0982    | 0.1918     | 0.2002    | 0.7884 *** | 1          |         |
| Stage 6 | −0.0824    | 0.1401     | 0.1783    | 0.7602 *** | 0.9828 *** | 1       |

**: $p \leq 0.05$; ***: $p \leq 0.01$.

A numerical example is presented in this paper, in which it was proposed that the travel restrictions were lifted on the designed date of 27 June 2020; $ES$, $S_f$, $S_0$, and $\Delta t$ were calculated according to Equation (2) for these 23 countries, and the results are listed in Table 4, where $S_f$ and $S_0$ are measured by cases per 100,000 persons, $\Delta t$ in days, and $ES$ by cases per 1,000,000 persons. The ranking of each country listed in Table 4 is based on the value of epidemic stability ($ES$).

Table 4 indicates that India has the lowest value of $S_0$ (PCCP in 105 days), amounting to 5.65 cases per 100,000 persons, a slightly lower value than that of China (5.81 cases per 100,000 persons). In contrast, Spain and Saudi Arabia have the highest values of $S_0$, amounting to 492.32 and 379.30 cases per 100,000 persons, respectively, which are much higher than the average of 172.19 cases per 100,000 persons. However, the ranking of the PCCP on 27 June 2020 ($S_f$) changes very much. China ranks at the top with the lowest $S_f$, amounting to 5.92 cases per 100,000 persons. The PCCP in India increases very much from 5.65 at $S_0$ to 36.88 cases per million at $S_f$. The USA has the highest value at $S_f$, amounting to 727.37 cases per 100,000 persons.

Table 4 also demonstrates that the $ES$ in China, Japan, Korea, and Australia is much better than that in the other countries, amounting to 0.01, 0.46, 0.68, and 0.89 cases per million persons per day, respectively, during the period between the last day of Stage 6 and 27 June 2020. In contrast, the $ES$ in Brazil, Saudi Arabia, South Africa, and the USA reaches 143.67, 93.97, 85.78, and 71.92 cases per million persons per day, respectively. Based on the values of $ES$, it is suggested that the future trends regarding the pandemic in Brazil, Saudi Arabia, South Africa, and the USA are not optimistic and are full of challenges.

Table 4. The epidemic stability for each country by rank.

| DMU | $S_0$ | $S_f$ | $\Delta t$ | ES | Rank |
|---|---|---|---|---|---|
| China | 5.81 | 5.92 | 74 | 0.01 | 1 |
| Japan | 12.04 | 14.47 | 59 | 0.46 | 2 |
| Korea | 21.07 | 24.68 | 54 | 0.68 | 3 |
| Australia | 27.11 | 29.78 | 30 | 0.89 | 4 |
| Nigeria | 7.06 | 11.3 | 15 | 2.83 | 5 |
| Indonesia | 13.99 | 18.74 | 12 | 3.95 | 6 |
| Germany | 203.51 | 230.64 | 46 | 5.90 | 7 |
| Italy | 368.99 | 396.88 | 43 | 6.49 | 8 |
| India | 5.65 | 36.88 | 44 | 7.10 | 9 |
| Spain | 492.32 | 530.22 | 42 | 9.02 | 10 |
| France | 209.24 | 239.23 | 30 | 10.00 | 11 |
| Turkey | 227.25 | 230.63 | 2 | 16.92 | 12 |
| Canada | 180.16 | 271.9 | 47 | 19.52 | 13 |
| Pakistan | 54.12 | 90.04 | 16 | 22.45 | 14 |
| UK | 348.69 | 455.71 | 42 | 25.48 | 15 |
| Iran | 191.32 | 259.22 | 21 | 32.33 | 16 |
| Mexico | 103.91 | 157.41 | 14 | 38.21 | 17 |
| Argentina | 72.54 | 116.07 | 10 | 43.53 | 18 |
| Russia | 186.41 | 430.09 | 42 | 58.02 | 19 |
| USA | 360.56 | 727.36 | 51 | 71.92 | 20 |
| South Africa | 141.45 | 210.07 | 8 | 85.78 | 21 |
| Saudi Arabia | 379.3 | 501.46 | 13 | 93.97 | 22 |
| Brazil | 347.9 | 577.77 | 16 | 143.67 | 23 |

$S_0$: epidemic stability on the designated date (27 June 2020); $S_f$: the last day of Stage 6; $\Delta t$: the period between the designated date and the last day of Stage 6; ES: epidemic stability.

## 4. Discussion

The DEA in this paper shows that Korea, Australia, and Japan had better mitigation efficiency by 27 June 2020, while the USA, Brazil, and Russia performed less efficiently and were ranked at the bottom. Ahn [26] suggested that the successful experience in Korea to counter COVID-19 spread may be attributed to the mass testing and effective contact tracking system. Individuals testing positive for the infection after viral tests were hospitalized at special facilities. The people who had been in contact with the infected were to remain self-quarantined for 14 days. The availability of personal protective equipment was ensured to have a sufficient supply to avoid further infection at the onset of COVID-19 in Korea. In contrast, the testing capacity has not been sufficient to support the policies of a gradual reopening of the economy planned in many US states [27].

### 4.1. The Trend Patterns in Efficiency Ranks

The trend patterns in efficiency ranks also revealed information about future trends regarding epidemic mitigation. Type (1) and Type (2) countries may have more optimistic chances regarding recovery from the spread of COVID-19, as the efficiency ranks of Type (1) and Type (2) countries were high in Stage 6.

The Type (1) countries included the following seven countries: Korea, China, Italy, Spain, the UK, Germany, and France.

In addition to Korea, the other countries implemented effective responsive strategies, including extensive viral tests, lockdowns, social distancing, temporary cessation of sports events, school closures, and wearing of masks. In China, testing policies were promoted by expanding the testing of individuals from persons with symptoms to the open public on 12 February 2020, and all levels of school were closed on 26 January 2020 [28,29]. China has successfully slowed the transmission of COVID-19 through a combination of lockdowns, viral tests, contacting tracing, and other minor strategies, including street sanitization, school closures, and wearing of masks. Strict lockdowns and strict checks to avoid close contact between people were implemented in China after the outbreak. In less than three months, China gradually eased the strict policy of the lockdown and started to motivate the opening of economic activities. The strict lockdowns, wearing of masks, and social distancing implemented in China may be the major contributors to the effective prevention of transmission in a short time.

In contrast, the response of European countries such as Italy was not as prompt and urgent as that in Korea or China, and their efficiency ranks after Stage 4 were worse. For example, schools in Italy closed on 2 March 2020, and people were asked to stay at home, with exceptions for daily exercise and grocery shopping, on 23 February 2020. However, the testing policy adopted in Italy focused on testing anyone with COVID-19 symptoms after 26 February [28,29]. However, the efficiency ranks for the UK in the later stages (Stages 4–6) were much worse than those of other European countries. In March 2020, the UK attempted to reduce the impact of COVID-19 by means of herd immunity, but later, it denied the claims of herd immunity and argued that herd immunity is a natural by-product of an epidemic [30]. Given this situation, the strategy to fight against the epidemic was delayed, and thus, the effect was reduced.

Type (2) countries consisted of only Japan and Australia, with overall efficiency ranks of first and third place, respectively. In the middle stages, the efficiency ranks initially improved and then grew worse. A possible cause for these changes in efficiency ranks may be the low levels of viral testing in the earlier stages.

Extensive viral tests were performed in Australia and amounted to nearly 1000 tests per 100,000 people in the population by 31 March 2020 [31]. This number continued to increase and reached 2081 tests per 100,000 people on 28 April 2020 and 3119 tests per 100,000 people on 9 May 2020 (the final observation point in Stage 6 for Australia). The high testing rate in Australia may have been a major factor in mitigating the increase in new cases and leading it to have the best overall efficiency among these 23 countries.

In contrast, the trend in efficiency ranks for Type (3) countries showed a continual deterioration in mitigation efficiency. Compared to other countries, the coronavirus testing rate per capita in India was very low, reaching a total of 144,910 tests in a population with more than 1.3 billion people by 9 April 2020 [32]. On 14 May 2020 (the final observation point in Stage 6 for India), the viral testing rate was only 1.41 tests per 1000 people [29]. The low testing rate may be a key factor in explaining the good performance based on the high-efficiency ranking from Stage 1 to Stage 4. Without testing, no data are generated; thus, higher efficiency scores are obtained. As of 27 June 2020, the total number of confirmed cases in India reached 508,953, which was about 6.5 times the total number of confirmed cases of 78,003 during the entire period as of 14 May 2020.

At the onset of the outbreak, Russia announced a temporary ban on Chinese citizens from entering Russia on 20 February 2020 [25]. This strategy may have been effective in preventing infection through imported cases from China in Stage 1 and Stage 2. Extensive testing had been conducted in Russia, including 0.32 tests per 1000 people on 5 March 2020, 1.12 tests per 1000 people on 22 March 2020, 4.38 tests per 1000 people on 4 April 2020, 11.06 tests per 1000 people on 16 April 2020, 27.04 tests per 1000 people on 2 May 2020, and 45.61 tests per 1000 people on 16 May 2020 (the last day of Stage 6). However, Russia's health department admitted that the test kits were often wrong and provided false-negative results. Therefore, the tested people with the virus were allowed to go home and thus infected other people. Thus, the real number of infected individuals was more than triple the official figure [33]. The ineffective tests may explain the continual deterioration in efficiency scores for Russia.

Type (4) countries contained the following nine countries: the USA, Iran, Turkey, Canada, Indonesia, Pakistan, South Africa, Argentina, and Brazil. If the current trends for these countries continue into the future, the outcomes do not look optimistic regarding the epidemic, and these countries need to devote more effort to improving mitigation in newly confirmed cases as their efficiency ranks were poor in the final stages. Some Type (4) countries lacked testing capacity in the earlier stages of the pandemic, and thus, the amount of testing that was performed was much lower than needed. Due to having less viral testing than the actual need, underestimation of newly confirmed cases may have taken place and led to the illusion of efficiency improvement, but eventually, efficiency ranks dropped in the final stages.

In the USA, the total number of tests performed relative to the size of the population before 7 March 2020 was very low, at less than 0.01 tests per 1000 people, and the situation gradually improved in March 2020 (in Stage 3). The testing rate increased to 0.23 tests per 1000 people by the end of March 2020 (in Stage 4) and then quickly increased to 10.43 tests per 1000 people on 16 April 2020 (in Stage 5). On the day of the final observation point in Stage 6 (7 May 2020), the testing rate rose to 24.63 tests per 1000 people, which seems to be a good figure compared to that of other countries. However, several experts have criticized the fact that the testing levels were not sufficient to meet the need for a gradual reopening by 1 May 2020 [27]. In addition, existing flaws in other response strategies also blocked improvements in the efficiency rank for the USA. For example, the US Centers for Disease Control and Prevention (CDC) emphasized the importance of mask-wearing, but Donald Trump continued to reject being photographed in public wearing a mask [34]. Some experts have suggested that the guidelines for mask-wearing have been confusing. Thus, many protesters across the country are described as people who refuse to wear a mask [35].

In fact, the USA has not been positively and seriously prepared for epidemic mitigation since the first confirmed case occurred on 23 January 2020. On 23 April 2020, Trump suggested injecting a powerful disinfectant into coronavirus patients as a possible cure for COVID-19. This news resulted in criticism from many scholars and reporters and disbelief and derision worldwide [36].

The trends in efficiency ranks for Type (5) countries, including Mexico, Nigeria, and Saudi Arabia, fluctuated more than those of the other country types. The testing rate in Mexico ranged from 0.01 to 3.1 tests per 1000 people during the whole period, which was much lower than that in other countries. Thus, the mitigation efficiency of Mexico ranked 17th among the 23 countries in Stage 5 and Stage 6. On 13 June 2020 (the final day of Stage 6 for Nigeria), the testing rate was 0.44 tests per 1000 people. Nigeria had a lower testing rate than Mexico, but the efficiency ranks for Nigeria were not bad. Thus, we reasonably suspect that the high-efficiency ranks of Nigeria may have been caused by an underestimation due to low viral testing rates.

*4.2. The Correlation of Efficiency Ranks among Various Stages*

Table 3 indicates that the correlation coefficient between two adjacent stages was higher than that between two non-adjacent stages. The correlation coefficients between Stage 1 and each stage after Stage 3 were low and negative. The negative or near-zero correlation coefficients between Stage 1 and Stages 4–6 imply that the efficiency ranking of the sampled countries at Stages 4–6 had been reorganized and completely differed from that at Stage 1. This implies that at Stage 1, some countries started to implement effective response strategies such as extensive viral testing, lockdowns, wearing of masks, etc., to prevent the spread of COVID-19 and thus created improved effects at Stages 4–6. In contrast, some countries purposely neglected the serious and emergent impacts arising from COVID-19 spread and failed to take any measures in response to the emergence of the epidemic. On the other hand, the high correlation coefficients between Stage 4 and Stage 5, Stage 4 and Stage 6, and Stage 5 and Stage 6 imply that the relative efficiency ranks among these countries became stable because their response strategies had stabilized.

The efficiency ranks in some countries showed a high degree of fluctuation across stages, especially the Type (5) countries. The high fluctuation in efficiency ranks implied that good efficiency rankings at a particular stage were only temporary and may have deteriorated in the next stage. The mitigation efficiency rankings for Type (3) countries continually worsened from Stage 1 to Stage 6. Thus, the Type (3) countries could not recover from the attack of COVID-19 in a short time and would have to adopt stricter response policies to mitigate the spread of COVID-19. Type (4) countries showed a U-shaped pattern, demonstrating temporarily improved ranks in the middle stages, but eventually, the ranking regressed in the final stages.

Both the inverted U-shaped (Type 1) and inverted N-shaped (Type 2) patterns in the trends in efficiency ranks seemed to be a good sign of improvement, as the efficiency ranks increased in the last stages. The probability of recovering from the attack of COVID-19 for Type (1) and (2) patterns is higher than that for other patterns. Nevertheless, the overall efficiency was calculated based on the whole period covering 105 days since the first confirmed case. The efficiency obtained was only temporary and could change for the better or worse if the assessment stage was extended to cover more days.

### 4.3. The Epidemic Stability

At the beginning of June 2020, the infectious disease COVID-19 remained a high risk in the world, but many countries have since attempted to lift the state of lockdown, restart the economy, and take action, as their governments have considered that the number of confirmed cases was greatly reduced and that newly diagnosed cases may be considered sporadic cases. For example, Trump attempted to end the lockdown and the stay-at-home order and to reopen schools at the beginning of June 2020 [37].

There was a high correlation between the efficiency scores in two adjacent stages, but it was still difficult to predict the epidemic stability of the next stage based on that of the previous stage. Thus, the data of the newly confirmed cases for the current dates are only for reference to determine the timing of restarting the economy. This paper suggests that an epidemic stability indicator in combination with a trend pattern of efficiency ranks such as Type (1) or (2) may be employed to judge the appropriateness of any measures to ease the response strategies such as travel restrictions, stay-at-home orders, and mask-wearing.

Low values of epidemic stability imply that the trend regarding the epidemic has attained a stable state and approached zero confirmed cases. Thus, China, Japan, Korea, and Australia seem to have recovered from the attack of COVID-19, while Brazil, Saudi Arabia, South Africa, and the USA remain engaged in the battle against COVID-19 and are required to devote more effort to create new opportunities. On 27 June 2020, China, Japan, Korea, and Australia had 24, 100, 51, and 37 daily new confirmed cases [1], respectively, being much lower than the peak of daily new confirmed cases for each country. In contrast, at the end of June 2020, Brazil and the USA continually set new records for daily new confirmed cases. The number of newly confirmed cases on 27 June 2020 was 39,483, 3938, 6215, and 40,526 cases for Brazil, Saudi Arabia, South Africa, and the USA, respectively [1].

On 30 June 2020, the European Council announced the easing of travel restrictions from 1 July 2020 for residents of recommended countries, including Australia, Japan, Korea, China, and Canada [38]. As indicated in Table 4, China, Japan, Korea, and Australia ranked first to fourth in epidemic stability. Canada was slightly behind in 13th place. To examine the appropriateness of lifting the travel restrictions at the external borders for residents of these countries, we used the data for 27 June 2020 as an example. On that day, the number of newly confirmed cases in China, Japan, Korea, Australia, and Canada was 24, 100, 51, 37, and 380, respectively, equivalent to a stability of 0.0168, 0.791, 0.995, 1.451, and 10.068 cases per million per day. The *ES* on 27 June 2020 in China, Japan, Korea, and Australia was much lower than the value of Germany's *ES* (Table 4). This implies that the spread of COVID-19 had been controlled in these countries and was more stable than in Germany. The *ES* value on 27 June 2020 for Canada was nearly the same as that for France, as indicated in Table 4. However, Canada showed a U-shaped pattern for the trend in efficiency ranks, and it is suggested that the EU wait and observe the efficiency trend and the newly confirmed cases for Canada. Thus, the results suggest that the lifting of travel restrictions for these countries, with the exception of Canada, is quite reasonable based on the indicator of epidemic stability and the trends in efficiency ranking presented in this paper.

## 4.4. The Effect of Vaccination on Changes in Efficiency Ranks

Since the outbreak of the epidemic, many countries have devoted efforts to develop vaccines for COVID-19 to mitigate the transmission of the virus. As of April 2021, several vaccines were authorized by many countries for public use, including Pfizer-BioNTech, Moderna, BBIBP-CorV, CoronaVac, Covaxin, Sputnik V, AstraZeneca, and Johnson & Johnson [39]. By the end of May 2021, 1.17 billion doses of COVID-19 vaccines had been administered in the world [40]. The starting data of vaccination for these 23 countries and the cumulative vaccination rate by 25 May 2021 are listed in Table 5, according to which China and Russia started vaccinations earlier than other countries did, starting from 15 December 2020. Nigeria was the last country to start the vaccination program on 24 March 2021 among these 23 countries.

Table 5. The vaccination starting date, cumulative vaccination rates by 25 May 2021, and efficiency ranking in the weeks of 4–10 January (Rank1) and 17–23 May 2021 (Rank2).

| Country | Vaccination Starting Date | Vaccination Rates [#] by 25 May 2021 | Rank1 | Rank2 |
|---|---|---|---|---|
| UK | 2021/1/3 | 91.32 | 23 | 9 |
| USA | 2020/12/20 | 86.48 | 21 | 13 |
| Canada | 2020/12/16 | 58.13 | 13 | 17 |
| Germany | 2020/12/27 | 56.52 | 14 | 16 |
| Spain | 2021/1/4 | 54.07 | 22 | 14 |
| Italy | 2020/12/27 | 53.54 | 17 | 15 |
| France | 2021/1/5 | 49.85 | 19 | 20 |
| China | 2020/12/15 | 39.37 | 1 | 1 |
| Saudi Arabia | 2021/1/6 | 38.49 | 3 | 8 |
| Turkey | 2021/1/14 | 33.81 | 15 | 10 |
| Brazil | 2021/1/19 | 30.38 | 18 | 22 |
| Argentina | 2020/12/31 | 25.07 | 16 | 23 |
| Mexico | 2020/12/27 | 21.49 | 11 | 7 |
| Russia | 2020/12/15 | 18.92 | 12 | 12 |
| Australia | 2021/2/23 | 14.88 | 2 | 3 |
| India | 2021/1/16 | 14.38 | 7 | 21 |
| Korea | 2021/2/26 | 11.79 | 6 | 4 |
| Indonesia | 2021/1/22 | 9.43 | 8 | 6 |
| Japan | 2021/2/22 | 8.38 | 9 | 11 |
| Iran | 2021/3/19 | 3.74 | 10 | 18 |
| Pakistan | 2021/3/14 | 2.43 | 5 | 5 |
| South Africa | 2021/2/19 | 1.18 | 20 | 19 |
| Nigeria | 2021/3/24 | 0.94 | 4 | 2 |

[#] unit: doses per 100 people.

Typically, individuals need two weeks after a one-dose vaccine or after vaccination of the second dose of a two-dose vaccine to have full protection against the COVID-19 virus [41]. Thus, the analysis of the effect of vaccination on efficiency change started from the beginning of 2021. The ranking of mitigation efficiency in the period of 4–17 January 2021 across countries was compared with that in the period of 10–23 May 2021.

As of 25 May 2021, the UK and the USA had the highest cumulative vaccination rate, reaching 91.32 doses and 86.48 doses per 100 people indicated in Table 5, much more than that of other countries. In contrast, Nigeria and South Africa had only 0.94 doses and 1.18 doses per 100 people, ranking at the bottom. Table 5 also lists the mitigation efficiency rank for these countries in the period of 4–17 January 2021 (in terms of Rank1) and in the period of 10–23 May 20 (in terms of Rank2). Among these 23 countries, the efficiency rankings of the UK and the USA changed the most. After the start of the vaccination program, the efficiency of the UK and of the USA was greatly improved, from 23rd and 21st place in the period of 4–17 January 2021 to 9th and 13th place in the period of 10–23 May 2021, respectively.

The improvement in the ranking of mitigation efficiency in the United Kingdom and the United States can be explained by the substantial reduction in newly confirmed cases in these two countries. The reduction rate of newly confirmed cases in the UK was 97%, from 417,620 cases in the week of 4–10 January 2021 to 12,466 cases in the week of 17–23 May 2021. The newly confirmed case number in the USA decreased from 1,786,773 cases in the week of 4–10 January 2021 to 188,410 cases in the week of 17–23 May 2021, with a reduction rate of 89.45%. This implies that the vaccination programs implemented in these two countries have made a great contribution to protecting the public from infection.

In contrast, the country with the most regressive efficiency ranking was India, which dropped from 7th place in the period of 4–17 January 2021 to 21st place in the period of 10–23 May 2021. The major reason for the efficiency drop in India may be the rapid increase in newly confirmed cases from 126,319 daily cases in the week of 4–10 January 2021 to 1,846,055 cases in the week of 17–23 May 2021. A possible cause for the surge in COVID-19 includes the easing of social distancing and mask-wearing as well as more human contacts due to mass political rallies for recent elections and religious events [42]. Compared to other countries, the vaccination rates in India were not bad, reaching 14.38 doses per 100 people, although this was much lower than the required herd immunity threshold of 65–70% vaccine coverage rates [43], equivalent to about 130–140 doses per 100 people. The case of the pandemic in India shows that the surge of the epidemic in a country is possible even if vaccination programs have been started.

Compared with the UK and the USA, the cumulative vaccination rate of European countries and Canada as of 25 May 2021, shown in Table 5, is 49.85 to 58.13 doses per 100 people, which is about 33–44% lower than that of the UK and the USA. However, the improvement in the mitigation efficiencies in these European countries and Canada is not so obvious as in the UK and the USA. This paper suggests that only when a country's vaccination rate reaches a certain level can the spread of the epidemic be slowed down.

## 5. Conclusions

At the onset of the COVID-19 infection in different populations, mass testing programs and effective tracing systems on infected people were implemented in some countries, such as China and Korea. Based on the trends in efficiency ranks and the epidemic stability indicators, China, Korea, Japan, and Australia have performed better than other countries have. Thus, this paper suggests that mass testing together with other strategies such as contact tracing, lockdowns, mask-wearing, and social distancing are significantly effective in mitigating the transmission of COVID-19. Testing suspected persons identified through contact tracing and reducing interpersonal contacts through complete or partial lockdown also play important roles in reducing the number of confirmed cases. Castillo et al. [44] examined the effect of the stay-at-home policy on COVID-19 infection rates and found that the infection rate decreased from 0.113/day pre-policy to 0.047/day post-policy. Ferguson et al. [45] found that a lockdown may result in an average reduction in COVID-19 transmission by 50%, school closure by 20%, and other measures by approximately 10% (cited from Willis et al. [46]). Some other studies have also presented the same conclusions that non-pharmaceutical interventions may effectively prevent the spread of infection [47,48].

Pearson's correlation tests were also performed in this paper to examine the impact of efficiency at earlier stages on that in subsequent stages and showed that the efficiency ranks for each country dramatically changed across stages. Due to insufficient testing facilities, the number of confirmed cases may be underestimated at the initial stages. Thus, the mitigation efficiency scores in the earlier stage might be less accurate. The main contribution of this paper is first that it demonstrates the relative mitigation efficiencies of various countries in various stages of the pandemic. Secondly, this paper integrates epidemic stability indicators with the obtained efficiency trends to judge the appropriateness of reopening the economy. While having not reached an appropriate level of epidemic stability, economic reopening may damage the anti-epidemic achievements from the earlier stages and lead to a second wave of the epidemic with exponential growth in the number of newly confirmed cases. In the future, a model needs to be developed to ensure the reliability of data on the number of confirmed cases reported by each country. In addition, the role of vaccines in affecting the spread of diseases may be worthy of attention.

**Author Contributions:** Conceptualization, E.C.-Y.S., C.-H.H., Y.-T.C., and S.-H.Y.; methodology, Y.-T.C. and S.-H.Y.; software, Y.-T.C. and C.-H.H.; formal analysis, E.C.-Y.S., C.-H.H., Y.-T.C., and S.-H.Y.; writing—original draft preparation, E.C.-Y.S. and Y.-T.C.; writing—review and editing, Y.-T.C., C.-H.H. and S.-H.Y. All authors have read and agreed to the published version of the manuscript.

**Funding:** This study was funded in part by the Ministry of Science and Technology (MOST) in Taiwan under grant number MOST 108-2410-H-227-008 to Yi-Tui Chen.

**Institutional Review Board Statement:** Not applicable.

**Informed Consent Statement:** Not applicable.

**Data Availability Statement:** The data for COVID-19 confirmed cases and vaccination rates can be found in WHO (https://www.who.int/emergencies/diseases/novel-coronavirus-2019/situation-reports, accessed on 18 June 2021) and Our World in Data (https://ourworldindata.org/covid-vaccinations, accessed on 18 June 2021), respectively.

**Conflicts of Interest:** The authors declare no conflict of interest.

## References

1. WHO (World Health Organization). Novel Coronavirus (2019-nCoV) Situation Reports. 2021. Available online: https://www.who.int/emergencies/diseases/novel-coronavirus-2019/situation-reports (accessed on 17 June 2021).
2. Ding, A.W.; Li, S. National response strategies and marketing innovations during the COVID-19 pandemic. *Bus. Horiz.* **2021**, *64*, 295–306. [CrossRef]
3. Patrikar, S.; Poojary, D.; Basannar, D.R.; Faujdar, D.S.; Kunte, R. Projections for novel coronavirus (COVID-19) and evaluation of epidemic response strategies for India. *Med. J. Armed Forces India* **2020**, *76*, 268–275. [CrossRef] [PubMed]
4. Chen, Y.T.; Yen, Y.F.; Yu, S.H.; Su, E.C. An Examination on the Transmission of COVID-19 and the Effect of Response Strategies: A Comparative Analysis. *Int. J. Environ. Res. Public Health* **2020**, *17*, 5687. [CrossRef]
5. Yaya, S.; Xi, C.; Xiaoyang, Z.; Meixia, Z. Evaluating the efficiency of China's healthcare service: A weighted DEA-game theory in a competitive environment. *J. Clean. Prod.* **2020**, *270*, 122431. [CrossRef]
6. Cavalieri, M.; Guccio, C.; Rizzo, I. On the role of environmental corruption in healthcare infrastructures: An empirical assessment for Italy using DEA with truncated regression approach. *Health Policy* **2017**, *121*, 515–524. [CrossRef] [PubMed]
7. Balitskiy, S.; Bilan, Y.; Strielkowski, W.; Štreimikienė, D. Energy efficiency and natural gas consumption in the context of economic development in the European Union. *Renew. Sustain. Energy Rev.* **2016**, *55*, 156–168. [CrossRef]
8. Da Cruz, N.; Carvalho, P.; Marques, R.C. Disentangling the cost efficiency of jointly provided water and wastewater services. *Util. Policy* **2013**, *24*, 70–77. [CrossRef]
9. Vazhayil, J.P.; Balasubramanian, R. Optimization of India's power sector strategies using weight-restricted stochastic data envelopment analysis. *Energy Policy* **2013**, *56*, 456–465. [CrossRef]
10. Oggioni, G.; Riccardi, R.; Toninelli, R. Eco-efficiency of the world cement industry: A data envelopment analysis. *Energy Policy* **2011**, *39*, 2842–2854. [CrossRef]
11. Mousavi-Avval, S.H.; Rafiee, S.; Mohammadi, A. Optimization of energy consumption and input costs for apple production in Iran using data envelopment analysis. *Energy* **2011**, *36*, 909–916. [CrossRef]
12. Mohammadi, A.; Rafiee, S.; Mohtasebi, S.S.; Avval, S.H.M.; Rafiee, H. Energy efficiency improvement and input cost saving in kiwifruit production using Data Envelopment Analysis approach. *Renew. Energy* **2011**, *36*, 2573–2579. [CrossRef]

13. Egilmez, G.; Kucukvar, M.; Tatari, O. Sustainability assessment of U.S. manufacturing sectors: An economic input output-based frontier approach. *J. Clean. Prod.* **2013**, *53*, 91–102. [CrossRef]
14. Khushalani, J.; Ozcan, Y.A. Are hospitals producing quality care efficiently? An analysis using Dynamic Network Data Envelopment Analysis (DEA). *Socio-Econ. Plan. Sci.* **2017**, *60*, 15–23. [CrossRef]
15. Deily, M.E.; McKay, N.L. Cost inefficiency and mortality rates in Florida hospitals. *Health Econ.* **2006**, *15*, 419–431. [CrossRef] [PubMed]
16. The World Bank. World Urbanization Prospects. 2020. Available online: https://data.worldbank.org/indicator/SP.URB.TOTL.IN.ZS?end=2018&start=1987 (accessed on 30 June 2020).
17. Charnes, A.; Cooper, W.W.; Rhodes, E. Measuring the efficiency of decision making units. *Eur. J. Oper. Res.* **1978**, *2*, 429–444. [CrossRef]
18. Farrell, M.J. The measurement of productive efficiency. *J. R. Stat. Soc. Ser. A (Gen.)* **1957**, *120*, 253–281. [CrossRef]
19. Cooper, W.W.; Seiford, L.M.; Tone, K. Data envelopment analysis: A comprehensive text with models, applications, references and DEA-solver software. *J.-Oper. Res. Soc.* **2001**, *52*, 1408–1409.
20. Hawdon, D. Efficiency, performance and regulation of the international gas industry—A bootstrap DEA approach. *Energy Policy* **2003**, *31*, 1167–1178. [CrossRef]
21. Neiderud, C.-J. How urbanization affects the epidemiology of emerging infectious diseases. *Infect. Ecol. Epidemiol.* **2015**, *5*, 27060. [CrossRef] [PubMed]
22. Lienhardt, C. From Exposure to Disease: The Role of Environmental Factors in Susceptibility to and Development of Tuberculosis. *Epidemiol. Rev.* **2001**, *23*, 288–301. [CrossRef]
23. Hayward, A.C.; Darton, T.; Van-Tam, J.N.; Watson, J.M.; Coker, R.; Schwoebel, V. Epidemiology and control of tuberculosis in Western European cities. *Int. J. Tuberc. Lung Dis.* **2003**, *7*, 751–757. [PubMed]
24. Worldometer. Countries in the World by Population. 2020. Available online: https://www.worldometers.info/world-population/population-by-country/6 (accessed on 17 June 2020).
25. Garda World. 2020. Available online: https://www.garda.com/crisis24/news-alerts/315171/russia-chinese-citizens-to-be-barred-entry-into-russia-from-february-20-update-7 (accessed on 2 July 2020).
26. Ahn, M. How South Korea Flattened the Coronavirus Curve with Technology. 2020. Available online: https://theconversation.com/how-south-korea-flattened-the-coronavirus-curve-with-technology-136202 (accessed on 21 April 2020).
27. Ferrier, K.; Hwang, S. How South Korea is Building Influence through COVID-19 Testing Kits. 2020. Available online: https://thediplomat.com/2020/04/how-south-korea-is-building-influence-through-covid-19-testing-kits/ (accessed on 30 April 2020).
28. Ritchie, H.; Ortiz-Ospina, E.; Beltekian, D.; Hasell, J.; Roser, M. Policy Responses to the Coronavirus Pandemic. 2020. Available online: https://ourworldindata.org/policy-responses-covid (accessed on 17 June 2020).
29. Ritchie, H.; Ortiz-Ospina, E.; Beltekian, D.; Mathieu, E.; Hasell, J.; Macdonald, B.; Giattino, C.; Appel, C.; Rodés-Guirao, L.; Roser, M.; et al. Statistics and Research: Coronavirus (COVID-19) Testing. *Our World in Data*. 2020. Available online: https://ourworldindata.org/coronavirus-data (accessed on 17 June 2020).
30. Barr, S. Coronavirus: What Is Herd Immunity and Is It a Possibility for the UK? 2020. Available online: https://www.independent.co.uk/life-style/health-and-families/coronavirus-herd-immunity-meaning-definition-what-vaccine-immune-covid-19-a9397871.html (accessed on 15 April 2020).
31. Tadros, E.; McIlroy, T.; Margo, J. Australia's Virus Testing Rate Leads World. 2020. Available online: https://www.afr.com/politics/federal/australia-s-testing-is-key-to-slower-infection-rate-20200401-p54fx7 (accessed on 10 July 2020).
32. Vaidyanathan, G. People Power: How India Is Attempting to Slow the Coronavirus. Without Enough Test Kits, the 1.3-Billion-Person Country Is Using a Gigantic Surveillance Network to Trace and Quarantine Infected People. 2020. Available online: https://www.nature.com/articles/d41586-020-01058-5 (accessed on 12 April 2020).
33. Tsvetkova, M. False Negative: Officials Say Russian Virus Tests Often Give Wrong Result. 2020. Available online: https://www.reuters.com/article/us-health-coronavirus-russia-tests/false-negative-officials-say-russian-virus-tests-often-give-wrong-result-idUSKBN22J347 (accessed on 8 May 2020).
34. Wibawa, T. Wearing a Mask in the United States is Political, But Republicans Are Speaking out as Coronavirus Cases Grow. 2020. Available online: https://www.abc.net.au/news/2020-07-01/coronavirus-masks-are-political-in-us-donald-trump-rejects-them/12403962 (accessed on 10 July 2020).
35. Coronavirus: Why Is There a US Backlash to Masks? Available online: https://www.bbc.com/news/world-us-canada-52540015 (accessed on 10 July 2020).
36. Eaton, M.; Borden King, A.; Emma, K.; Seigler, A. Trump Suggested 'Injecting' Disinfectant to Cure Coronavirus? We're Not Surprised. 2020. Available online: https://www.nytimes.com/2020/04/26/opinion/coronavirus-bleach-trump-autism.html (accessed on 26 April 2020).
37. NDTV. Trump Calls for Shift in COVID-19 Strategy to Allow End of US Lockdown. 2020. Available online: https://www.ndtv.com/world-news/coronavirus-president-donald-trump-calls-for-shift-in-covid-19-strategy-to-allow-end-of-us-lockdown-2241532 (accessed on 10 June 2020).
38. European Council. Council Agrees to Start Lifting Travel Restrictions for Residents of Some Third Countries. 2020. Available online: https://www.consilium.europa.eu/en/press/press-releases/2020/06/30/council-agrees-to-start-lifting-travel-restrictions-for-residents-of-some-third-countries/ (accessed on 30 June 2020).

39. Wikipedia. History of COVID-19 Vaccine Development. 2021. Available online: https://en.wikipedia.org/wiki/History_of_COVID-19_vaccine_development (accessed on 26 May 2021).
40. Our World in Data. Coronavirus (COVID-19) Vaccinations. 2021. Available online: https://ourworldindata.org/covid-vaccinations (accessed on 26 May 2021).
41. Colburn, N. How Long Does It Take for the COVID-19 Vaccine to Work? 2021. Available online: https://wexnermedical.osu.edu/blog/how-long-for-covid-vaccine-to-work (accessed on 26 May 2021).
42. Thiagarajan, K. Why Is India Having a Covid-19 Surge? *BMJ 2021*. 2021. Available online: https://www.bmj.com/content/373/bmj.n1124 (accessed on 29 May 2021).
43. BBC News. Covid: Israel May Be Reaching Herd Immunity. 2021. Available online: https://www.bbc.com/news/health-56722186 (accessed on 8 May 2021).
44. Castillo, R.C.; Staguhn, E.D.; Weston-Farber, E. The effect of state-level stay-at-home orders on COVID-19 infection rates. *Am. J. Infect. Control* **2020**, *48*, 958–960. [CrossRef] [PubMed]
45. Ferguson, N.; Laydon, D.; Nedjati Gilani, G.; Imai, N.; Ainslie, K.; Baguelin, M.; Bhatia, S.; Boonyasiri, A.; Cucunuba Perez, Z.; Cuomo-Dannenburg, G. Report 9: Impact of non-pharmaceutical interventions (NPIs) to reduce COVID19 mortality and healthcare demand. *Imp. Coll. Lond.* **2020**, *10*, 491–497.
46. Willis, M.J.; Diaz, V.H.G.; Prado-Rubio, O.A.; von Stosch, M. Insights into the dynamics and control of COVID-19 infection rates. *Chaos Solitons Fractals* **2020**, *138*, 109937. [CrossRef]
47. Aledort, J.E.; Lurie, N.; Wasserman, J.; A Bozzette, S. Non-pharmaceutical public health interventions for pandemic influenza: An evaluation of the evidence base. *BMC Public Health* **2007**, *7*, 208. [CrossRef]
48. Torner, N.; Soldevila, N.; Garcia-Garcia, J.J.; Launes, C.; Godoy, P.; Castilla, J.; Domínguez, A. Effectiveness of non-pharmaceutical measures in preventing pediatric influenza: A case-control study. *BMC Public Health* **2015**, *15*, 543. [CrossRef]

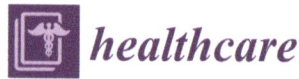 

*Article*

# Shedding Light on the Direct and Indirect Impact of the COVID-19 Pandemic on the Lebanese Radiographers or Radiologic Technologists: A Crisis within Crises

Rasha Itani [1], Mohammed Alnafea [2], Maya Tannoury [1], Souheil Hallit [3,4] and Achraf Al Faraj [1,*]

1. Department of Radiologic Sciences, Faculty of Health Sciences, American University of Science and Technology (AUST), Beirut 1100, Lebanon; Rasha_Itani@outlook.com (R.I.); mtannoury@aust.edu.lb (M.T.)
2. Department of Radiological Sciences, College of Applied Medical Sciences, King Saud University, Riyadh 11433, Saudi Arabia; alnafea@ksu.edu.sa
3. Faculty of Medicine and Medical Sciences, Holy Spirit University of Kaslik (USEK), Jounieh 1200, Lebanon; souheilhallit@hotmail.com
4. INSPECT-LB: National Institute of Public Health, Clinical Epidemiology and Toxicology, Beirut 1100, Lebanon
* Correspondence: achraf.alfaraj@gmail.com or aalfaraj@aust.edu.lb

**Citation:** Itani, R.; Alnafea, M.; Tannoury, M.; Hallit, S.; Al Faraj, A. Shedding Light on the Direct and Indirect Impact of the COVID-19 Pandemic on the Lebanese Radiographers or Radiologic Technologists: A Crisis within Crises. *Healthcare* 2021, 9, 362. https://doi.org/10.3390/healthcare9030362

Academic Editors: Eduardo Tomé, Thomas Garavan and Ana Dias

Received: 4 February 2021
Accepted: 21 March 2021
Published: 23 March 2021

**Publisher's Note:** MDPI stays neutral with regard to jurisdictional claims in published maps and institutional affiliations.

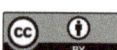

**Copyright:** © 2021 by the authors. Licensee MDPI, Basel, Switzerland. This article is an open access article distributed under the terms and conditions of the Creative Commons Attribution (CC BY) license (https://creativecommons.org/licenses/by/4.0/).

**Abstract:** With the novel coronavirus disease 2019 (COVID-19) pandemic, the need for radiologic procedures is increasing for the effective diagnosis and follow-up of pulmonary diseases. There is an immense load on the radiographers' shoulders to cope with all the challenges associated with the pandemic. However, amidst this crisis, Lebanese radiographers are also suffering from a socioeconomic crisis and record hyperinflation that have posed additional challenges. A cross-sectional study was conducted among registered Lebanese radiographers to assess the general, workplace conditions, health and safety, mental/psychologic, financial, and skill/knowledge development impacts. Despite applying an adapted safety protocol, institutions are neither providing free RT-PCR testing to their staff nor showing adequate support for infected staff members, thus causing distress about contracting the virus from the workplace. Aggravated by the deteriorating economic situation that affected the radiographers financially, they additionally suffer from severe occupational physical and mental burnout. Regardless of that, they used their free time during the lockdown for skill/knowledge development and have performed many recreational activities. This cross-sectional study highlighted the different ways the pandemic has impacted the radiographers: physically, psychologically, and financially. It aimed to shed light on what these frontline heroes are passing through in the midst of all these unprecedented crises.

**Keywords:** COVID-19; radiographers; radiology and medical imaging; safety protocols; social and economic consequences

## 1. Introduction

The outbreak of the SARS-CoV-2 virus in December 2019 through the increasing number of patients suffering from a new form of "viral pneumonia" and the declaration of the coronavirus disease 2019 (COVID-19) pandemic by the World Health Organization (WHO) have flipped the entire world upside down [1]. Despite having less fatality rate (3.4%) and milder symptoms than its precursors, SARS-CoV (9.6%) and MERS-CoV (35%), the new SARS-CoV-2 has faster human-to-human transmission [2], which has been clearly shown by its ability to infect over 83 million people around the globe within its first year [3]. By the end of the year 2020, several potential vaccines (i.e., Pfizer/BioNTech, Moderna, Oxford-AstraZeneca, Sputnik V, etc.) have cleared phase III trials and were approved by health authorities for emergency use [4]. Many countries around the globe have already started their vaccination campaigns, with high hopes of slowing down the spread of the disease. Despite showing more than 90% efficiency in clinical trials, there has been no concrete evidence thus far concerning possible adverse effects and long term immunity, as well as the mechanism of action in the elderly and those suffering from underlying health conditions [5]. Additionally, the sudden emergence of numerous strains worldwide, such as the B.1.1.7 (United Kingdom) and B.1.1.28 (South Africa) linages, added to their divergent mutations, the little known information about their severity, transmission, and resistance have all put the fate of the newly proposed treatments and vaccines at stake [6,7].

In addition to the frightening infection and deaths worldwide, COVID-19 has taken its toll on the global economy. With increasing infections and multiple forced lockdowns, many businesses, manufacturing companies, and organizations reduced their activities, sales, and overall productions, which, in turn, slowed down the global economy until it almost came into a "freeze" [8]. The global economic knockout has drastically affected healthcare workers, particularly the radiology department. With the increasing need of intensive care unit (ICU) beds, medications, and personal protective equipment (PPE) on one hand, and the reduction in admissions on the other hand due to fear of contracting the virus, hospitals are struggling to maintain their revenues [9]. Radiology departments worldwide are experiencing a significant drop in imaging volumes, especially screening services for breast and lung cancer, after the American College of Radiology (ACR) and Centers for Disease Control and Prevention (CDC) implemented several guidelines, some of which included postponing and rescheduling non-urgent patient visits [10].

As for Lebanon, a 10,452 $Km^2$ country located in the Middle East, the battle with controlling the viral spread is strenuous. With the first COVID-19 infection reported on 21 February 2020, Lebanon has faced many obstacles that hindered the ability to slow the spread of the virus among its inhabitants [11]. Despite the fact that Lebanon was not the pioneer in healthcare according to the WHO's report in 2000, holding the rank 91 [12], the country underwent various changes, reforms, and advancements to be ranked as the 23rd country worldwide in 2018 according to Bloomberg's Healthcare Efficiency Index [13]. However, according to the same index, the country has later on declined and ranked 48th in 2020 amid the pandemic, since Lebanon was less prepared for such a pandemic compared to other countries. Unfortunately, this efficient healthcare system is not free for its citizens. This has led many Lebanese people suffering from COVID-19 symptoms to skip performing necessary diagnostic tests and avoid hospital admission simply because they cannot afford the cost. In addition, in spite of having some of the most advanced hospitals, Lebanon, like many other countries, was not prepared for such pandemic due to the limited number of beds in the ICUs and the significant shortage in ventilators. Therefore, in spite of all efforts to "flatten the curve", Lebanon has recorded an exponential drastic increase in the daily number of cases and deaths. The reason behind that was the massive explosion that occurred at the Port of Beirut on 4 August 2020. The explosion killed over 200 people, injured more than 6000 others, and left around 300,000 people homeless [14], causing chaos in hospitals as well as a spike in the reported COVID-19-positive cases. Following the explosion, various essential hospitals in the capital were completely destroyed, thus putting more weight on the medical staff, especially the radiology department.

On top of that, due to political problems, Lebanon is suffering from a critically deteriorating economic crisis. The national currency, the Lebanese pound (LBP), is falling stiff against the United States dollar (USD). It lost about 80% of its value, thus causing a severe inflation in the country [15]. With inflation reaching terrifyingly high levels, Lebanon is currently ranked second worldwide in terms of hyperinflation according to the Hanke's Annual Inflation Rate model [16]. Besides increasing poverty level to 55% (compared to 28% in 2019) [17], this inflation negatively impacts the healthcare system as all products needed are imported in foreign currency (i.e., USD or EUR). Most healthcare institutions in the country are private hospitals and/or medical centers and laboratories. Therefore, there is a huge difficulty in coping with the increasing prices of materials and equipment, thus posing a risk to the staff's health and safety as institutions administrators can no longer afford adequate and/or good quality PPE and disinfecting/cleaning agents. This increases the threat to healthcare members, especially radiographers, of contracting the virus from the workplace and transmitting it to their family and/or loved ones. The worsening economic situation does not only strike the healthcare systems and staff in Lebanon financially, but also drains them of all energy and hospital beds by escalating the daily number of COVID-19-reported cases. Lebanese people are forced to break all lockdown rules and open their shops/businesses in order to put food on their tables and feed their families, a phenomenon accompanied by the absence of social distancing and precautions, thus reflecting a soar in COVID-19 cases and more pressure on the healthcare system.

Following international guidelines, thoracic imaging, especially chest radiography and chest Computed Tomography (CT), are being laboriously used in all hospitals and imaging centers in Lebanon as powerful tools for the diagnosis, detection of complications, and follow-up of COVID-19 patients [18]. Various studies have proven the importance of chest CT in detecting SARS-CoV-2 in patients with negative reverse transcription polymerase chain reaction (RT-PCR) results [19]. One study involving 1014 patients showed that chest CT scan had a higher sensitivity (97%) compared to RT-PCR [20]. In addition, a recent study proved the practicability of magnetic resonance imaging (MRI) in the detection of pulmonary changes and damage caused by COVID-19, thus proposing a potential radiation-free alternative to chest CT, especially when periodic, repetitive scans are required for follow-up [21]. Furthermore, the newly emerging artificial intelligence (AI)-based algorithms that have the ability to detect COVID-19 pneumonia on chest CT with approximately 90.8% accuracy, 84% sensitivity, and 93% specificity [22], can consequently enhance the paramount role radiographers and medical imaging play during the COVID-19 pandemic.

The huge workload on radiology departments in Lebanon, specifically on Lebanese radiographers or radiologic technologists, due to the ongoing pandemic, as well as the worsening economic situation, have led to many adverse effects such as irregular and disturbed shifts, loss of work, increased radiation exposure, deteriorating mental and physical health. There are currently no studies conducted in the region to point out the critical situation radiographers or radiologic technologists are going through. This study aimed to shed light on what the frontline heroes are going through in the midst of all these unprecedented crises, and evaluate factors associated with stress from contracting the COVID-19 virus from the workplace among radiography technicians.

## 2. Methods

### 2.1. Study Design

A cross-sectional study was conducted among radiographers or radiologic technologists registered in the Lebanese Society of Radiographers (LSR) in multiple hospitals and medical centers all over the country. They were requested to fill out an electronic survey specifically tailored to inquire how the pandemic affected them, their work, and their overall wellbeing, directly and indirectly. The study was conducted from 3 December 2020 until 17 December 2020.

### 2.2. Minimal Sample Size Calculation

On the basis of a population size of 325 active radiography technicians, and a 75.4% expected frequency of workplace-related stress after the outbreak [23], we found that the minimal sample size needed for bivariate and multivariable analysis was 152 according to the Epi-info software (Centers for Disease Control and Prevention, Atlanta, GA, USA) [24].

### 2.3. Questionnaire and Variables

The online survey, proposed in 3 languages (English, Arabic, and French), was distributed to all LSR registered members via the social network platforms (i.e., official WhatsApp groups of the syndicate). The survey was composed of 26 questions organized into 6 sections (general, workplace conditions, health and safety, mental/psychologic, financial, and skill/knowledge development questions). The first section aimed to study the demographical and educational status of the radiographers: age, gender, marital status, degree, and workplace type. The second section aimed to assess the changes made in the workplace: variability in shifts, overall changes in department workload, workflow, protocols, and safety measures (PPE use, disinfection, compulsory mask use). The next section discussed the impact of the virus on technologists' health and safety with questions evaluating whether they have contracted the virus, its severity, its transmission, and the need for any hospital admission. The following section analyzed the mental or psychologic outcome, with questions inquiring about the presence and severity of workplace-related stress, its impact on them and their family/loved ones, and the support received. The fifth section aimed to determine the financial impact of the pandemic on Lebanese radiographers by including questions concerning the monthly salary, the extent of modifications done to that salary, and whether the radiographers are considering quitting their jobs. The last section estimated a rather positive impact of the pandemic, especially during the lockdown periods and decreased shifts, in terms of skills and/or knowledge development with questions evaluating the use of free time in beneficial, recreational activities and the preferred type of activities.

*2.4. Statistical Analysis*

Descriptive, bivariate, and multivariable statistical analyses were conducted using Statistical Package for the Social Sciences (SPSS) v.25 (Armonk, NY, USA). The quantitative variables were expressed as percentages and comparisons were made using the chi-squared test. A multinomial regression was conducted, taking the stress/worry about contracting COVID-19 from the workplace categories (strongly disagree/disagree, agree/strongly agree, and neutral) as the dependent variable. The neutral group was taken as reference. The Nagelkerke pseudo $R^2$ values were also calculated to determine the variance explained by each independent variable of the outcome variable. Significance was set at $p < 0.05$.

## 3. Results

A total of 212 survey responses that accounted for 32.5% of overall registered radiologic technologists or 65.3% of active members was received. Out of the three survey languages available, the Arabic language was preferred by almost 46.23% ($n = 98$) of radiographers, then the English language with 39.62% ($n = 84$) submissions, followed by the French language with 14.15% ($n = 30$) submissions (Figure 1). As for the rest of the survey questions, the results of the three survey languages were combined.

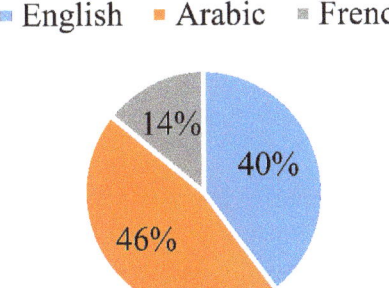

**Figure 1.** Pie chart showing the percentage distribution of the three languages: English, Arabic, and French (the percentages were rounded to the nearest whole number).

*3.1. General Questions*

Responses were received mainly from radiographers that belonged to the 20–29 age group (47.17%) and the 30–39 age group (31.13%), while only 1.89% of radiographers were above 60 years old. Concerning the gender distribution of radiographers, responses were almost equally distributed between males and females, with the percentage of males being slightly greater than that of females (51.42% vs. 48.58%, respectively). As for the marital status, results showed that 52.36% of participants were married, 38.21% were single, 8.02% were engaged, and only 1.41% were divorced. Concerning the highest degree in the field, participants held a T.S./L.T. (technical degrees) in Radiography with 36.32% submissions, 16.98% had a university diploma, 33.96% earned their Bachelor of Science (B.S.) degree, 8.02% had a Master of Science (M.S.) degree, and only 4.72% chose the "other" option and relied mainly on practical experience. Regarding the distribution of work locations, most of the participants (71.23%) worked in private hospitals, 14.62% in imaging centers, and only 10.83% in public hospitals. Table 1 summarizes the questions, answers, and percentages for this section.

**Table 1.** Table summarizing the questions, choices, and percentages concerning the general questions section.

| Question | Choices and Percentages | | | | |
|---|---|---|---|---|---|
| Age | 20–29 47.17% | 30–39 31.13% | 40–49 11.79% | 50–59 8.02% | 60+ 1.89% |
| Gender | Males 51.42% | | | Females 48.58% | |
| Marital Status | Single 38.21% | Engaged 8.02% | | Married 52.36% | Divorced 1.41% |
| Highest Degree | T.S./L.T. 36.32% | Diploma 16.98% | B.S. 33.96% | M.S. 8.02% | Others 4.72% |
| Work Location | Private Hospital 71.23% | Public Hospital 10.85% | | Lab/Medical Imaging Center 14.62% | Others 3.30% |

*3.2. Workplace Conditions during the Pandemic*

A total of 69.81% of participants agreed that the workload in the department was affected by the pandemic (agree (45.28%), strongly agree (24.53%)). Similarly, the highest percentage of participants (58.49%) agreed (agree (37.74%), strongly agree (20.75%)) that their shift duration and distribution were impacted by the pandemic. While voting for the modality that received the most workload, the most selected choices were CT and X-ray, with 47.87% and 38.53%, respectively. Participants were given the chance to select more than one option resulting in a total of 353 votes, 169 for CT and 136 for X-ray. When asked whether the institution is applying an adapted safety protocol for COVID-19 patients, 67.45% of votes agreed (agree (47.17%), strongly agree (20.28%)). In the same sense, most radiographers agreed that their institution is providing PPE and/or cleaning/disinfecting agents with around 69.81% of the votes (agree (43.87%), strongly agree (25.94%)). Likewise, 88.68% of the participants agreed (agree (32.08%), strongly agree (56.60%)) that their institution is forcing all patients, visitors, and staff to wear face masks. Figure 2 summarizes the questions, answers, and percentages for this section.

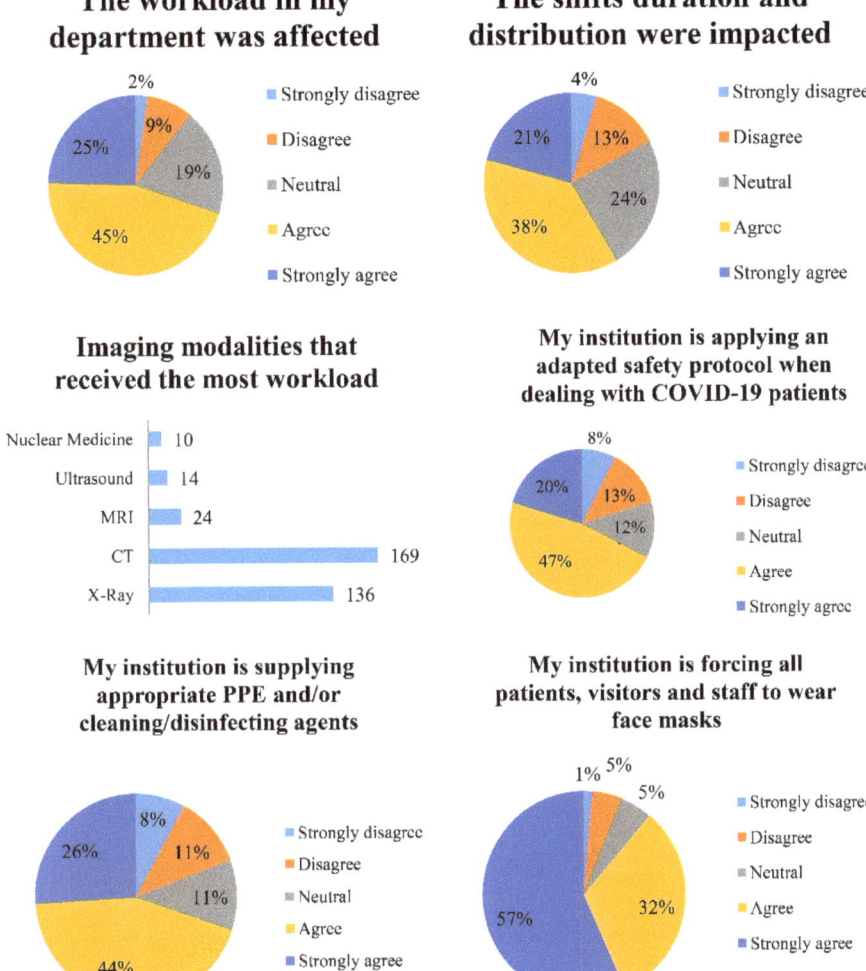

**Figure 2.** Pie charts summarizing the questions, choices, and percentages concerning the workplace conditions section.

*3.3. Health and Safety*

Responses showed that 64.15% of radiographers disagreed (disagree (25.00%), strongly disagree (39.15%)) that their institution is providing regular/periodic, free PCR testing for the staff, while only 25.94% agreed. The highest percentage of participants 74.53% did not contract the virus. Out of the 12.26% radiographers who caught the virus, 61.54% got it from the workplace, 34.62% suffered from mild symptoms, and 92.31% were not admitted to the hospital. Only 30.77% of infected radiologic technologists transmitted the virus to family members/friends/colleagues, while 50.00% did not, and 19.23% were not sure. Table 2 summarizes the questions, answers, and percentages for this section.

**Table 2.** Table summarizing the questions, choices, and percentages concerning the health and safety section.

| Question | Choices and Percentages | | | | |
|---|---|---|---|---|---|
| My institution is providing regular/periodic, free PCR testing for staff. | Strongly Disagree 39.15% | Disagree 25.00% | Neutral 9.91% | Agree 16.04% | Strongly Agree 9.90% |
| Have you contracted the virus? | Yes 12.26% | | No 74.53% | | I am not sure 13.21% |
| Is it from the workplace? | Yes 61.54% | | No 11.54% | | I am not sure 26.92% |
| What was the severity of the disease? | No symptoms 7.69% | | Mild symptoms 34.62% | Moderate symptoms 30.77% | Severe symptoms 26.92% |
| Were you admitted to the hospital? | | Yes 8.02% | | No 25.94% | |
| Did you transmit the virus to any family member/friend/colleague? | Yes 30.77% | | No 50.00% | | I am not sure 19.23% |

### 3.4. Financial Questions

Participants were asked to give an estimate (in LBP) of their original monthly salary provided by the institution, according to the work contract (Figure 3).

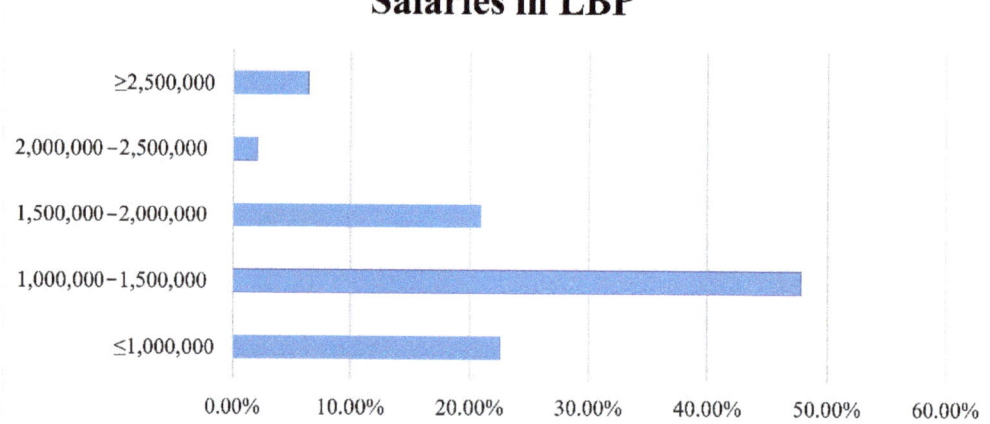

**Figure 3.** Bar graph presenting the percentages of salary ranges as disclosed by the participants.

While 60.85% of radiologic technologists had no change in their salary, 30.19% disclosed that they had 25–50% or even more than 50% reductions in their salary, whereas 4.24% were not getting paid their monthly salary. Moreover, 61.11% of participants disagreed (disagree (36.42%), strongly disagree (24.69%)) on leaving their job/staying home, while 35.80% had a different opinion. Table 3 summarizes the questions, answers, and percentages for this section.

**Table 3.** Table summarizing the questions, choices, and percentages concerning the financial questions section.

| Question | Choices and Percentages | | | | |
|---|---|---|---|---|---|
| To what extent did the institution modify/decrease the monthly salary provided to you in accordance with the economic situation? | Severely (>50% reduction) 6.13% | Moderately (25–50% reduction) 24.06% | No Change 60.85% | My salary was modified but what was reduced will be paid later on 4.72% | I am not getting paid my monthly salary 4.24% |
| I am considering leaving job/staying home, as it is not worth it. | Strongly Disagree 24.69% | Disagree 36.42% | Neutral 3.09% | Agree 25.31% | Strongly Agree 10.49% |

### 3.5. Mental/Psychological Questions

Concerning mental/psychological questions, 60.85% of radiographers agreed (agree (35.85%), strongly agree (25.00%)) that they were feeling stressed/worried about contracting the virus from the workplace. Similarly, 67.92% agreed (agree (45.75%), strongly agree (22.17%)) that their family members, friends, and/or loved ones were affected by this work-related stress. Furthermore, 43.86% of surveyors disagreed (disagree (20.75%), strongly disagree (23.11%)) that their institution is showing adequate social, psychological, and/or financial care/follow up for staff members who contracted the virus. Half of the participants disagreed (disagree (25.47%), strongly disagree (24.53%)) about thinking/planning to change the field of work and leave the healthcare system; 69.81% of responders agreed (agree (25.00%), strongly agree (44.81%)) about leaving the country to seek a better opportunity abroad, while only 16.04% voted for the opposite. Figure 4 summarizes the questions, answers, and percentages for this section.

### 3.6. Skill/Knowledge Development

More than half of the participants (65.09%) used their free time during the lockdown for skill development and/or knowledge expansion. Numerous options were selected regarding the kind of activities done, and many of the participants chose the "other" option. For simplicity, the kinds of activities done are summarized in the bar graph below (Figure 5).

### 3.7. Bivariate Analysis

A significantly higher percentage of persons who had a neutral opinion about the workload being affected by the pandemic agreed/strongly agreed that they are stressed and worried about contracting COVID-19 from the workplace (Table 4). No significant association was found between all other variables and the stress/worry about contracting COVID-19 from the workplace.

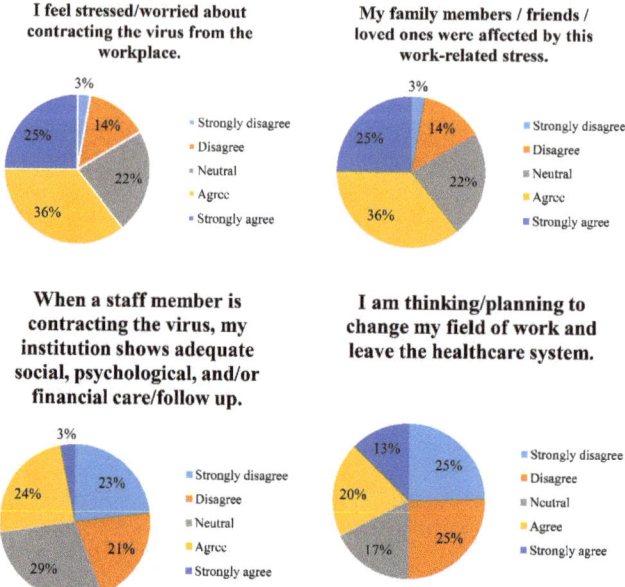

**Figure 4.** Pie charts summarizing the questions, choices, and percentages concerning the mental/psychological questions section.

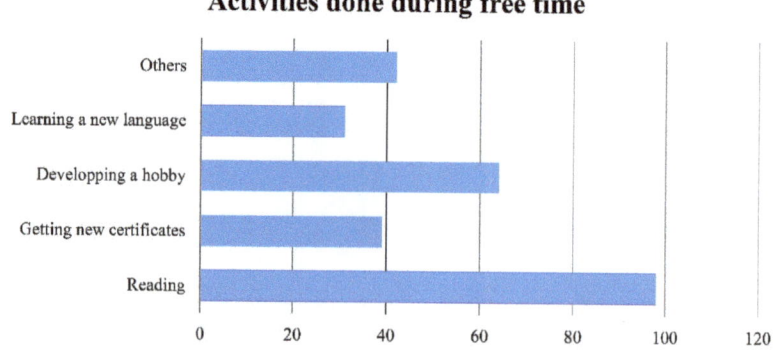

**Figure 5.** Bar graph summarizing the various types of recreational activities done by the participants during their free time in the lockdown.

Table 4. Bivariate analysis of factors associated with stress categories.

| Variable | Stress/Worry about Contracting COVID-19 from the Workplace | | | p |
|---|---|---|---|---|
| | Neutral | Strongly Disagree/Disagree | Agree/Strongly Agree | |
| **Age categories (in years)** | | | | 0.145 |
| 20–29 | 27 (26.5%) | 22 (21.6%) | 53 (52.0%) | |
| 30–39 | 16 (24.2%) | 9 (13.6%) | 41 (62.1%) | |
| 40–49 | 4 (16.0%) | 3 (12.0%) | 18 (72.0%) | |
| 50 and above | 1 (4.8%) | 3 (14.3%) | 17 (81.0%) | |
| **Gender** | | | | 0.238 |
| Male | 29 (26.6%) | 20 (18.3%) | 60 (55.0%) | |
| Female | 19 (18.1%) | 17 (16.2%) | 69 (65.7%) | |
| **Marital status** | | | | 0.841 |
| Single/engaged/divorced | 25 (24.3%) | 17 (16.5%) | 61 (59.2%) | |
| Married | 23 (20.7%) | 20 (18.0%) | 68 (61.3%) | |
| **Workload affected by the pandemic** | | | | **0.034** |
| Strongly disagree/disagree | 12 (29.3%) | 6 (14.6%) | 23 (56.1%) | |
| Neutral | 0 (0%) | 5 (21.7%) | 18 (78.3%) | |
| Agree/strongly agree | 36 (24.0%) | 26 (17.3%) | 88 (58.7%) | |
| **Shift duration distribution impacted during the pandemic** | | | | 0.204 |
| Strongly disagree/disagree | 12 (23.5%) | 4 (7.8%) | 35 (68.6%) | |
| Neutral | 8 (21.6%) | 5 (13.5%) | 24 (64.9%) | |
| Agree/strongly agree | 28 (22.2%) | 28 (22.2%) | 70 (55.6%) | |
| **Institution applies adapted safety protocol** | | | | 0.268 |
| Strongly disagree/disagree | 4 (15.4%) | 2 (7.7%) | 20 (76.9%) | |
| Neutral | 8 (18.6%) | 6 (14.0%) | 29 (67.4%) | |
| Agree/strongly agree | 36 (24.8%) | 29 (20.0%) | 80 (55.2%) | |
| **Institution supplying cleaning agents** | | | | 0.224 |
| Strongly disagree/disagree | 4 (17.4%) | 4 (17.4%) | 15 (65.2%) | |
| Neutral | 6 (14.6%) | 4 (9.8%) | 31 (75.6%) | |
| Agree/strongly agree | 38 (25.3%) | 29 (19.3%) | 83 (55.3%) | |
| **Institution forces mask wearing** | | | | 0.083 |
| Strongly disagree/disagree | 4 (36.4%) | 0 (0%) | 7 (63.6%) | |
| Neutral | 0 (0%) | 2 (15.4%) | 11 (84.6%) | |
| Agree/strongly agree | 44 (23.2%) | 35 (18.4%) | 111 (58.4%) | |

Numbers in bold indicate significant p-values.

### 3.8. Multivariable Analysis

The results of the regression, taking stress/worry about contracting COVID-19 from the workplace (agree/strongly disagree vs. neutral*) as the dependent variable, showed that having 50 or more years vs. 20–29 years (adjusted odds ratio (aOR) = 9.53; $p = 0.036$) was significantly associated with higher odds of agreeing/strongly agreeing about having stress/worry about contracting COVID-19 from the workplace (Table 5).

Table 5. Multinomial regression.

| Stress/Worry About Contracting COVID-19 from the Workplace (Agree/Strongly Agree vs. Neutral) | | | |
|---|---|---|---|
| Variable | aOR | p | 95% CI |
| Age categories (in years) | | 0.182 | |
| 20–29 | 1 | | |
| 30–39 | 1.28 | 0.531 | 0.59–2.79 |
| 40–49 | 1.69 | 0.407 | 0.49–5.81 |
| 50 and above | 9.53 | **0.036** | 1.16–78.30 |

Numbers in bold indicate significant p-values.

None of the variables were significantly associated with disagreeing/strongly disagreeing about having stress/worry about contracting COVID-19 from the workplace compared to neutral.

Variables entered in the model: workload affected by the pandemic, institution forces mask wearing, age categories (Nagelkerke pseudo $R^2$ = 21.3%); Nagelkerke pseudo $R^2$ for the variable workload affected by the pandemic = 6.9%; Nagelkerke pseudo $R^2$ for the variable institution forces mask wearing = 6.4%; Nagelkerke pseudo $R^2$ for the variable age categories = 6.8%; numbers in bold indicate significant $p$-values ($p < 0.05$).

## 4. Discussion

Radiology, especially chest X-ray and CT examinations, has played a crucial role and proven its effectiveness in the diagnosis and follow-up of pneumonia in COVID-19 patients, in addition to assessing better treatment protocols, including measurement of disease changes and predicting prognosis [25]. Radiologic technologists stand equal to, and side by side with, all doctors and nurses who are fighting hand-in-hand in this pandemic, deserving the title "frontline heroes". With the radiology department being the primary destination to all Emergency Room (ER) patients suffering from respiratory problems and suspected to be COVID-19-positive, the radiographers' roles and direct contact with these patients weigh no less than those of their medical colleagues.

This distinctive study is the first of its kind in the region and aimed to assess the direct and indirect impact of the ongoing COVID-19 pandemic on radiographers in a country severely affected by the COVID-19 pandemic, in addition to political and economic crisis.

Most radiologic technologists in the country are relatively young (belonging to the 20–29 age group), with the genders almost equally distributed between males and females. Institutions all over the country are facing a decrease in imaging volumes, as shown by the large number of radiographers who agreed/strongly agreed that the workload in their department and shifts were impacted. Similarly, many hospitals and imaging centers around the globe have also seen significant drops in non-urgent outpatient visits, imaging, and services, even below baseline values. Nevertheless, thoracic imaging volumes involving X-ray and CT were not severely impacted by the pandemic [26]. The results clearly show the vital role of X-ray and CT scan in this management, as they received the greatest amount of votes regarding the modalities, with most workload reflecting the important role of thoracic imaging in managing patients during the pandemic by detecting signs of COVID-19 pneumonia [27]. Most healthcare systems are implementing and adapted safety protocol when dealing with COVID-19 patients and are supplying the staff with the appropriate PPEs (i.e., masks, face shields, gloves, etc.) and cleaning/disinfecting agents. The strict rules concerning the compulsory use of face masks by patients, visitors, and staff also reflect the efficiency of institutions' efforts in controlling disease spread, a vital strategy that is implemented around the globe for disease handling and protection of the staff from infections [28]. Proven effective, a very high number of participants did not contract the virus. Those who did, on the other hand, suffered from mild to moderate symptoms and did not require hospital admission.

As for the financial aspect, the median monthly income of the Lebanese radiographers is 1661,125 LBP, which is relatively low compared to the high hyperinflation levels the country is suffering from and the fall of the Lebanese currency compared to foreign currencies, especially in black markets. The radiographer's average monthly salary that used to be equivalent to around 1096 USD pre-hyperinflation (official exchange rate 1 USD = 1515 LBP) now barely equals 144 USD (black market 1 USD = 11,500 LBP). Despite the economic crisis, more than half of the participants reported no change in their monthly income, yet a considerable number of radiographers are suffering from a 20 to 50% reduction in their salary. A struggle that reflects the fact that the middle-income level of the Lebanese population is shrinking. Regardless of all challenges and reductions, radiographers disagreed quitting their job and/or staying home, as they strongly hold onto their humane role and life-saving duties at all costs. The proceeding pandemic has affected Lebanese radiographers, not only physically, but mentally as well, with most radiologic technologists reporting increased stress and/or anxiety regrading contracting the virus from the workplace. This stress has also impacted their families, friends, and/or loved ones too. This stress and "burnout" does not only apply to Lebanese radiographers and their families, as it is also reported by countless radiographers universally who most suffer constant distress concerning the high risk of contracting the virus from COVID-19-positive patients when exposed to them without appropriate PPE [29]. Various studies and publications have heavily discussed how stress, especially at times of a pandemic such as COVID-19, may be a valuable variable in preventing the spread of the virus. Those suffering constant stress, mainly the elderly as shown in the statistical analysis, have an aggravated fear of getting infected by the virus, added to the fear of believing false information found online. These fears have a positive impact on these individuals, forcing them to constantly search for legitimate and scientific information and avoid false theories. Moreover, this "beneficial stress" may lead to the correct and efficient application of protection methods and the adoption of correct hygienic practices. However, the adverse effects of stress, especially over prolonged period the pandemic has been going as well as the forced lockdowns and frightening death toll, may outweigh the benefits. Prolonged exposure to stress can negatively impact body function, leading to morphological and functional changes in various parts of the brain like such as hippocampus (leading to memory and learning disorders), as well as amygdala and temporal lobe (resulting in cognitive, behavioral, and mood disorders). In addition, it was proven that stress can impair the immune system, thus leading to more illnesses [30]. Lebanese radiographers are passing through a highly stressful period, whether it be through physical, mental, financial, and/or work-related strain. Unfortunately, institutions in Lebanon do not show adequate social, psychological, and/or financial care or follow-up to the infected staff members, which, in turn, add up to the deteriorating mental health of radiographers in the country. In spite of that, they disagree on changing their field of work and leaving the healthcare system but, in turn, are planning to leave the country in hopes of seeking a better opportunity abroad.

In defiance of all the negative direct and indirect impacts COVID-19 had on the Lebanese radiographers, a significant number benefited from their free time during the lockdown to develop their skills, expand their knowledge, and engage in positive recreational activities. With learning a new language, developing a hobby, getting new certificates, and reading being the most frequent types of activities reported by the participants.

## 5. Conclusions

The unprecedented COVID-19 pandemic has adversely impacted the world—travel, tourism, the economy, etc., were all shaken and frozen. The greatest impact, however, struck the unprepared healthcare systems that are struggling with the rapid spread of this virus. Worn out and exhausted, frontline heroes do not hesitate when it comes to emergency situations and always answer their humane call. With the heavy workload falling on members of the radiology department, radiographers and radiologists had to cope with irregular shifts, increased radiation exposure, and serious risk of contracting the virus. Following international guidelines and adapting some of their own, the Lebanese radiographers spare no efforts when it comes to narrowing the viral spread in the country and saving lives. However, it is clear that radiographers in Lebanon are suffering from deteriorating physical and psychological health due to the constant stress, absence of any support from their healthcare instructions, added to the country's collapsing economy and increasing hyperinflation levels. With such tension and strain, not only the radiographers but any other member in the healthcare system passing through the same conditions cannot continue with the same productivity, motivation, enthusiasm, and power, and thus will collapse later on. This cross-sectional study highlighted all the obstacles, dangers, and challenges that radiographers or radiologic technologists in Lebanon are combatting whether physically, mentally, and/or financially. It also aims to provide better and safer workplace conditions together with more specifically adapted and robust workflow to fight not only the ongoing pandemic, but also future ones as well. Finally, with radiology being the "eye of medicine", radiographers should be appreciated just like other healthcare members as the pandemic warriors that wear lead aprons instead of capes.

**Author Contributions:** Conceptualization, R.I., M.T., and A.A.F.; methodology, M.A. and A.A.F.; validation, R.I., M.T., and A.A.F.; formal analysis, S.H., M.A., and M.T.; writing—original draft preparation, R.I. and A.A.F.; writing—review and editing, M.T., M.A., S.H., and A.A.F. All authors have read and agreed to the published version of the manuscript.

**Funding:** This research received no external funding.

**Institutional Review Board Statement:** Not applicable.

**Informed Consent Statement:** Not applicable.

**Data Availability Statement:** The data presented in this study are available on request from the corresponding author.

**Acknowledgments:** The authors would like first to salute all the radiographers and radiologic technologists, the "frontline heroes" in the ongoing fight against COVID-19, who participated in the survey. A special thanks to Paul Makdessi, the president of the Lebanese Syndicate of Radiographers, for his support and hard work in the midst of these crises.

**Conflicts of Interest:** The authors declare no conflict of interest.

## References

1. Sohrabi, C.; Alsafi, Z.; O'Neill, N.; Khan, M.; Kerwan, A.; Al-Jabir, A.; Iosifidis, C.; Agha, R. World Health Organization declares global emergency: A review of the 2019 novel coronavirus (COVID-19). *Int. J. Surg.* **2020**, *76*, 71–76. [CrossRef] [PubMed]
2. Fani, M.; Teimoori, A.; Ghafari, S. Comparison of the COVID-2019 (SARS-CoV-2) pathogenesis with SARS-CoV and MERS-CoV infections. *Future Virol.* **2020**. [CrossRef]
3. World Health Organization. *Novel Coronavirus (2019-nCoV) Situation Reports-Weekly Epidemiological Update-5 January 2021*; World Health Organization: Geneva, Switzerland, 2021.
4. Mishra, S.K.; Tripathi, T. One year update on the COVID-19 pandemic: Where are we now? *Acta Trop.* **2020**, *214*, 105778. [PubMed]
5. Chung, J.Y.; Thone, M.N.; Kwon, Y.J. COVID-19 vaccines: The status and perspectives in delivery points of view. *Adv. Drug Deliv. Rev.* **2021**, *170*, 1–25. [CrossRef] [PubMed]
6. Andrew Rambaut, N.L.; Pybus, O.; Barclay, W.; Barrett, J.; Carabelli, A.; Connor, T.; Peacock, T.; Robertson, D.L.; Volz, E. Preliminary Genomic Characterisation of an Emergent SARS-CoV-2 Lineage in the UK Defined by a Novel Set of Spike Mutations. Available online: https://virological.org/t/preliminary-genomic-characterisation-of-an-emergent-sars-cov-2-lineage-in-the-uk-defined-by-a-novel-set-of-spike-mutations/563 (accessed on 1 February 2021).
7. Volz, E.; Hill, V.; McCrone, J.T.; Price, A.; Jorgensen, D.; O'Toole, Á.; Southgate, J.; Johnson, R.; Jackson, B.; Nascimento, F.F.; et al. Evaluating the Effects of SARS-CoV-2 Spike Mutation D614G on Transmissibility and Pathogenicity. *Cell* **2021**, *184*, 64–75.e11. [CrossRef] [PubMed]
8. Nicola, M.; Alsafi, Z.; Sohrabi, C.; Kerwan, A.; Al-Jabir, A.; Iosifidis, C.; Agha, M.; Agha, R. The socio-economic implications of the coronavirus pandemic (COVID-19): A review. *Int. J. Surg.* **2020**, *78*, 185–193. [CrossRef]
9. Cavallo, J.J.; Forman, H.P. The Economic Impact of the COVID-19 Pandemic on Radiology Practices. *Radiology* **2020**, *296*, E141–E144. [CrossRef]
10. Azam, S.A.; Myers, L.; Fields, B.K.K.; Demirjian, N.L.; Patel, D.; Roberge, E.; Gholamrezanezhad, A.; Reddy, S. Coronavirus disease 2019 (COVID-19) pandemic: Review of guidelines for resuming non-urgent imaging and procedures in radiology during Phase II. *Clin. Imaging* **2020**, *67*, 30–36. [CrossRef]
11. Kerbage, A.; Matta, M.; Haddad, S.; Daniel, P.; Tawk, L.; Gemayel, S.; Amine, A.; Warrak, R.; Germanos, M.; Haddad, F.; et al. Challenges facing COVID-19 in rural areas: An experience from Lebanon. *Int. J. Disaster. Risk Reduct.* **2021**, *53*, 102013. [CrossRef]
12. Tandon, A.; Murray, C.; Lauer, J.; Evans, D. Measuring Overall Health System Performance for 191 Countries. Available online: https://www.who.int/healthinfo/paper30.pdf (accessed on 1 February 2021).
13. Miller, L.; Lu, W. These Are the Economies With the Most (and Least) Efficient Health Care. *Bloomberg*, 19 September 2018.
14. Devi, S. Lebanon faces humanitarian emergency after blast. *Lancet* **2020**, *396*, 456. [CrossRef]
15. Abouzeid, M.; Habib, R.R.; Jabbour, S.; Mokdad, A.H.; Nuwayhid, I. Lebanon's humanitarian crisis escalates after the Beirut blast. *Lancet* **2020**, *396*, 1380–1382. [CrossRef]
16. Hanke, S.H. Hanke's Inflation Dashboard: Measurements vs. Forecasts-Lebanon Hyperinflates. Available online: https://www.cato.org/publications/commentary/hankes-inflation-dashboard-measurements-vs-forecasts (accessed on 1 February 2021).

17. The United Nations Economic and Social Commission for Western Asia (ESCWA). Poverty in Lebanon: Solidarity is Vital to Address the Impact of Multiple Overlapping Shocks. Available online: https://www.unescwa.org/sites/www.unescwa.org/files/20-00268_pb15_beirut-explosion-rising-poverty-en.pdf (accessed on 1 February 2021).
18. Kwee, T.C.; Kwee, R.M. Chest CT in COVID-19: What the Radiologist Needs to Know. *Radiographics* **2020**, *40*, 1848–1865. [CrossRef] [PubMed]
19. Long, C.; Xu, H.; Shen, Q.; Zhang, X.; Fan, B.; Wang, C.; Zeng, B.; Li, Z.; Li, X.; Li, H. Diagnosis of the Coronavirus disease (COVID-19): rRT-PCR or CT? *Eur. J. Radiol.* **2020**, *126*, 108961. [CrossRef]
20. Ai, T.; Yang, Z.; Hou, H.; Zhan, C.; Chen, C.; Lv, W.; Tao, Q.; Sun, Z.; Xia, L. Correlation of Chest CT and RT-PCR Testing for Coronavirus Disease 2019 (COVID-19) in China: A Report of 1014 Cases. *Radiology* **2020**, *296*, E32–E40. [CrossRef] [PubMed]
21. Heiss, R.; Grodzki, D.M.; Horger, W.; Uder, M.; Nagel, A.M.; Bickelhaupt, S. High-performance low field MRI enables visualization of persistent pulmonary damage after COVID-19. *Magn. Reson. Imaging* **2020**, *76*, 49–51. [CrossRef] [PubMed]
22. Harmon, S.A.; Sanford, T.H.; Xu, S.; Turkbey, E.B.; Roth, H.; Xu, Z.; Yang, D.; Myronenko, A.; Anderson, V.; Amalou, A.; et al. Artificial intelligence for the detection of COVID-19 pneumonia on chest CT using multinational datasets. *Nat. Commun.* **2020**, *11*, 4080. [CrossRef] [PubMed]
23. Akudjedu, T.N.; Botwe, B.O.; Wuni, A.R.; Mishio, N.A. Impact of the COVID-19 pandemic on clinical radiography practice in low resource settings: The Ghanaian radiographers' perspective. *Radiography* **2020**. [CrossRef]
24. Centers for Disease Control and Prevention. Epi Info™. Available online: https://www.cdc.gov/epiinfo/index.html (accessed on 1 February 2021).
25. Tan, B.S.; Dunnick, N.R.; Gangi, A.; Goergen, S.; Jin, Z.-Y.; Neri, E.; Nomura, C.H.; Pitcher, R.D.; Yee, J.; Mahmood, U. RSNA International Trends: A Global Perspective on the COVID-19 Pandemic and Radiology in Late 2020. *Radiology* **2020**, 204267. [CrossRef]
26. Shi, J.; Giess, C.S.; Martin, T.; Lemaire, K.A.; Curley, P.J.; Bay, C.; Mayo-Smith, W.W.; Boland, G.W.; Khorasani, R. Radiology Workload Changes During the COVID-19 Pandemic: Implications for Staff Redeployment. *Acad. Radiol.* **2021**, *28*, 1–7. [CrossRef]
27. Rubin, G.D.; Ryerson, C.J.; Haramati, L.B.; Sverzellati, N.; Kanne, J.P.; Raoof, S.; Schluger, N.W.; Volpi, A.; Yim, J.J.; Martin, I.B.K.; et al. The Role of Chest Imaging in Patient Management During the COVID-19 Pandemic: A Multinational Consensus Statement From the Fleischner Society. *Chest* **2020**, *158*, 106–116. [CrossRef]
28. Yu, J.; Ding, N.; Chen, H.; Liu, X.-J.; He, W.-j.; Dai, W.-c.; Zhou, Z.-G.; Lin, F.; Pu, Z.-h.; Li, D.-f.; et al. Infection Control against COVID-19 in Departments of Radiology. *Acad. Radiol.* **2020**, *27*, 614–617. [CrossRef] [PubMed]
29. Foley, S.J.; O'Loughlin, A.; Creedon, J. Early experiences of radiographers in Ireland during the COVID-19 crisis. *Insights Imaging* **2020**, *11*, 104. [CrossRef] [PubMed]
30. Yaribeygi, H.; Panahi, Y.; Sahraei, H.; Johnston, T.P.; Sahebkar, A. The impact of stress on body function: A review. *EXCLI J.* **2017**, *16*, 1057–1072. [CrossRef] [PubMed]

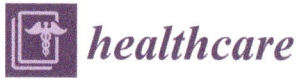 

*Article*

# Nationwide Lockdown, Population Density, and Financial Distress Brings Inadequacy to Manage COVID-19: Leading the Services Sector into the Trajectory of Global Depression

Donglei Yu [1], Muhammad Khalid Anser [2,*], Michael Yao-Ping Peng [3], Abdelmohsen A. Nassani [4], Sameh E. Askar [5], Khalid Zaman [6], Abdul Rashid Abdul Aziz [7], Muhammad Moinuddin Qazi Abro [4], Sasmoko [8] and Mohd Khata Jabor [9]

1. School of Political Science and Public Administration, Wuhan University, Wuhan 430000, China; yudonglei@163.com
2. School of Public Administration, Xi'an University of Architecture and Technology, Xi'an 710000, China
3. School of Economics & Management, Foshan University, Foshan 528000, China; s91370001@mail2000.com.tw
4. Department of Management, College of Business Administration, King Saud University, Riyadh 11587, Saudi Arabia; Nassani@ksu.edu.sa (A.A.N.); qaziabro@gmail.com (M.M.Q.A.)
5. Department of Statistics and Operations Research, College of Science, King Saud University, Riyadh 11587, Saudi Arabia; saskar@ksu.edu.sa
6. Department of Economics, University of Haripur, Haripur 22620, Pakistan; khalid.zaman@uoh.edu.pk
7. Faculty of Leadership and Management, University Sains Islam Malaysia, Nilai 71800, Negeri Sembilan, Malaysia; rashid@usim.edu.my
8. Primary Teacher Education Department, Faculty of Humanities, Bina Nusantara University, Jakarta 11480, Indonesia; sasmoko@binus.edu
9. Faculty of Social Sciences & Humanities, Universiti Teknologi Malaysia (UTM), Johor 81310, Malaysia; mkhata@utm.my
* Correspondence: mkhalidrao@xauat.edu.cn

**Citation:** Yu, D.; Anser, M.K.; Peng, M.Y.-P.; Nassani, A.A.; Askar, S.E.; Zaman, K.; Abdul Aziz, A.R.; Qazi Abro, M.M.; Sasmoko; Jabor, M.K. Nationwide Lockdown, Population Density, and Financial Distress Brings Inadequacy to Manage COVID-19: Leading the Services Sector into the Trajectory of Global Depression. *Healthcare* **2021**, *9*, 220. https://doi.org/10.3390/healthcare9020220

Academic Editors: Eduardo Tomé, Thomas Garavan, Ana Dias and Tao-Hsin Tung

Received: 6 December 2020
Accepted: 14 February 2021
Published: 17 February 2021

**Publisher's Note:** MDPI stays neutral with regard to jurisdictional claims in published maps and institutional affiliations.

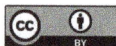

**Copyright:** © 2021 by the authors. Licensee MDPI, Basel, Switzerland. This article is an open access article distributed under the terms and conditions of the Creative Commons Attribution (CC BY) license (https://creativecommons.org/licenses/by/4.0/).

**Abstract:** The service industry provides distributive services, producer services, personal services, and social services. These services largely breakdowns due to restrictions on border movements, confined travel and transportation services, a decline in international tourists' visitation, nationwide lockdowns, and maintaining social distancing in the population. Although these measures are highly needed to contain coronavirus, it decreases economic and financial activities in a country, which requires smart solutions to globally subsidize the services sector. The study used different COVID-19 measures, and its resulting impact on the services industry by using world aggregated data from 1975 through 2020. The study benefited from the Keynesian theory of aggregate demand that remains provided a solution to minimize economic shocks through stringent or liberalizing economic policies. The COVID-19 pandemic is more severe than the financial shocks of 2018 that affected almost all sectors of the globalized world, particularly the services sector, which has been severally affected by COVID-19; it is a high time to revisit economic policies to control pandemic recession. The study used quantiles regression and innovation accounting matrix to obtain ex-ante and ex-post analysis. The quantile regression estimates show that causes of death by communicable diseases, including COVID-19, mainly decline the share of services value added to the global GDP at different quantiles distribution. In contrast, word-of-mouth helps to prevent it from the transmission channel of coronavirus plague through information sharing among the general masses. The control of food prices and managing physical distancing reduces suspected coronavirus cases; however, it negatively affects the services sector's value share. The smart lockdown and sound economic activities do not decrease coronavirus cases, while they support increasing the percentage of the services sector to the global GDP. The innovation accounting matrix suggested that smart lockdown, managing physical distancing, effective price control, and sound financial activities will help to reduce coronavirus cases that will further translate into increased services value-added for the next ten years. The social distancing will exert a more considerable variance error shock to the services industry, which indicates the viability of these measures to contained novel coronavirus over a time horizon. The study used the number of proxies to the COVID-19 measures on the service sector that can be continued with real-time variables to obtain more inferences.

**Keywords:** COVID-19; services value-added; lockdown; word-of-mouth; social distancing; quantile regression

## 1. Introduction

The novel coronavirus leads to novel global depression, as it spread at an exponential rate and increases death tolls accordingly. The current comprehensive statistics of coronavirus cases are, to date, at 62,564,449 and death tolls at 1,458,112. The active cases are 17,917,632, and critical severe cases are 105,238. The USA economy mainly suffers from the coronavirus pandemic and it has added 21.7% registered cases globally. India, Brazil, Russia, and France have been added by 15%, 10.5%, 3.58%, and 3.53%, respectively. The share of Europe in registered cases relative to world economy reached 27%, followed by North America, i.e., 25.3%, Asia, i.e., 26.38%, South America, i.e., 17.67%, Africa, i.e., 3.4%, and Oceania, i.e., 0.07% [1].

The effects of coronavirus are not limited to any single sector, affecting the overall global economy. This study focused on the services sector, as it contributes a share of more than 60% of the world GDP. The percentage of the services sector is more significant in high-income countries (i.e., more than 70%), followed by middle-income countries (i.e., more than 50%) and low-income countries (more than 45%). The services sector provides distributive services (that are related to transportation, means of communications, storage, wholesale businesses, retail businesses, hotels, and restaurants businesses), producer services (referred to financial activities), personal services (related to mass entertainment, recreation activities, ownership, and dwelling), and social services (as compared to public administration, defiance, provision of education, health, and other community services) [2].

The impact of coronavirus (COVID-19) on the services industry is evident, mainly because of the high risk associated with spreading coronavirus; thus, the globalized world has already taken several precautionary steps as per WHO available guidelines, among which few of them are presented, as follows, i.e., maintaining physical distancing between the residents. Therefore, all Giga shopping malls should have been closed; complete and partial lockdowns the streets; school/colleges/universities closures; travel and transport restrictions; international flights cancelled; borders closed; banned massive gatherings; and, limited recreational activities and community services. All of these COVID-19 measures directly affect the services value-added, which is essential in given circumstances. Governments put many efforts into contain coronavirus through national and international strategic unified policies and going towards smart lockdowns to keep relaxing the COVID-19 measures where required. In a short period, many scholarly writings were available on the effects of COVID-19 on different sectors of the economy. The study focused on the impacts of COVID-19 measures on the services industry, as it is considered to be a globalized world's backbone. The study used some different Boolean operators to assess how many scholarly writings have been carried out for COVID-19 and the services industry via using the Google Scholar search engine. The advanced search is used to limit the given words in the 'title of the article'. Table 1 shows the presented statistics for ready reference.

The given searched results confirmed the need to explore the impacts of COVID-19 measures on the services industry, as minimal work has been carried out in the given sector. The critical literature has been cited to understand the direction of earlier researches on the stated topic; for instance, Gössling et al. [3] discussed the impact of COVID-19 on international tourism. They argued that the recent pandemic affects the massive global population, due to international travel bans, and it is projected that more than one-quarter of international tourism will be affected relative to 2019. The greater need for strategic policies is desirable for the transportation industry to maintain its growth rate with safety measures. Thams et al. [4] found that the COVID-19 epidemic mainly affected the international tourism industry in the form of the suspended tourism value chain, including restrictions on travel and transportation services within and outside the countries, not to allow tourists for visitation, hotels closure, stopped airlines, cruise lines, and retailers' activities, which substantially decline the country's revenue streams. The fair chance is to contain coronavirus through unified tourism policies and make them safer and healthier globally. Ruiz Estrada et al. [5] evaluated the impact of COVID-19 on the Chinese economies into four different sectors, including international tourism, air travel industry, foreign trade, and energy markets. They found that, except for energy markets, the rest of the three sectors negatively contribute to the country's economic growth while increasing the demand for electricity consumption due to high medical services and quarantine usage will likely perform high in stock market indices. Thus, it has ultimately contributed to the country's economic growth. Foremny et al. [6] surveyed Spain's sizeable population regarding public health preferences and their willingness to acquire healthcare services. The results show that the low-income group is mostly disturbed by this pandemic, and their mental health is mainly deteriorating due to continuous lockdown. They require healthcare provision and early recovery, so they could reduce their sufferings, both mentally and financially. Goodell [7] discussed the vulnerability of COVID-19 on global economic and financial structure, and argued that, due to the massive increase in healthcare expenditures for identification and prevention of susceptible coronavirus patients, the cost of medical instruments, protective gadgets, and much other healthcare-related infrastructure put enormous pressure on the global economy, which has to be subsidized by the financial sector. However, banking sectors face many challenges regarding the loan disbursement and loan recoveries that put more stress on the other economic areas. Zhao et al. [8] investigated the outbreak of coronavirus pandemic in Wuhan China through the transmission channel of mainly travel by train. The high need for making a 'command and control travel system' may limit the outbreak of COVID-19 to the other cities and the world.

**Table 1.** Assessment of Scholarly Writings on COVID-19 and Services Industry.

| Words Operators | Searching Statistics | Words Operators | Searching Statistics | Words Operators | Searching Statistics |
|---|---|---|---|---|---|
| COVID-19 and Services Industry | No results found | COVID-19 and Hotel Business | No results found | Coronavirus and Defense | No results found |
| Coronavirus and Services Industry | No results found | COVID-19 and Restaurant Business | No results found | Coronavirus and Education | 12 results |
| COVID-19 and Tourism | 13 results | COVID-19 and Finance | 2 results | Coronavirus and Health | 134 results |
| COVID-19 and Transportation | 8 results | COVID-19 and Entertainment | 1 result | Coronavirus and Community Services | No results found |
| COVID-19 and Wholesale Business | No results found | COVID-19 and Recreational Activities | No results found | Total number of studies = 172 | |
| COVID-19 and Retail Business | No results found | Coronavirus and Public Administration | 2 results | | |

Zheng et al. [9] further concluded that private and public transportation provides a transmission carrier of coronavirus pandemics from one city to another. A positive association was found between the different transportation channels and increased COVID-19 cases from Wuhan China to other cities. A negative correlation was found between the more considerable distances between the Wuhan city and the other cities in spreading coronavirus. Public transportation provides a carrier to transmits coronavirus from Wuhan to nearby cities; thus, the Wuhan city's complete lockdown was enviable in reducing the coronavirus outbreak to the other cities and the world. Basch et al. [10] concluded that social media could significantly minimize the COVID-19 impacts through knowledge sharing and awareness regarding the pandemic to use prevention measures to the contain pandemic. YouTube is considered to be the most inspiring way to share the coronavirus pandemic and improve community health services. Peyrav et al. [11] considered a case of Iran's economy that has been negatively affected by the coronavirus, and the sizeable number of registered cases is increasing day-by-day. The Iranian government has worked dedicatedly to contain the coronavirus through massive public education programs and electronic awareness campaigns, while, on the other side, the country is conducting research workshops, training, and increasing healthcare budgets to the control the pandemic. The need for word-of-mouth campaigns regarding coronavirus prevention is vital to promote country resilience. Sahu [12] suggested several policy measures to contain the coronavirus among the students and teaching/administrative staff, as high risk is associated with the educational institutes through close contacts. As per WHO guidelines, the closure of all educational institutes is deemed to be desirable for such an indefinite period until the virus can be controlled accordingly. Nevertheless, these positive measures negatively impact the mental health of students and academic staff. Thus, the need for proper counselling, online teaching courses, assessments, and evaluation is highly desirable in improving students and academic staff's psychological health. Bhalekar [13] argued that the Indian economy was mainly affected by the coronavirus pandemic due to a random lockdown in a country that increases the daily wagers' miseries, which led to increasing the source of virus in a country. The COVID-19 affects all major sectors of the Indian economy, not limited to the labor market, educational institutes, electronic commerce, and overall economic growth. The high need for strategic thinking, unified global policies, smart lockdowns, emergency relief packages to the poor laborer, and stable financial markets would help control to the coronavirus resourcefully. Zheng [14] suggested the need for psychological treatment of healthcare workers directly exposed to the coronavirus, and they are more likely concerned about their families and friends. This family support for health care workers is desirable for working with sound health. Sanità di Toppi et al. [15] confined their findings on a more important aspect of spreading coronavirus pandemic related to the airborne particulate, providing a channel to carry coronavirus into the human respiratory system. The urgent need is for making sustainable policies to limit particulate matters and limit the virus accordingly. Musselwhite et al. [16] suggested that public transportation could be a carrier of coronavirus spread, as people are either sitting or standing in a closed environment, while coughing, touching, and sneezing may transmit the microorganism from one to others. The doors, ticket machines, windows, elevators, seats, and many other areas could be possible places of the infectious disease. Deng and Peng [17] found that the case-fatality ratio is mainly evident with the following symptoms of coronavirus, including high fever, too much coughing, shortness of breath, and chest pain, while other comorbidities of the fatality cases, including high stress, heart patients, diabetes, cerebral infarction, and chronic bronchitis. These healthcare concerns that are required more good policies to reduce the case fatality ratio, while symptomatic treatment is provided to the coronavirus patients until the possible medication and the vaccine is not invented. Anser et al. [18] considered a panel of 76 countries using time series data from 2010–2019 to evaluate the impact of COVID-19 measures on global poverty, and found that population density, lack of necessary sanitation facilities, environmental challenges, and death by communicable diseases put a significant burden on the low-income group, which could be minimized by increasing public healthcare expenditures across countries. The need for pro-poor growth policies will support the breakdown of the vicious cycle of poverty that would be further translated into sustained economic growth.

The significant discussion that is based on earlier literature emphasized the need to evaluate the possible impacts of COVID-19 measures on services industries while using an aggregated world data level. Fewer studies on the stated topic give room to investigate to select the specified area, which would provide more policy insights for analyzing the services industry's response against the COVID-19 measures. The objectives of the study are as follows:

(I) To examine the possible impacts of COVID-19 measures on the global services industry.

(II) To investigate the direct effect of communicable diseases, including COVID-19, on services value-added.

(III) To determine the role of word-of-mouth against the coronavirus pandemic and its possible impact on the services industry and

(IV) To observe the effects of lockdown, social distancing, price control, and financial activities on the services industry.

Different countries have widely adopted these measures against the coronavirus that analyzed in the study of the services sector. The study used quantile regression estimates to analyze the predictors' different variations on the response variable at different quantiles distribution. This technique is better in a given scenario that will provide robust inferences.

## 2. Data Sources and Methodological Framework

There are some COVID-19 measures that have been used to control the pandemic at a global scale, and a few of them are listed below, i.e.,

(I) Information Sharing: the right information with correct facts and figures are the responsibility of every government to share with their residents, while, at an international platform, the WHO and other international agencies have to prepare the policy documents regarding prevention from novel coronavirus and spread it through different information channels. The national and international agencies have already provided the right information through various communication channels, and it is now a duty to respond to the general masses to act like a civilized person. The 'word-of-mouth' mostly used the word in marketing the specified products where information is shared from one person to another through oral communication [19]. The adult literacy rate played a vital role in promoting communication channels to reach the right customers. Based on the above discussion, this study used the adult literacy rate (% of people ages 15 and above) as a correct variable for information sharing about coronavirus, and considers it as word-of-mouth (as denoted by WOM) information novel coronavirus among the general masses in this study. The rationale for using this proxy is that the literate person would effectively use all kinds of communication among agents. Hence, this proxy would leave the impact on the literature of network awareness.

(II) Lockdown: the lockdowns, either partial or complete, depend upon the severity of the new coronavirus outbreak in any country. This strategy used almost every country in their perspectives to prevent their ordinary peoples from the deadly disease. The evidence indicates that lockdown is not successful in many parts of the world due to the high incidence of poverty and hunger, which were later funded by the government's emergency reliefs' packages for the needy peoples [20]. The law enforcement agencies played an essential role in lockdown in the city, as per Federal government instructions [21]. The people did not usually follow the government instructions due to ignorance, a lack of information, and other social issues; for this call, law enforcement agencies can handle this situation. Thus, this study used 'armed forces personnel' (in total) for a nearby LOCKDOWN proxy to restrict free mobility. Measuring "lockdowns" by armed forces personnel is used to show a stringent government policy that, using 'power and control' to contain widespread coronavirus cases by the forceful imposition of standard operating procedures (SOPs) regarding coronavirus prevention, likely shows a better proposition than the 'Oxford stringency index' or 'Google mobility series'.

(III) Social Distancing: according to the WHO guidelines regarding preventing and controlling the coronavirus pandemic, it avoids massive gatherings and maintains physical distancing among the residents. This strategy is mostly applied uniformly across the globe. Physical distancing helps to minimize the risk of coronavirus incidence as it is a transmitted disease, and its spread from close contacts [22]. The population compactness could be one reason that provides a channel to carry one person to another [18]. This study used 'population density', as per square km of land area, as a nearby proxy for the social distancing (denoted by SOCDIS) to obtain some conclusive findings in this regard. The study measures "social distancing" by population density, rather than using % of the urban population because, the higher the population compact in the country, the greater will be the chances to spread coronavirus cases, irrespective of rural and urban spheres. The study did not limit population density to the urban population while it used the overall population compactness, as coronavirus cases are spreading uniformly in rural and urban regions.

(IV) Price Control: due to the coronavirus outbreak, the globalized world's most critical concern is the 'price control' of the food items especially. As the news about the COVID-19 outbreak transmitted across the globe, mass panic spread among ordinary people, and they rushed at food items to store in their homes. Every time, the governments give confidence to the familiar people and the producers and retailers to keep calm and remain easy so that food challenges can be resolved. In this regard, governments make food control price committees in a different part of the world to provide a free flow of food supply at lower prices [23]. The present study used the 'consumer price index-inflation' (%) as a proxy of food price control in the sense that the coronavirus pandemic increases the prices of food items due to the shortage of the food supply chain. Thus, the need to assess the price hikes can be used through CPI values for making an effective price control strategy.

(V) Financial and Economic Activities: the outbreak of novel coronavirus negatively affects the global stock market index. It is crushed in many parts of the world, due to full travel restrictions, lockdowns, and other preventive measures, which directly hit the local and international businesses [24]. The study used 'broad money supply', as % of GDP and 'GDP per capita' in constant 2010 US$ as nearby proxies of financial activities (denoted by FACT) and economic activities (EACT), respectively, to assess the country's economic and financial situation amid the coronavirus pandemic. The rationale to use both of the factors is that money supply is considered to be one of the vital factors of financial development indicators that mostly viewed in the relation of COVID-19 pandemic. Similarly, economic activities can be better checked with the country's per capita income that mainly affected the pandemic recession. Thus, these proxies would be helpful in tracing the real problem of the pandemic recession across countries.

(VI) Causes of Death by Communicable Diseases: the study used the data of 'causes of death by communicable diseases' (as % of total) (denoted by COMD) as a reference point to analyze the death toll by a coronavirus.

(VII) Services Value Added: the service's value added (% of GDP) (as denoted by SVAD) comprises distributive services, producer services, personal services, and social services, which is used in this study as a response variable.

The COVID-19 measures are considered to be explanatory variables of the study, while the value of the service added is served as the explained variable. The world aggregated data are used for empirical analysis, covering a period of 1975–2020. The missing information is filled by the preceding and succeeding value of the respective variables where required. The data were obtained from the World Bank [25].

The study benefited from the Keynesian theory of aggregate demand, which argued that aggregate demand could be affected by any prevailing shocks in the economies, which need to be stabilized through economic policies. Similarly, the COVID-19 crisis is more severe than the financial depression of 2008 shocks that captured the whole world, which declined world economic growth. The COVID-19 crisis has affected the economies' supply and demand simultaneously; for instance, social distancing creates distancing between the one person and another. It reduces productive labor hours that lower the supply, which increases the marginal cost of production [26,27]. Significantly, the services sector is majorly affected through social distancing, as its closely connected with the hospitality and recreational activities that are banned due to the high risk of spreading COVID-19 cases. Services value-added is a substantial part of economic growth, as its GDP share is more than 60% worldwide. The services sector is used as a reference point that analyzed its performance in the world's GDP that is most affected by COVID-19 pandemic, which can be viewed by the suggested empirical equation, i.e.,

$$\ln(SVAD) = \alpha_0 + \alpha_1 \ln(COMD) + \alpha_2 \ln(WOM) + \alpha_3 \ln(LOCKDOWN) + \alpha_4 \ln(FACT) + \alpha_5 \ln(EACT) + \alpha_6 \ln(PCONT) + \alpha_7 \ln(SOCDIS) + \varepsilon$$

$$\therefore \frac{\partial \ln(SVAD)}{\partial \ln(COMD)} < 0, \frac{\partial \ln(SVAD)}{\partial \ln(WOM)} > 0, \frac{\partial \ln(SVAD)}{\partial \ln(LOCKDOWN)} < 0, \frac{\partial \ln(SVAD)}{\partial \ln(FACT)} < 0, \frac{\partial \ln(SVAD)}{\partial \ln(EACT)} < 0, \quad (1)$$

$$\frac{\partial \ln(SVAD)}{\partial \ln(PCONT)} < 0, \frac{\partial \ln(SVAD)}{\partial \ln(SOCDIS)} < 0.$$

where SVAD shows the services value-added, COMD shows communicable diseases, WOM shows word-of-mouth, LOCKDOWN shows lockdown, FACT shows financial activities, EACT shows economic activities, PCONT shows price control, SOCDIS shows social distancing, and $\varepsilon$ shows the error term.

Equation (1) shows that the stated factors influence service value-added. It is likely that the causes of death by communicable diseases, including COVID-19, will decrease service value-added, whereas improving the communication means of information sharing, including word-of-mouth about coronavirus pandemic, would be helpful in maintaining service value-added share relative to GDP. Although it is not favorable to the value of the functions added in managing their GDP share, the temporary or complete lockdown is not favorable. However, it is deemed to be desirable to control coronavirus on a global scale. The financial and economic activities suppressed with the COVID-19 pandemic negatively influenced services value-added. The price hikes in food items needed efficient price control to facilitate the needy community members, which subsidized the services sector to charge a smaller price, thus maintaining reasonable profit. Finally, social distancing is the remedial measure to contain coronavirus; however, it negatively affects service value-added. Figure 1 shows the research framework of the study.

Figure 1 shows the impacts of COVID-19 measures on the services industry and identified some significant determinants that negatively affect global service value added. These COVID-19 measures are highly required for the controlled pandemic; however, it decreases services share relative to its country GDP. The following research hypotheses have been developed to analyze it during estimation, i.e.,

**Hypothesis 1 (H1).** *Communicable diseases, including COVID-19, will likely decrease the share of services value-added relative to the country's GDP.*

**Hypothesis 2 (H2).** *Word-of-mouth of coronavirus pandemic would likely to be helpful for the prevention of virus and increases services value-added, and*

**Hypothesis 3 (H3).** *Lockdown, population compactness, and financial instability will likely decrease services share in total GDP.*

The study utilized a quantile regression apparatus to obtain parameter estimates. It works under different assumptions. It gives a more trending analysis of the said parameters at different quantiles distribution, which other available regression apparatuses would be powerless to perform, such as time-series cointegration techniques, instrumental regression techniques, and robust regression. These techniques would perform well in their domain, but these are ineffective in analyzing trending regression estimates over 10th quantiles to 90th quantiles. The given procedure would give greater leverage to express the parameter estimates for sound inferences. Equation (2) shows the empirical illustration of different quantiles distribution of the stated parameters for ready reference, i.e.,

$$\ln(SVAD)_{\tau 10} = \alpha_0 + \alpha_1 \ln(COMD)_{\tau 10} + \alpha_2 \ln(WOM)_{\tau 10} + \alpha_3 \ln(LOCKDOWN)_{\tau 10} + \alpha_4 \ln(FACT)_{\tau 10}$$
$$+ \alpha_5 \ln(EACT)_{\tau 10} + \alpha_6 \ln(PCONT)_{\tau 10} + \alpha_7 \ln(SOCDIS)_{\tau 10} + \varepsilon_{\tau 10}$$
;
$$\ln(SVAD)_{\tau 25} = \alpha_0 + \alpha_1 \ln(COMD)_{\tau 25} + \alpha_2 \ln(WOM)_{\tau 25} + \alpha_3 \ln(LOCKDOWN)_{\tau 25} + \alpha_4 \ln(FACT)_{\tau 25}$$
$$+ \alpha_5 \ln(EACT)_{\tau 25} + \alpha_6 \ln(PCONT)_{\tau 25} + \alpha_7 \ln(SOCDIS)_{\tau 25} + \varepsilon_{\tau 25}$$
:
$$\ln(SVAD)_{\tau 50} = \alpha_0 + \alpha_1 \ln(COMD)_{\tau 50} + \alpha_2 \ln(WOM)_{\tau 50} + \alpha_3 \ln(LOCKDOWN)_{\tau 50} + \alpha_4 \ln(FACT)_{\tau 50} \quad (2)$$
$$+ \alpha_5 \ln(EACT)_{\tau 50} + \alpha_6 \ln(PCONT)_{\tau 50} + \alpha_7 \ln(SOCDIS)_{\tau 50} + \varepsilon_{\tau 50}$$
:
$$\ln(SVAD)_{\tau 75} = \alpha_0 + \alpha_1 \ln(COMD)_{\tau 75} + \alpha_2 \ln(WOM)_{\tau 75} + \alpha_3 \ln(LOCKDOWN)_{\tau 75} + \alpha_4 \ln(FACT)_{\tau 75}$$
$$+ \alpha_5 \ln(EACT)_{\tau 75} + \alpha_6 \ln(PCONT)_{\tau 75} + \alpha_7 \ln(SOCDIS)_{\tau 75} + \varepsilon_{\tau 75}$$
:
$$\ln(SVAD)_{\tau 90} = \alpha_0 + \alpha_1 \ln(COMD)_{\tau 90} + \alpha_2 \ln(WOM)_{\tau 90} + \alpha_3 \ln(LOCKDOWN)_{\tau 90} + \alpha_4 \ln(FACT)_{\tau 90}$$
$$+ \alpha_5 \ln(EACT)_{\tau 90} + \alpha_6 \ln(PCONT)_{\tau 90} + \alpha_7 \ln(SOCDIS)_{\tau 90} + \varepsilon_{\tau 90}$$

where $\tau_{10}$ to $\tau_{90}$ show quantiles regression estimates from 10th quantiles to 90th quantile distribution.

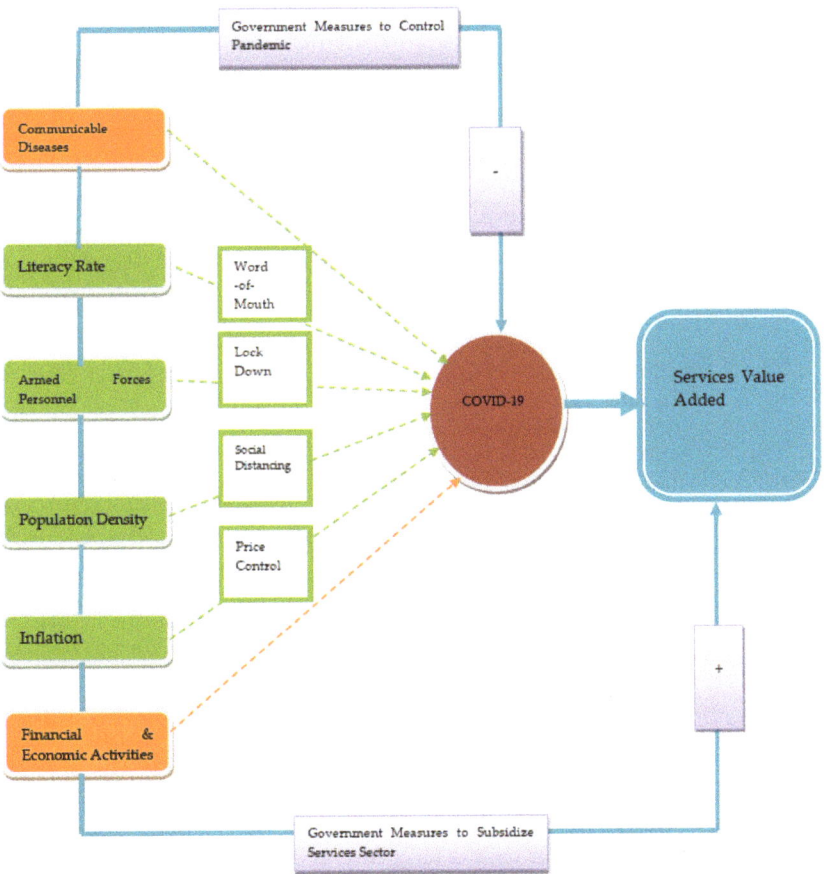

**Figure 1.** Research Framework of the Study. Source: Author's extract.

The study further used impulse response function (IRF) and variance decomposition analysis (VDA) for analyzing the parameter estimates in the forecasting framework for the next ten year time period.

## 3. Results

Table 2 shows the descriptive statistics of the candidate variables. The share of service value that is added to world GDP has reached a maximum of 65.26%, minimum at 54.24%, and mean 58.47%. The causes of death by communicable diseases, on average, are entered at 27.29% of total world death. Word-of-mouth is measured by an adult literacy rate with a minimum value of 65.19%, a maximum amount of 87.30%, and an average value of 77.30%. Armed forces personnel are used as a proxy for lockdown, which shows that the global world needed 25,744,314 armed forces personnel to keep successful lockdown to some specified area on average. The financial and economic activities are measured by broad money supply and GDP per capita, with an average value of 92.75% of GDP and US$8,007.36, respectively. The price control is measured by changes in the price level with an average value of 6.39%. Finally, social distancing is observed by population compactness, which has an average value of 45.95 people per square m of land area. The given descriptions of the candidate variables showed a trend analysis over the past 45 years.

Table 2. Descriptive Statistics.

| Methods | SVAD | COMD | WOM | LOCKDOWN | FACT | EACT | PCONT | SOCDIS |
|---|---|---|---|---|---|---|---|---|
| Mean | 58.47710 | 27.29407 | 77.30327 | 25744314 | 92.75388 | 8007.362 | 6.394944 | 45.95990 |
| Maximum | 65.26177 | 30.90569 | 87.30101 | 30196640 | 125.0989 | 10892.00 | 12.47161 | 59.63624 |
| Minimum | 54.24299 | 20.17717 | 65.19396 | 22209230 | 62.15986 | 5681.743 | 1.431611 | 31.91508 |
| Std. Dev. | 4.384618 | 4.428943 | 7.039300 | 2934139 | 18.24449 | 1571.258 | 3.560119 | 8.506539 |
| Skewness | 0.212882 | −0.521528 | −0.341577 | −0.087964 | −0.073547 | 0.346740 | 0.464993 | −0.013921 |
| Kurtosis | 1.326914 | 1.512059 | 1.738246 | 1.402185 | 2.251956 | 1.834101 | 1.970756 | 1.779506 |

Source: World Bank [25]. Note: SVAD shows services value-added, COMD shows communicable disease, WOM shows word-of-mouth, LOCKDOWN shows lockdown, FACT shows financial activity, EACT shows economic activity, PCONT shows price control, and SOCIDIS shows social distancing.

Table 3 shows the correlation estimates and found that communicable diseases, including COVID−19 and price control, negatively correlate with service value-added. In contrast, the other variables, including word-of-mouth, lockdown, financial and economic activities, and social distancing, positively associate services value-added. The result implies that services value-added exposed an increased risk of coronavirus pandemic, while strict price control further decreases services value-added across the globe. The government's measures to controlled coronavirus would be primarily supported services value added to run their businesses during a relaxed time as per governments' provision to open their markets. The word-of-mouth for coronavirus pandemic to the general masses would help keep residents at their homes to become safe from the virus, while, for successful operating lockdowns, the increasing number of armed forces personnel is desirable. Financial and economic activities allow general masses to start their businesses under strict government safety measures at their business site. Finally, social distancing is the only step that helps the broad population to keep away from the coronavirus; thus, avoiding massive gatherings and close contacts would enable peoples to do their work under the safety parameters. All of this positivity would support services value-added on a global scale.

Table 4 shows the ADF unit root estimates and found that, except SOCDIS, the remaining variables exhibit the first difference stationary, while SOCDIS does not show either I(0) or I(1) characteristics, thus it does not confirm the order of integration at the level or first difference. Based on the estimates, the study moves towards quantile regression estimates to show the variations of variables at different quantiles distribution.

Table 3. Correlation Matrix.

| Variables | SVAD | COMD | WOM | LOCKDOWN | FACT | EACT | PCONT | SOCDIS |
|---|---|---|---|---|---|---|---|---|
| SVAD | 1 | | | | | | | |
| | — | | | | | | | |
| COMD | −0.925 | 1 | | | | | | |
| | (0.000) | — | | | | | | |
| WOM | 0.912 | −0.834 | 1 | | | | | |
| | (0.000) | (0.000) | — | | | | | |
| LOCKDOWN | 0.726 | −0.543 | 0.821 | 1 | | | | |
| | (0.000) | (0.000) | (0.000) | — | | | | |
| FACT | 0.857 | −0.809 | 0.953 | 0.708 | 1 | | | |
| | (0.000) | (0.000) | (0.000) | (0.000) | — | | | |
| EACT | 0.946 | −0.927 | 0.955 | 0.703 | 0.943 | 1 | | |
| | (0.000) | (0.000) | (0.000) | (0.000) | (0.000) | — | | |
| PCONT | −0.832 | 0.734 | −0.894 | −0.716 | −0.887 | −0.832 | 1 | |
| | (0.000) | (0.000) | (0.000) | (0.000) | (0.000) | (0.000) | — | |
| SOCDIS | 0.931 | −0.887 | 0.987 | 0.772 | 0.964 | 0.986 | −0.875 | 1 |
| | (0.000) | (0.000) | (0.000) | (0.000) | (0.000) | (0.000) | (0.000) | — |

Note: Small bracket shows probability value. SVAD shows services value-added, COMD shows communicable disease, WOM shows word-of-mouth, LOCKDOWN shows lockdown, FACT shows financial activity, EACT shows economic activity, PCONT shows price control, and SOCIDIS shows social distancing.

Table 4. Unit Root Estimates.

| Variables | Level | | First Difference | |
|---|---|---|---|---|
| | Constant | Constant with Trend | Constant | Constant with Trend |
| SVAD | −0.062 | −2.152 | −5.892 | −5.879 |
| | (0.947) | (0.503) | (0.000) | (0.000) |
| COMD | −0.264 | −2.196 | −6.178 | −6.741 |
| | (0.921) | (0.479) | (0.000) | (0.000) |
| WOM | −1.542 | −0.631 | −4.663 | −4.922 |
| | (0.503) | (0.971) | (0.000) | (0.001) |
| LOCKDOWN | −1.617 | −2.073 | −7.663 | −7.579 |
| | (0.465) | (0.545) | (0.000) | (0.000) |
| FACT | −0.386 | −2.016 | −5.932 | −5.859 |
| | (0.902) | (0.576) | (0.000) | (0.000) |
| EACT | 1.214(0.997) | −1.332 | −5.028 | −5.255 |
| | | (0.866) | (0.000) | (0.000) |
| PCONT | −1.757 | −3.107 | −7.776 | −7.718 |
| | (0.396) | (0.117) | (0.000) | (0.000) |
| SOCDIS | −0.972 | −0.930 | −0.730 | −0.147 |
| | (0.754) | (0.943) | (0.828) | (0.992) |

Note: small bracket shows probability values. SVAD shows services value-added, COMD shows communicable disease, WOM shows word-of-mouth, LOCKDOWN shows lockdown, FACT shows financial activity, EACT shows economic activity, PCONT shows price control, and SOCIDIS shows social distancing.

Table 5 shows the quantile regression estimates and found that communicable diseases hurt the services value added at different quantiles distribution with a minimum impact of −0.068% and maximum impact of −0312%, while an increasing one per cent increase in services value-added share to the globe GDP. The results are interpreted in light of the novel coronavirus. Kim et al. [28] argued that community health is mainly influenced by the coronavirus outbreak that has increased the healthcare burden in national healthcare bills. The case study of New York city developed some protocols for the outpatient service department to minimize the risk of coronavirus pandemic, including a first stage, the possible test of coronavirus is performed on the susceptible patients. If found to be positive, then the second step is to give symptomatic treatments. The third stage is to track the patients once during at least five consecutive days, and, finally, teach them how to isolate in-home or elsewhere under prescribed medical guidelines. Samarathunga [29] discussed the possible challenges of the coronavirus pandemic on international tourism in Sri Lanka. The results show that the coronavirus pandemic negatively affects the country's tourism sector, as it adversely affects the source markets, local tourism resources, and travel industry. The suspension of transportation modes, partial and complete lockdowns, and maintaining the distance between humans all decline tourism income. However, these measures are essential in containing coronavirus in a country. Yang et al. [30] concluded that, due to the high health risk of coronavirus pandemics to the national and international tourists, the tourism demand decreases through government institute bans on human mobility. Further, travel restrictions that are imposed by the government exacerbate adverse outcomes from the tourism sector. Thus, social welfare is the subject matter and prime responsibility of the government. Any strict policies regarding their prevention are desirable. However, the governments should subsidize the tourism sector to improve tourism sites; once the pandemic vanishes, an enormous amount of tourism revenue could be generated. Wanjala [31] argued that novel coronavirus negatively affects a country's economic growth via low international trade and tourism transmission mechanisms. The travel and transportation restrictions for possible caution to take care of the humans from coronavirus are desirable, being substituted by the specific government-initiated reforms packages to the tourism and trade to maintain economic activities countrywide.

Table 5. Quantile Regression Estimates.

| Quantiles | $\tau_{10}$ | $\tau_{20}$ | $\tau_{30}$ | $\tau_{40}$ | $\tau_{50}$ | $\tau_{60}$ | $\tau_{70}$ | $\tau_{80}$ | $\tau_{90}$ |
|---|---|---|---|---|---|---|---|---|---|
| LOG(COMD) | −0.310 (0) | −0.313 (0) | −0.283 (0) | −0.262 (0.012) | −0.115 (0.008) | −0.105 (0.026) | −0.084 (0.064) | −0.068 (0.158) | −0.162 (0.017) |
| LOG(WOM) | 0.699 (0.001) | 0.860 (0.001) | 0.711 (0.006) | 0.750 (0.022) | 0.327 (0.605) | 0.243 (0.705) | 0.170 (0.794) | 0.201 (0.777) | 0.343 (0.704) |
| LOG(LOCKDOWN) | 0.027 (0.484) | 0.010 (0.823) | 0.043 (0.470) | 0.056 (0.472) | 0.247 (0.011) | 0.239 (0.028) | 0.231 (0.051) | 0.208 (0.114) | 0.243 (0.137) |
| LOG(FACT) | −0.112 (0) | −0.138 (0) | −0.127 (0.001) | −0.129 (0.008) | −0.072 (0.350) | −0.097 (0.289) | −0.122 (0.234) | −0.155 (0.201) | −0.118 (0.405) |
| LOG(EACT) | 0.220 (0.026) | 0.178 (0.118) | 0.165 (0.208) | 0.222 (0.181) | 0.418 (0.031) | 0.392 (0.037) | 0.397 (0.027) | 0.420 (0.030) | 0.261 (0.218) |
| LOG(PCONT) | −0.027 (0.002) | −0.029 (0.008) | −0.032 (0.010) | −0.032 (0.037) | −0.030 (0.009) | −0.030 (0.005) | −0.026 (0.017) | −0.027 (0.023) | −0.022 (0.171) |
| LOG(SOCDIS) | −0.442 (0.008) | −0.451 (0.018) | −0.374 (0.062) | −0.439 (0.083) | −0.447 (0.282) | −0.346 (0.354) | −0.252 (0.480) | −0.239 (0.518) | −0.256 (0.557) |
| Constant | 1.834 (0.170) | 1.959 (0.212) | 1.741 (0.366) | 1.020 (0.678) | −2.875 (0.071) | −2.435 (0.076) | −2.343 (0.034) | −2.239 (0.041) | −1.839 (0.100) |
| Statistical Tests | | | | | | | | | |
| Slope Equality Test | Wald Test | $\chi^2$-statistic: 37.055 | | $\chi^2$-statistic degree of freedom = 14 | | | Probability value: 0.000 | | |
| Symmetric Quantiles Test | Wald Test | $\chi^2$-statistic: 13.616 | | $\chi^2$-statistic degree of freedom = 8 | | | Probability value: 0.092 | | |

Note: Small bracket shows probability value. SVAD shows services value-added, COMD shows communicable disease, WOM shows word-of-mouth, LOCKDOWN shows lockdown, FACT shows financial activity, EACT shows economic activity, PCONT shows price control, and SOCDIS shows social distancing.

The sound financial activities, price control measures, and social distancing have proven to be the best strategy to control coronavirus; however, these measures negatively impact services value-added, leading to a global depression. The positive impact of word-of-mouth, lockdown, and sound economic activities decreases the risk of coronavirus pandemic and supports the services share into the world GDP. These results have been shown at different quantiles distribution. Brodeur et al. [32] discussed the vulnerability of the COVID-19 pandemic at a mass scale across the globe. The government put many efforts to restrain coronavirus through multiple strategies. However, the unified adopted policy included lockdown, which bears multifaceted mental health challenges to population well-being that are not limited to boredom, loneliness, sadness, worry, suicidal thoughts, stress, and divorce. The need for smart lockdowns and information sharing among the masses to stay safe in homes would be desirable, while the government should engage their population in some online group tasks to reduce mental health challenges. Wong [33] described the real situation of the coronavirus pandemic in the Malaysian context, where the physical distancing along with the national lockdowns were enforced with the one order command that local population from international travels, not allowing foreigners to visit a country, temporary shut down of businesses, closure of schools, colleges, and other institutions. At the same time, only essential services have been permitted under safety measures. These measures affect industries, including the services industry, which may cause a global depression. Barro et al. [34] found that the coronavirus pandemic and Spanish flu increase mortality and economic contraction, mostly low real returns on stocks and short-term government bills. Gómez-Ríos et al. [35] concluded that the coronavirus pandemic was mainly out of control due to the imported number of cases from uncontrolled air travellers. Social distancing avoids massive gatherings and restricts international travelling to maintain the decreasing trend in the infections trend. Yezli and Khan [36] argued that, besides the socio-economic, political, and religious challenges faced by the Kingdom of Saudi Arabia, the country took bold steps to restrain coronavirus through social distancing and complete lockdown. The country suddenly closed due to the high epidemic curve because of its social and religious norms hosting massive religious gatherings. These measures are essential in containing the virus, although at the cost of a severe economic crisis. The services industry mainly suffers due to restrictions being imposed on the travel and tourism sector, businesses shut down, closure of educational and other institutions, and maintaining social distancing; all of these measures would help to restrain the country's epidemic curve. Figure 2 shows the quantile process estimates for ready reference.

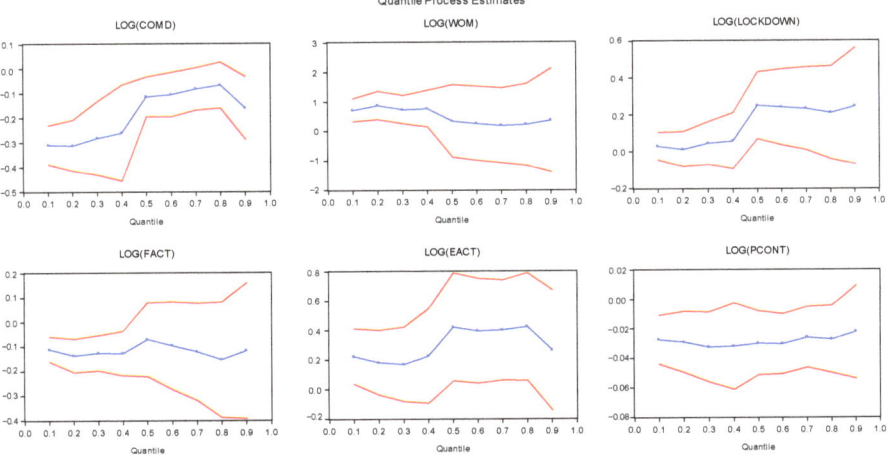

**Figure 2.** *Cont.*

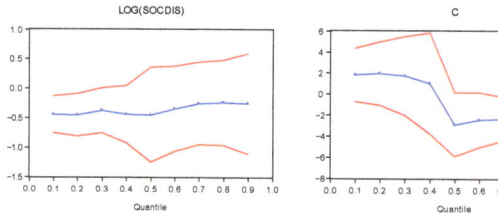

**Figure 2.** Quantile Process Estimates. Source: Authors' estimates. Note: SVAD shows services value-added, COMD shows communicable disease, WOM shows word-of-mouth, LOCKDOWN shows lockdown, FACT shows financial activity, EACT shows economic activity, PCONT shows price control, and SOCIDIS shows social distancing. LOG shows natural logarithm. C shows constant. Red lines shows the critical region. Blue line shows the estimated value.

## 4. Discussion

Table 6 shows the endogeneity test results that were performed through quantile median regression. Financial development generally works as a growth proxy; thus, evaluating the possible endogeneity in the given model, the study performs the three-step procedure. The first step is to use ln (FACT) as a dependent variable that is replaced by ln (SVAD), while the remaining variables are exogenous variables and obtained its residual value (i.e. res_01). In the second step, ln (SVAD) is used again as a primary endogenous variable, while res_01 and other variables, except for ln (FACT), are used as regressors and obtain coefficient estimates. In the final step, the Wald coefficient restrictions are applied on the given res_01 term and found the statistically insignificant results of t-statistics, F-statistics, and Chi-square statistics. The results confirmed that there are no possible endogeneity issues in the quantile regression estimates. Thus, the results are valid and reliable.

**Table 6.** Endogeneity Test performed by Quantiles Median Regression.

| Variables | First Step: ln (SVAD) | | | | Second Step: ln (FACT) | | | | Final Step: ln (SVAD) | | | |
|---|---|---|---|---|---|---|---|---|---|---|---|---|
| | Coefficient | Std. Error | t-Statistic | Prob. | Coefficient | Std. Error | t-Statistic | Prob. | Coefficient | Std. Error | t-Statistic | Prob. |
| C | −2.875 | 1.550 | −1.854 | 0.071 | 6.848 | 4.894 | 1.399 | 0.169 | −3.374 | 1.741 | −1.937 | 0.064 |
| ln(FACT) | −0.072 | 0.077 | −0.946 | 0.350 | N/A | N/A | N/A | N/A | N/A | N/A | N/A | N/A |
| ln(COMD) | −0.115 | 0.041 | −2.789 | 0.008 | 0.434 | 0.175 | 2.469 | 0.018 | −0.146 | 0.030 | −4.818 | 0.000 |
| ln(WOM) | 0.327 | 0.628 | 0.520 | 0.605 | −1.080 | 1.638 | −0.659 | 0.513 | 0.406 | 0.679 | 0.598 | 0.553 |
| ln(lockdown) | 0.247 | 0.092 | 2.674 | 0.011 | −0.355 | 0.218 | −1.627 | 0.112 | 0.273 | 0.072 | 3.764 | 0.000 |
| ln(EACT) | 0.418 | 0.186 | 2.240 | 0.031 | −0.005 | 0.538 | −0.011 | 0.991 | 0.419 | 0.187 | 2.240 | 0.031 |
| ln(PCONT) | −0.030 | 0.011 | −2.717 | 0.009 | −0.078 | 0.032 | −2.427 | 0.020 | −0.024 | 0.009 | −2.477 | 0.017 |
| ln(SOCDIS) | −0.447 | 0.410 | −1.090 | 0.287 | 1.880 | 1.118 | 1.681 | 0.100 | −0.584 | 0.480 | −1.217 | 0.231 |
| Res_01 | N/A | N/A | N/A | N/A | N/A | N/A | N/A | N/A | −0.072 | 0.077 | −0.946 | 0.350 |
| Adjusted R² | 0.852 | | | | 0.779 | | | | 0.852 | | | |
| S.E. of regression | 0.018 | | | | 0.044 | | | | 0.018 | | | |
| Quantile dependent variable | 4.080 | | | | 4.537 | | | | 4.080 | | | |
| Sparsity | 0.023 | | | | 0.119 | | | | 0.023 | | | |
| | Wald Coefficient Restrictions | | | | | | | | | | | |
| Wald Test | t-statistic: −0.946, $p > 0.090$ | | | | F-statistics: 0.896, $p > 0.090$ | | | | Chi-square statistic: 0.895, $p > 0.090$ | | | |

Note: SVAD shows services value-added, COMD shows communicable disease, WOM shows word-of-mouth, LOCKDOWN shows lockdown, FACT shows financial activity, EACT shows economic activity, PCONT shows price control, res_01 shows residual term, and SOCIDIS shows social distancing. N/A shows not applicable.

Table 7 shows the IRF estimates and suggested that smart lockdown services will positively influence services value-added, sound financial and economic activities, price control, and social distancing. In contrast, word-of-mouth and communicable diseases largely influenced services value-added that required a substantial information sharing system and increased healthcare expenditures to control the coronavirus pandemic and improve the share of services value added to the global GDP a time horizon.

Table 7. Impulse Response Function (IRF) Estimates.

| Period | Response of SVAD | | | | | | | |
|---|---|---|---|---|---|---|---|---|
| | SVAD | COMD | WOM | LOCKDOWN | FACT | EACT | PCONT | SOCDIS |
| 2020 | 0.487233 | 0 | 0 | 0 | 0 | 0 | 0 | 0 |
| 2021 | 0.190553 | 0.015831 | 0.083155 | 0.166405 | 0.048038 | −0.142270 | −0.020177 | −0.128719 |
| 2022 | 0.046358 | 0.217748 | 0.246702 | 0.549362 | −0.124709 | −0.177730 | −0.186485 | −0.423154 |
| 2023 | −0.281975 | 0.376039 | 0.442166 | 0.222861 | −0.044556 | −0.308266 | −0.105952 | −0.891468 |
| 2024 | −0.984015 | 0.843134 | 1.169902 | −0.028800 | −0.137800 | −1.591205 | −0.521476 | −2.367387 |
| 2025 | −2.808627 | 2.151347 | 3.273988 | −0.258479 | −0.563898 | −4.765879 | −1.940319 | −6.366720 |
| 2026 | −7.404040 | 5.685884 | 8.494693 | −0.770462 | −1.497330 | −12.39932 | −5.735708 | −16.45630 |
| 2027 | −18.24873 | 14.34690 | 20.75606 | −1.890141 | −3.522563 | −30.50206 | −14.81691 | −40.46431 |
| 2028 | −43.56493 | 34.82272 | 49.22016 | −4.514128 | −8.166525 | −72.90151 | −36.00114 | −96.68157 |
| 2029 | −102.6897 | 82.82517 | 115.3919 | −10.72818 | −18.99123 | −171.9555 | −85.43064 | −228.0026 |

Note: SVAD shows services value-added, COMD shows communicable disease, WOM shows word-of-mouth, LOCKDOWN shows lockdown, FACT shows financial activity, EACT shows economic activity, PCONT shows price control, and SOCIDIS shows social distancing.

Table 8 shows the VDA estimates and suggested that social distancing would exert a more significant magnitude to influence services value-added with a variance error shock of 43.3%, followed by economic activity, word-of-mouth, price control, communicable diseases, and financial business with variance errors of 24.6%, 11.1%, 6.0%, 5.6%, and 0.302%, respectively. The least variance error shock of service value-added services will be lockdown with an estimated variance error shock of 0.09%.

Table 8. Variance Decomposition Analysis (VDA) Estimates.

| Period | Variance Decomposition of SVAD | | | | | | | | |
|---|---|---|---|---|---|---|---|---|---|
| | SE | SVAD | COMD | WOM | LOCKDOWN | FACT | EACT | PCONT | SOCDIS |
| 2020 | 0.487233 | 100.0000 | 0.000000 | 0.000000 | 0.000000 | 0.000000 | 0.000000 | 0.000000 | 0.000000 |
| 2021 | 0.589989 | 78.63170 | 0.072003 | 1.986502 | 7.955115 | 0.662960 | 5.814880 | 0.116955 | 4.759883 |
| 2022 | 1.010587 | 27.01061 | 4.667119 | 6.636374 | 32.26216 | 1.748787 | 5.074869 | 3.445038 | 19.15504 |
| 2023 | 1.546070 | 14.86678 | 7.909779 | 11.01467 | 15.86205 | 0.830233 | 6.143777 | 1.941547 | 41.43116 |
| 2024 | 3.723758 | 9.545757 | 6.490126 | 11.76918 | 2.740337 | 0.280061 | 19.31862 | 2.295818 | 47.56011 |
| 2025 | 10.22254 | 8.815312 | 5.290159 | 11.81905 | 0.427555 | 0.341449 | 24.29885 | 3.907338 | 45.10029 |
| 2026 | 26.90904 | 8.843002 | 5.228243 | 11.67120 | 0.143684 | 0.358904 | 24.73920 | 5.107267 | 43.90850 |
| 2027 | 67.05981 | 8.829139 | 5.418946 | 11.45926 | 0.102580 | 0.333716 | 24.67216 | 5.704278 | 43.47992 |
| 2028 | 161.4784 | 8.801253 | 5.585035 | 11.26718 | 0.095839 | 0.313321 | 24.63691 | 5.954317 | 43.34614 |
| 2029 | 382.2614 | 8.787153 | 5.691285 | 11.12292 | 0.095867 | 0.302734 | 24.63175 | 6.057192 | 43.31110 |

Note: SVAD shows services value-added, COMD shows communicable disease, WOM shows word-of-mouth, LOCKDOWN shows lockdown, FACT shows financial activity, EACT shows economic activity, PCONT shows price control, and SOCIDIS shows social distancing. SE shows standard error.

## 5. Conclusions

The novel coronavirus is transmitted from one person to another through close contacts, coughing, sneezing, and touching. Hence, the governments adopted several policy instruments to contain coronavirus across the globe. The COVID-19 prevention measures are essential for breaking down the transmission channels, which would ultimately support the vanished coronavirus pandemic. In the recent crisis of the increased epidemic curve, the services sector is mainly affected due to lockdowns, travel, tourism, transport-related restrictions, business shutdown, and meagre economic and financial activities on a global scale. This study examined the possible impacts of COVID-19 measures on the services industry by using aggregated world data between 1975 and 2019. The results show that the causes of death by communicable diseases, including COVID-19, low financial activities, price control, and maintaining physical distancing, negatively affected the services value-added. In contrast, increased word-of-mouth regarding coronavirus pandemic in general masses, and smart lockdowns subsidized the services sector's value across the globe. The study evaluated the COVID-19 pandemic's impacts on the service industry in the inter-temporal forecasting relationship and suggested that smart lockdowns, sound economic policies, efficient price control mechanisms, and physical distancing will largely control the coronavirus, which leads to an increase in services share relative to the world GDP, over a time horizon. In this regard, the study proposed the following policy implications for a healthier contribution in the research community at a global scale, i.e.,

(I) There is a high need to control the possible transmission channels through which coronavirus is sustained for at least 14 days in the human body and found to uphold another carrier. It could mostly be contained through an improved information-sharing mechanism, which works as a word-of-mouth campaign through social media, print media, and other controlled information sources to spread knowledge regarding the deadly disease and suggest the ways to escape out from this pandemic. We have to think more strategically and look to new, innovative channels that are supposed to restrain coronavirus activities at a large scale, for instance, to promote subsidized nutritional supplements to the large population to obtain an increase in their immunity system and give emphasis to take healthy diets along with the supplements to produce resistance against the virus. Further, vigorous exercise workouts, brainstorming puzzles, indoor activities, and free internet and calling facilities may reduce the boredom and make them the excitement that encourages staying at home out of safety. On the other side, the governments offer some incentive packages to the whole-sellers, retailers, hotels, and business owners, so that they may be able to survive in a time of crisis. The lockdowns could be relaxed for some hours in a day and keep monitoring the business activities, so the risk of spreading coronavirus should be limited. The transportation and means of communications are mainly disturbed during this unprecedented time, affecting logistics activities and service quality. The governments should allow goods transportation at night time, which can freely reach the destination.

(II) Financial transactions and economic activities mainly suffered due to limited business opportunities in the crisis period. The nationwide lockdowns, social distancing, and inefficient price monitoring system led to more financial sector problems regarding loan disbursement and recovery. The small-scale industries have already been closed due to low demand, a sizeable number of people have been unemployed, and the related industries are shut down; all of these problems require smart solutions to manage the crisis period. The easy economic policies may attract investors to obtain a loan at less interest rate. However, the governments should have to create a demand and allow for some international goods movement in the form of exports and imports to channelize the financial activities.

(III) The community-based services should be initiated by involving local public administration, armed forces, healthcare workers, and academicians to provide fresh food-for-thoughts to get out from the misery. The public administration should build a liaison with the other stakeholders and business owners to schedule their work under the adoption of safety measures. A few suggestions can be beneficial in this regard, i.e.,

- all of the employees have to be regularly checked by the physicians and get health certification, so the workers may go inside the production unit and work accordingly;

- provide healthy, nutritious food in a meal to the employees to keep energy during the work process;
- maintaining the social distancing, as it is the root cause of spreading the pandemic;
- keep monitoring employees' health and provide healthcare awareness to escape out from this pandemic; and,
- take care of their employees and motivate them through incentive-based work.

The armed forces can be effectively used to conduct lockdowns during the scheduled times. The healthcare workers played a decisive role in spreading mass awareness regarding methods of home isolation and their SOPs, while academics should have to teach students online at their homes and find a way to conduct assignments and quizzes, so the students get involved in their studies and obtain exam marks accordingly.

The COVID-19 measures to prevent the general masses from the deadly disease are the governments' prime responsibility, while its impact should be regularly monitored to sustain economic activities in a country. The international tourism infrastructure is mainly damaged during the crisis period. It is a suggestion to make quarantine into tourists' destination point, so the hotels and restaurants can utilize some subsidized payments, which helps to restore employment in this sector. The free flow of goods movement within and outside the country needed international SOPs and trading guidelines, so every country could get an equal opportunity. The smart lockdowns, accessible investment opportunities, charging low-interest rates, easy schedule of returning loans, food pricing control, maintaining physical distance in air-railways-road transportation, proper seating arrangement in keeping the gap between the seats and passengers, and tax rebates to the general public and industries could lessen the intensity of the coronavirus pandemic to support business-related activities across countries. The government should have to liberalize its economic policies to permit economic activities to maintain COVID-19 SOPs and monitor economic activities. Expansionary economic policies seem desirable for supporting vulnerable businesses. The second wave of coronavirus disease is exacerbated due to the failure of implementation in maintaining COVID-19 SOPs in highly dense cities and poor hygiene conditions, while the lack of a proper drainage system, garbage collection, and improper waste recycling system, as well of ignorance in adopting SOPs, make this pandemic more lethal. The COVID-19 vaccine would likely be available in the early or late 2021, although the priority is to infuse the vaccine to the healthcare physicians, staff, and older peoples, while, at a later stage, it will be available to the resident peoples. However, the government should adopt strict healthcare policies and COVID-19 SOPs to contain an enormous increase of COVID-19 cases for pandemic recovery. The study limited some suggested proxy factors that are closely linked to the government's actions to contain the COVID-19 pandemic. Further research can be extended by using some real-time factors, including information and communication technologies, Oxford Stringency Index, Google Mobility series, and stock market indices, to assess pandemic recession in the globalized data set.

**Author Contributions:** Conceptualization, D.Y., M.K.A., M.Y.-P.P., A.A.N. and S.E.A.; methodology, K.Z., A.R.A.A., M.M.Q.A., S. and M.K.J.; software, D.Y., M.K.A., M.Y.-P.P. and K.Z.; validation, K.Z., A.R.A.A., M.M.Q.A., S. and M.K.J.; formal analysis, D.Y., M.K.A., M.Y.-P.P., S. and M.K.J.; investigation, D.Y., M.K.A., M.Y.-P.P., A.A.N. and S.E.A.; resources, A.R.A.A., M.M.Q.A., S. and M.K.J.; data curation, S.E.A., K.Z., A.R.A.A., S. and M.K.J.; writing—original draft preparation, D.Y., M.K.A., M.Y.-P.P., A.A.N., S.E.A. and A.R.A.A.; writing—review and editing, D.Y., M.K.A., M.Y.-P.P., A.R.A.A., S. and M.K.J.; visualization, A.R.A.A., S. and M.K.J.; supervision, D.Y., M.K.A., A.A.N. and S.E.A. All authors have read and agreed to the published version of the manuscript.

**Funding:** Researchers Supporting Project number (RSP-2020/167), King Saud University, Riyadh, Saudi Arabia.

**Institutional Review Board Statement:** Not applicable.

**Informed Consent Statement:** Not applicable.

**Data Availability Statement:** The data is freely available at World Development Indicators published by World Bank [25] at https://databank.worldbank.org/source/world-development-indicators (accessed on 15 September 2020).

**Acknowledgments:** Researchers Supporting Project number (RSP-2020/167), King Saud University, Riyadh, Saudi Arabia.

**Conflicts of Interest:** The authors declare no conflict of interest.

## References

1. Worldometer. COVID-19: Coronavirus Pandemic. 2020. Available online: https://www.worldometers.info/coronavirus/ (accessed on 28 November 2020).
2. Ahmed, A.; Ahsan, H. *Contribution of Services Sector in the Economy of Pakistan*; Working Paper No. 79; Pakistan Institute of Development Economics: Islamabad, Pakistan, 2011; pp. 1–18.
3. Gössling, S.; Scott, D.; Hall, C.M. Pandemics, tourism and global change: A rapid assessment of COVID-19. *J. Sustain. Tour.* **2021**, *29*, 1–20. [CrossRef]
4. Thams, A.; Zech, N.; Rempel, D.; Ayia-Koi, A. *An Initial Assessment of Economic Impacts and Operational Challenges for the Tourism & Hospitality Industry Due to COVID-19*; IUBH Internationale Hochschule: Erfurt, Germany, 2020.
5. Ruiz Estrada, M.A.; Park, D.; Lee, M. The Evaluation of the Final Impact of Wuhan COVID-19 on Trade, Tourism, Transport, and Electricity Consumption of China. Tourism, Transport, and Electricity Consumption of China. 2020. Available online: https://papers.ssrn.com/sol3/papers.cfm?abstract_id=3551093 (accessed on 10 May 2020).
6. Foremny, D.; Sorribas-Navarro, P.; Vall Castelló, J. Living at the Peak: Health and Public Finance During the Covid-19 Pandemic. 2020. Available online: https://papers.ssrn.com/sol3/Papers.cfm?abstract_id=3578483 (accessed on 10 May 2020).
7. Goodell, J.W. COVID-19 and finance: Agendas for future research. *Financ. Res. Lett.* **2020**, *35*, 101512. [CrossRef]
8. Zhao, S.; Zhuang, Z.; Ran, J.; Lin, J.; Yang, G.; Yang, L.; He, D. The association between domestic train transportation and novel coronavirus (2019-nCoV) outbreak in China from 2019 to 2020: A data-driven correlational report. *Travel Med. Infect. Dis.* **2020**, *33*, 101568. [CrossRef]
9. Zheng, R.; Xu, Y.; Wang, W.; Ning, G.; Bi, Y. Spatial transmission of COVID-19 via public and private transportation in China. *Travel. Med. Infect. Dis.* **2020**, *34*, 10162. [CrossRef]
10. Basch, C.E.; Basch, C.H.; Hillyer, G.C.; Jaime, C. The Role of YouTube and the Entertainment Industry in Saving Lives by Educating and Mobilizing the Public to Adopt Behaviors for Community Mitigation of COVID-19: Successive Sampling Design Study. *JMIR Public Health Surveill.* **2020**, *6*, e19145. [CrossRef]
11. Peyravi, M.; Marzaleh, M.A.; Shamspour, N.; Soltani, A. Public Education and Electronic Awareness of the New Coronavirus (COVID-19): Experiences from Iran. *Disaster Med. Public Health Prep.* **2020**, *14*, e5–e6. [CrossRef]
12. Sahu, P. Closure of Universities Due to Coronavirus Disease 2019 (COVID-19): Impact on Education and Mental Health of Students and Academic Staff. *Cureus* **2020**, *12*, e7541. [CrossRef]
13. Bhalekar, V. Novel Coronavirus Pandemic-Impact on Indian Ecology, Economy, E-commerce, Education and Employment. 2020. Available online: https://papers.ssrn.com/sol3/papers.cfm?abstract_id=3580342 (accessed on 11 May 2020).
14. Zheng, W. Mental health and a novel coronavirus (2019-nCoV) in China. *J. Affect Disord.* **2020**, *269*, 201–202. [CrossRef]
15. Musselwhite, C.; Avineri, E.; Susilo, Y. Editorial JTH 16–The Coronavirus Disease COVID-19 and implications for transport and health. *J. Transp. Health* **2020**, *16*, 100853. [CrossRef]
16. Di Toppi, L.S.; Di Toppi, L.S.; Bellini, E. Novel Coronavirus: How Atmospheric Particulate Affects Our Environment and Health. *Challenges* **2020**, *11*, 6. [CrossRef]
17. Deng, S.-Q.; Peng, H.-J. Characteristics of and Public Health Responses to the Coronavirus Disease 2019 Outbreak in China. *J. Clin. Med.* **2020**, *9*, 575. [CrossRef]
18. Anser, M.K.; Yousaf, Z.; Khan, M.A.; Nassani, A.A.; Alotaibid, S.M.; Abro, M.M.Q.; Voe, X.V.; Zaman, K. Does communicable diseases (including COVID-19) may increase global poverty risk? A cloud on the horizon. *Environ. Res.* **2020**, *187*, 109668. [CrossRef]
19. Oraedu, C.; Izogo, E.E.; Nnabuko, J.; Ogba, I.E. Understanding electronic and face-to-face word-of-mouth influencers: An emerging market perspective. *Manag. Res. Rev.* **2020**. [CrossRef]
20. Chirisa, I.; Mutambisi, T.; Chivenge, M.; Mabaso, E.; Matamanda, A.R.; Ncube, R. The urban penalty of COVID-19 lockdowns across the globe: Manifestations and lessons for Anglophone sub-Saharan Africa. *GeoJournal* **2020**. [CrossRef] [PubMed]
21. Owa, F.T.; Yakmut, A.H.S.; Abubakar, I.A.; Onibiyo, E.R.; Olasupo, A.S. Impact of covid-19 on community relationship and technical preparedness of law enforcement agencies in Nigeria. *KOGJOURN* **2020**, *5*, 128–143.
22. Chu, D.K.; Akl, E.A.; Duda, S.; Solo, K.; Yaacoub, S.; Schünemann, H.J.; Reinap, M. Physical distancing, face masks, and eye protection to prevent person-to-person transmission of SARS-CoV-2 and COVID-19: A systematic review and meta-analysis. *Lancet* **2020**, *395*, 1973–1987. [CrossRef]
23. Islam, T.; Pitafi, A.H.; Arya, V.; Wang, Y.; Akhtar, N.; Mubarik, S.; Xiaobei, L. Panic buying in the COVID-19 pandemic: A multi-country examination. *J. Retail. Consum. Serv.* **2020**, *59*, 102357. [CrossRef]

24. Bahrini, R.; Filfilan, A. Impact of the novel coronavirus on stock market returns: Evidence from GCC countries. *Quant. Financ. Econ.* **2020**, *4*, 640–652. [CrossRef]
25. World Bank. *World Development Indicators*; World Bank: Washington, DC, USA, 2020.
26. Lopez, L.; Bianchi, G. Economic Theories on COVID-19's Impact on Hospitality and Tourism. 2020. EHL Insights. Available online: https://hospitalityinsights.ehl.edu/economic-theories-covid-impact-hospitality-tourism (accessed on 20 January 2021).
27. Gursoy, D.; Chi, C.G. Effects of COVID-19 pandemic on hospitality industry: Review of the current situations and a research agenda. *J. Hospit. Market. Manag.* **2020**, *29*, 527–529. [CrossRef]
28. Kim, J.; Kim, D.H.; Sancho-Torres, I.; Nwangwu, J.; Jiakponnah, N.N. An Approach to Outpatient Screening, Treatment, and Community Health Outreach during the Coronavirus Epidemic in New York City. *Adv. Infect. Dis.* **2020**, *10*, 1–5. [CrossRef]
29. Samarathunga, W. Post-COVID-19 Challenges and Way Forward for Sri Lanka Tourism. 2020. Available online: https://papers.ssrn.com/sol3/papers.cfm?abstract_id=3581509 (accessed on 13 May 2020).
30. Yang, Y.; Zhang, H.; Chen, X. Coronavirus pandemic and tourism: Dynamic stochastic general equilibrium modeling of infectious disease outbreak. *Ann. Tour. Res.* **2020**, *83*, 102913. [CrossRef]
31. Wanjala, K. The Economic Impact Assessment of the Novel Coronavirus on Tourism and Trade in Kenya: Lessons from Preceding Epidemics. *Financ. Econ. Rev.* **2020**, *2*, 1–10. [CrossRef]
32. Brodeur, A.; Clark, A.E.; Fleche, S.; Powdthavee, N. Assessing the impact of the coronavirus lockdown on unhappiness, loneliness, and boredom using Google Trends. *arXiv* **2020**, arXiv:2004.12129.
33. Wong, C.H. Malaysia: Coronavirus, political coup and lockdown. *Round Table* **2020**, *109*, 336–337. [CrossRef]
34. Barro, R.J.; Ursúa, J.F.; Weng, J. The Coronavirus and the Great Influenza Pandemic: Lessons from the "Spanish Flu" for the Coronavirus's Potential Effects on Mortality and Economic Activity (No. w26866). *Natl. Bur. Econ. Res.* **2020**. [CrossRef]
35. Gómez-Ríos, D.; Ramirez-Malule, D.; Ramirez-Malule, H. The effect of uncontrolled travelers and social distancing on the spread of novel coronavirus disease (COVID-19) in Colombia. *Travel Med. Infect. Dis.* **2020**, 101699. [CrossRef] [PubMed]
36. Yezli, S.; Khan, A. COVID-19 social distancing in the Kingdom of Saudi Arabia: Bold measures in the face of political, eco-nomic, social and religious challenges. *Travel Med. Infect. Dis.* **2020**, *37*, 101692. [CrossRef] [PubMed]

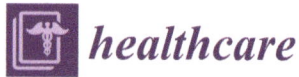 

*Review*

# Beyond COVID-19 Pandemic: An Integrative Review of Global Health Crisis Influencing the Evolution and Practice of Corporate Social Responsibility

Henry Asante Antwi [1,*], Lulin Zhou [1,2], Xinglong Xu [2] and Tehzeeb Mustafa [1]

1 Centre for Health and Public Policy Research, Jiangsu University, 301 Xuefu Road, Zhenjiang 212013, China; lulinzhou@yahoo.com (L.Z.); 5103140204@stmail.ujs.edu.cn (T.M.)
2 School of Management, Jiangsu University, 301 Xuefu Road, Zhenjiang 212013, China; 1000004932@ujs.edu.cn
* Correspondence: 5103150217@stmail.ujs.edu.cn

**Abstract: Background:** Global health crisis continues to drive the dynamics of corporate social responsibility (CSR) across industries with self-perpetuating momentum. From a historical point of view, more than a century of immense corporate fecundity has formed the ecological conditions and shaped current understanding of the effect of public health on CSR. This study sought to examine the extent to which companies are able to balance their business interest with social interest through health-related CSR and how knowledge of them can help explain the potential impact of COVID-19. **Method:** This study employs a narrative review of current literature; however, the integrative strategy was combined with the Preferred Reporting Items for Systematic reviews and Meta-Analyses (PRISMA) checklist to rigorously select the necessary articles for proper integrative synthesis. **Results:** We note that in the pursuit of their social responsibility, corporate enterprises struggle to balance the interest of society and their own interest. Genuine CSR activities such as donations are often undermined by unbridled and excessive desire to draw society on themselves to reap economic benefits are largely dominated by the need to advance. There are signals that enterprises might see COVID-19-related CSR as an entry door to increase corporate influence thereby commercializing the pandemic. **Conclusions:** The impact of COVID-19 on CSR is epochal. There is a moral obligation for enterprises to reform current risk assessments and collaborate more deeply with state agencies to invest in the health and safety inspections at the world place. CSR strategies must be proactive to endure other unknown pandemics with equal capacity to disrupt business operations. Companies must create innovative and regular activities to educate its stakeholders to become more committed to safeguarding future enterprise-based defense mechanism needed to diagnose, protect, treat, and rehabilitate victims and those threatened by pandemics and other emergencies that affect the stability of an organization to reduce its cost and protect revenue.

**Keywords:** CSR; implication; public; health; evolution; COVID-19

**Citation:** Asante Antwi, H.; Zhou, L.; Xu, X.; Mustafa, T. Beyond COVID-19 Pandemic: An Integrative Review of Global Health Crisis Influencing the Evolution and Practice of Corporate Social Responsibility. *Healthcare* **2021**, *9*, 453. https://doi.org/10.3390/healthcare9040453

Academic Editors: Eduardo Tomé, Thomas Garavan and Ana Dias

Received: 21 February 2021
Accepted: 1 April 2021
Published: 12 April 2021

**Publisher's Note:** MDPI stays neutral with regard to jurisdictional claims in published maps and institutional affiliations.

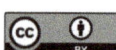

**Copyright:** © 2021 by the authors. Licensee MDPI, Basel, Switzerland. This article is an open access article distributed under the terms and conditions of the Creative Commons Attribution (CC BY) license (https://creativecommons.org/licenses/by/4.0/).

## 1. Introduction

Nowadays, an ever-increasing number of enterprises recognize the need to voluntarily donate to support society to meet some of its pervading challenges in one way or the other. There seems to be an urgent need among enterprises across the globe to hold fast to corporate social responsibility (CSR) as a synergistic platform to enhance corporate offer and competitiveness [1]. From a historical point of view, more than a century of immense corporate fecundity has formed the ecological conditions, shaped the current understanding of CSR, and made a profound impact on CSR research and practice across the globe [2]. Along this CSR evolutionary trajectory, different revolutionary occurrences of historical significance have serenaded the principles, theories, practices, mechanisms, approaches, driving dynamics and stratagems of corporate social responsibility [3].

The early theories of corporate social responsibility (CSR) advocacy that emerged in the 19th century provided conflicting evidence as to why a firm should support CSR or not. In his 'magnum opus' "the wealth of nations", renowned Scottish philosopher Adam Smith explained that consumers were "social sentinels" and must only support enterprises that are socially responsible. These are enterprises whose actions and inactions advance their interest without compromising the interest of the society [4]. According to Adam Smith as cited in Hedblom et al. [4], given the opportunity, an industry player will always pursue a selfish reason to satisfy its personal benefit at the expense of society. Smith believed that consumers are the best stakeholders to guard the welfare of society by ensuring that only goods and services of social companies are patronized.

However, there are many dissenting voices to this notion of corporate social responsibility. For example, Milton Friedman believed that business organizations are established just to satisfy the profit motives of their shareholders [4,5]. With time, more convincing CSR theories (e.g., social contract theory, stakeholder theory, etc.) have emerged and the field has so matured beyond being a simple corporate sidebar.

Several contemporary enterprises have gained a better appreciation of the need to develop a corporate conscience and stimulate socially responsible activities. This is the only way by which they can obtain social legitimacy and bolster brand value to safeguard its continuous existence and prosperity [6,7]. CSR has become a business strategy that is well established not only in the academic literature but also in practice.

Long before the industrial revolution and many years afterwards, several public and global health crises have driven and continue to drive changes in society and the workplace. Health crises are harder to understand as they are typically infrequent and unpredictable. Thus, health crises are akin to the black swan as they are unexpected yet have severe consequences. Since December 2019, the enormity of the impact of COVID-19 on corporate organizations and the global economy has triggered an unprecedented and unfathomable shift in corporate social responsibility paradigm and practices as the world battles to contain the corona virus [8]. Yet, long before COVID-19, the discombobulating effect of the Spanish flu, cholera, malaria, HIV-AIDS, environmental health crisis, H1N1, MES, ebola, obesity, and the opioid epidemics, etc., on corporate stability had catalyzed the incubation of public-health-led CSR strategies to advance the frontiers of corporate social responsibility.

Even though general literature on health-related CSR is dotted across different extant studies, a synthesis of how public health crises have shaped the past, present, and future of CSR is limited. Moreover, not every health pandemic has become an extremely topical issue to influence the cause of corporate social responsibility. This is because only a few of such epidemics manage to gain the attention of the global public, international organizations, and multinational corporations to elicit their interest, advocacy, and support. This is because the corporate world is profit oriented and only global health crises that have the potential to cause wide range disruptions in business or improve business interest of firms often get corporate social support [8]. This review explores the global health crises that have influenced the evolution of CSR practices and principles and how knowledge of them can help explain the potential impact of COVID-19 on CSR. Consequently, the following are the research questions this study seeks to answer:

(a) To compare how different global health crises influenced the evolution of corporate social responsibility practice.
(b) Whether business organizations are able to balance economic intentions and the need to support societal through CSR programs during global health crises.

The rest of the article is structured as follows. The Materials and Methods section is explained after this introductory section. Next, we discuss the findings from literature under five main topics. The conclusions and theoretical implications of the study are drawn. The limitations and future research directions are then outlined to conclude the paper.

## 2. Materials and Methods

The effect of global health on CSR is a complex issue but the debilitating effect of COVID-19 demands timely and accurate information to support enterprises. As such, an integrative review method was chosen but ideas were borrowed from the Preferred Reporting Items for Systematic reviews and Meta-Analyses (PRISMA) checklist to ensure that the reviewed scientific literature was not selected arbitrarily. Figure 1 shows the graphical representation of the selected activities. Consistent with the prior works of D'Aprile and Mannarini [9], corporate social responsibility was treated as a multidimensional construct and its mechanisms, processes, and evolution are driven by an ensemble of sophisticated intrinsic and extrinsic factors. These factors sometimes come closer and move apart. In other words, the context of CSR motivation and practice, theoretical expositions and assumptions, policy and regulatory framework are shaped by a matrix of socio-cultural and economic factors that evolves overtime. This makes CSR practice a dynamic and constantly and rapidly evolving endeavor for business organizations that wants to take advantage of its benefits. To this end, this research synthesized and evaluated the most current studies that highlight how health-related factors have shaped contemporary CSR practices and its future trend in the midst of COVID-19. Health drivers of corporate social responsibility were first extracted from available studies and clustered in accordance with evolution, purposes, diffusion into CSR practices, and effect of such diffusions.

### 2.1. Search Strategy

A total of 10 bibliographic databases were shortlisted for extended search based on initial screening on related contents between February 2019 and February 2021. This date was chosen to give enough time to understand the impact of the COVID-19 pandemic on enterprises after it emerged in December 2019. The databases were the Web of Science, EBSCO, SCOPUS, Pro-Quest, Directory of Open Access Journals, Digital Library of the Commons Repository, Education Resources Information Center, Social Science Research Network, Public Library of Science, and Social Science Research Network. These databases were chosen because of their credibility, volume of information they store, and impact factor of articles stored in them regarding CSR and public health. Even till today, there are several aspects of COVID-1 that remain unclear and research, knowledge about its impact on corporate practices is still developing. As such, most of the available studies are still deposited in pre-print databases awaiting peer review. For this reason, frequently cited pre-print databases such as arXiv e-Print Archive were consulted for additional information. For each database, distinct and hierarchical search cluster terms were defined i.e., main topic, subtopic, and specific theme.

Narrative search was used to select the articles. The search terms (public health interventions, health-related CSR, environmental health-related CSR, COVID-19-related CSR) were combined through Boolean operators such as AND/OR. The search terms were entered individually in English. Truncations as well as wildcard characters helped to improve the sensitivity and precision of the searches. The initial searches did not discriminate in terms of publication time frame, research design (qualitative/quantitative research, primary/secondary research), peer review criteria (essay or dissertation or academic paper). The initial search yielded 1763 articles and was supplemented with additional hand searches in Google Scholar and a cross-check of the reference lists of studies included for analysis. Through this process, 107 additional articles were retrieved and added to the selection process.

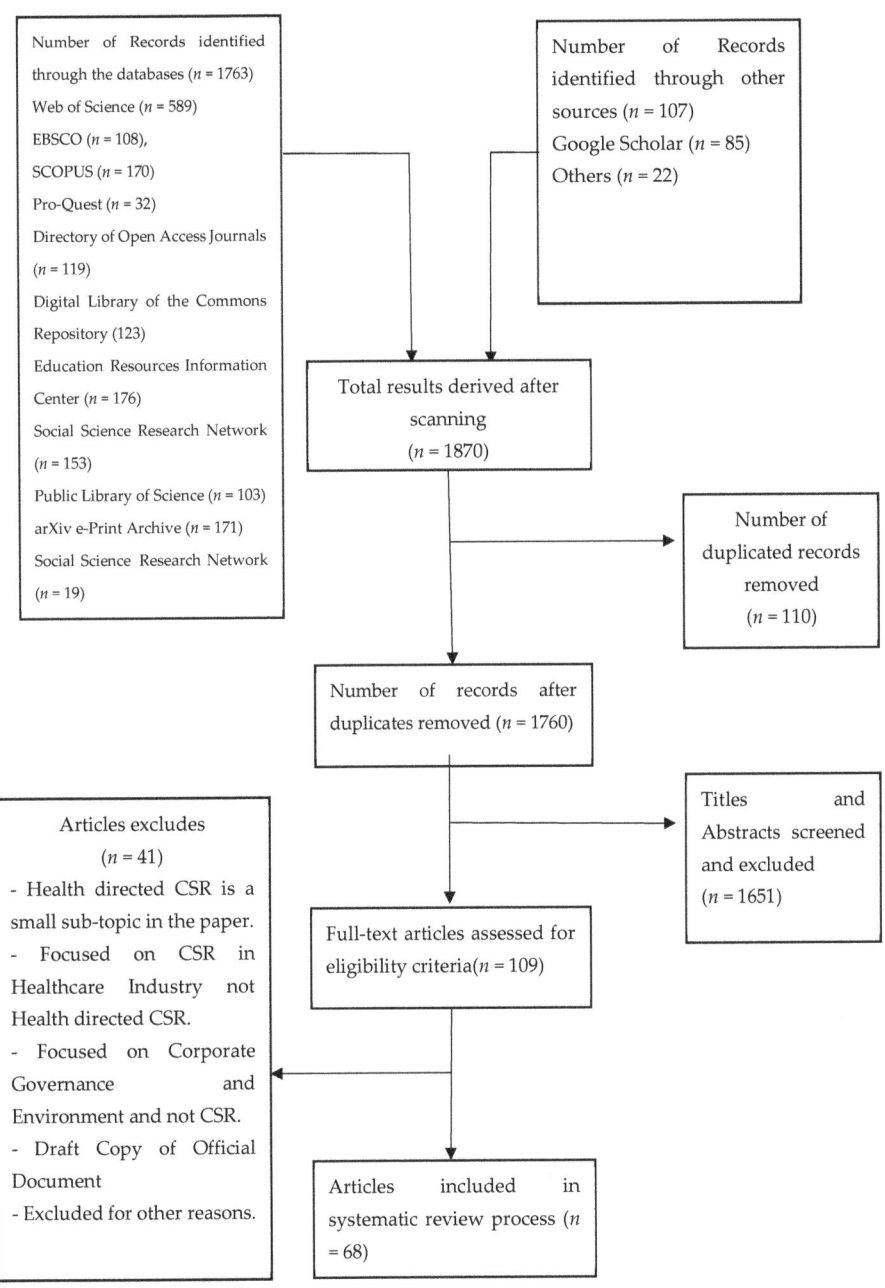

**Figure 1.** PRISMA model.

Table 1 presents the summary of the different types of global health crises that are of CSR concerned initially extracted from the articles in the databases and other sources. The difference in the number of cases per source and the total number of articles from each source stems from the fact that the cases overlapped across the articles. In other words, in some instances, a single article discussed more than a single global health issue that has affected CSR practice. Most importantly, three groups of global health epidemics emerged as dominantly discussed in the extant literature and they form the basis for the discussion in this paper. For example, in the initial search, environmental health crisis was reported 1316 times across the articles whereas the influence of HIV-AIDS on CSR was reported 1253 times in the studies. On the other hand, COVID-19 was reported 298 times whiles the opioid and obesity epidemics are represented in 283 and 163 studies, respectively.

**Table 1.** Summary of CSR-related global health crisis extracted from databases and other sources.

| Databases | HIV-AIDS Pandemic | Environment Health Pandemic | Spanish Flu | Cholera | Opioid Epidemic | Malaria | Obesity Epidemic | COVID-19 Pandemic |
|---|---|---|---|---|---|---|---|---|
| Web of Science | 204 | 342 | 17 | 35 | 32 | 109 | 21 | 25 |
| SCOPUS | 193 | 161 | 9 | 17 | 13 | 28 | 9 | 17 |
| EBSCO | 68 | 47 | 7 | 12 | 19 | 39 | 11 | 23 |
| Pro-Quest | 17 | 21 | 2 | 8 | 5 | 31 | 16 | 18 |
| Directory of Open Access Journals | 86 | 81 | 8 | 19 | 39 | 52 | 7 | 25 |
| Digital Library of the Commons Repository | 73 | 75 | 5 | 41 | 28 | | 31 | 23 |
| Education Resources Information Center | 101 | 108 | 18 | 23 | 20 | 38 | 4 | 32 |
| Social Science Research Network | 93 | 106 | 6 | 19 | 6 | 64 | 6 | 23 |
| Public Library of Science | 98 | 121 | 12 | 36 | 3 | 43 | 9 | 21 |
| arXiv e-Print Archive | 121 | 106 | 6 | 3 | 9 | | 6 | 19 |
| Social Science Research Network | 108 | 79 | 9 | 8 | 78 | 52 | 18 | 31 |
| Google Scholar | 74 | 54 | 4 | 13 | 23 | 19 | 15 | 29 |
| Others | 17 | 15 | 5 | 9 | 8 | 48 | 9 | 12 |

## 2.2. Screening

The articles were initially screened to remove duplicates in a two-step process. The entire list of articles was imported to four citation managers namely Mendeley, EndNote, Sciwheel, and Zotero. Four well-trained research assistants with expertise in library and archival reference management information system removed all duplications. This was strictly supervised by the author. The screened results from each of the four citation managers were carefully compared. After manually inspecting and validating the articles, the author compiled the final list of qualified articles. From this process, a total of 110 duplicate articles were removed from the list of 1870 articles, leaving a total of 1760 qualifying articles. These final articles were further validated by the author and the research assistants.

## 2.3. Eligibility

A strict eligibility criterion was used to determine qualifying articles for the final review. Firstly, the article should be available in English language. Secondly, the article must focus on healthcare issues in corporate social responsibility including any domain or topic-specific health-driven CSR studies. Thirdly, the article should be a peer reviewed academic paper. Where the paper is not a peer review paper, then it must be a document from a highly rated, international team or recognized professional group. Official CSR documents released by multinational enterprises, international organizations such as the United Nations, International Labour Organization, etc., and papers that offer insight into the historical evolution or unique information and context for conceptualizing and theorizing health-related CSR were included. Another criterion for inclusion and exclusion was that the selected article must document available health-related CSR practices, strategies, systems, corporate initiatives, successes, failures, and future changes.

Finally, a recent article that synthesizes CSR and COVID-19 was highly recommended. Articles published in relation to corporate responsibility and the obesity epidemic, CSR and Internet addiction, opioid addiction and CSR, which are not known contagious pathogenic health crisis but have been linked with CSR in the past, were included for analysis. Whether articles were included for full-text analysis was determined by the author with the assistance of trained literature search specialists depending on whether the articles fitted well with the eligibility criteria. Publications that were disputable were further validated through a snowballing of other relevant considerations and deliberations among the research team members until consensus was reached to accept or reject its inclusion.

*2.4. Data Extraction and Analysis*

A final set of 68 articles that summarized the major public health crisis that influences CSR were selected for full-text analysis based on the following reasons. Twenty-one of them contained information on HIV-AIDS and corporate social responsibility, while 26 of them contained information on environmental health catastrophe and corporate governance. Sixteen of them described the interplay between COVID-19 and corporate governance. Other studies that directly addressed the three shortlisted subjects were included in view of their current position on COVID-19 and the new insight they provide for the future of corporate social responsibility after COVID-19. All the sixty-eight articles were qualitatively evaluated and synthesized through a four-step inductive content analysis process. In the first place, the eligible articles were scanned definitions and conceptual models that were directly developed for the target group or adapted to it or included relevant perspectives on health literature as a whole.

Next, the definitions and models were coded and extracted by the research team based on an inductive approach. Definitions and models that overlapped from the same research groups were included on a single occasion. For non-related articles that explain the same health literature definitions or models, only the original reference was added and marked accordingly. In the third stage, important background data were declined and extracted into a matrix. Some of these data include age of target group, reason for studying the target group, whether the perspective of the target group was considered in developing the definition or model or in applicability and relevance of these and the settings for which they were developed. Finally, the articles' research design and methodological quality were assessed. Finally, the identified themes and dimensions were discussed with a whole research team in April 2020 and the feedback was integrated into the final analysis.

## 3. Results

The study selection flow diagram is illustrated in Figure 1. It summarizes the number of the studies recorded at each stage of the process. For example, the figure reveals that the initial search yielded 1760 potentially relevant citations and after screening abstract and titles, 109 were kept. Further screening of the citations led to the final set of 45 articles which have been presented for extended analysis in this report.

*3.1. Study Characteristics*

Table 2 presents the characteristics of the 68 shortlisted studies. About 27% of the results were focused on HIV-AIDs whereas 34% were focused largely on environmental health. Overlapping studies were also recorded. For example, 9% of the studies involved COVID-19 while 17% involved COVID-19 and HIV-AIDS. Further, 13% involved COVID-19 and environmental health while 11% involved environmental health and HIV-AIDS. In addition, 21% of the studies were primary qualitative research whereas 42% were secondary qualitative research. Further, 17% of the studies were primary quantitative research while 20% quantitative research studies. The settings of the study were widely variable. Additionally, 48.7% of the studies focused on the Sub-Saharan Africa while 19.3% focused on Europe. Further, 15% of the studies focused on South America and 9% were focused on the United States of America. The total number of studies that focused on Asia was 17% while focused on a global scale.

Table 2. Descriptive characteristics of extracted articles for systematic analysis.

| Study | Year of Publication | Methodological Design | Setting | Focus | Funding | Key Objectives |
|---|---|---|---|---|---|---|
| Gentilini | 2020 | Quantitative | Global | COVID/MES/Cholera | Yes | How countries and Multinational Companies (MNCs) are responding to the COVID-19 pandemic, Cholera/MES |
| Lindgreen et al. | 2009 | Quantitative | Botswana and Malawi | Global Health/COVID/MES | Yes | Economic benefits of health-related CSR practices |
| Amoako et al. | 2019 | Quantitative | Ghana | Environment and Health/Spanish Flu/opioid | Yes | Health-related CSR activities among the oil marketing companies |
| Makwara et al. | 2019 | Quantitative | Zimbabwe and South Africa | HIV-AIDS/Spanish Flu/Malaria/Cholera | Yes | Employee's HIV and AIDS-related corporate social responsibility (CSR) practices by small business based on experiences from the Spanish Flu/Malaria |
| Flanagan and Whiteman | 2007 | Quantitative | Brazil | HIV-AIDS/COVID/Spanish Flu/Malaria | Yes | Private and public Partnership to fight HIV-AIDS based on experiences from the Spanish Flu/Malaria |
| Utuk et al. | 2017 | Quantitative | Nigeria | HIV-AIDS/COVID/Spanish Flu/Malaria | Yes | Stigmatising attitudes towards co-workers with HIV in the workplace based on experiences from the Spanish Flu/Malaria |
| uduji et al. | 2019 | Quantitative | Nigeria | HIV-AIDS | Yes | Impact of CSR of multinational oil companies on HIV/AIDS prevalence in Nigeria based on experiences from Cholera/Malaria |
| Bowen et al. | 2014 | Qualitative | South Africa | HIV-AIDS/COVID/Spanish Flu/Malaria | Yes | Guidelines for effective workplace HIV/AIDS intervention management by construction firms based on experiences from Cholera/Malaria |
| Rampersad | 2013 | Qualitative | South Africa | HIV-AIDS/COVID/ | Yes | Moral and social responsibility of the corporate sector in its effort to deal with the issue of HIV/AIDS |
| Ferreira | 2002 | Qualitative | Global | HIV-AIDS | Yes | Access to affordable HIV/AIDS drugs: The human rights obligations of multinational pharmaceutical corporations based on experiences from Cholera/Malaria |
| Bolton | 2002 | Qualitative | South Africa | HIV-AIDS | Yes | How South African companies are taking action against HIV in ways that set new benchmarks |

Table 2. Cont.

| Study | Year of Publication | Methodological Design | Setting | Focus | Funding | Key Objectives |
|---|---|---|---|---|---|---|
| Mahajan et al. | 2007 | Qualitative | Southern Africa | HIV-AIDS | Yes | An overview of HIV/AIDS workplace policies and programmes in southern Africa based on experiences from Cholera/Malaria |
| Davis and Anderson | 2008 | Qualitative | Global | HIV-AIDS/COVID/Spanish Flu/Malaria | Yes | Demands faced by multinationals to assume greater responsibility for solving social problems large and small. |
| based on experiences from Cholera/Malaria Dufee | 2006 | Qualitative | Global | HIV-AIDS | Yes | Corporate Responsibility and the AIDS Catastrophe in Sub-Saharan Africa, Pharmaceutical companies |
| Stadler | 2004 | Qualitative | South Africa | HIV-AIDS | Yes | Health-related corporate social responsibility initiatives in commercial advertising agency |
| Rajak | 2010 | Qualitative | South Africa | HIV-AIDS | Yes | How relations between employer and employee are being transformed by corporate HIV programmes |
| Sharma and Kiran | 2012 | Qualitative | India | HIV-AIDS/COVID/Spanish Flu/Malaria | Yes | The status and progress and initiatives made by large firms of India in context to CSR policy framing and implementation |
| Orlitzky et al. | 2011 | Qualitative | Global | Environment and Health/opioid/obesity | Yes | Agenda for future research on strategic CSR and environmental sustainability based on experiences from Cholera/Malaria |
| Lyon and Maxwell | 2008 | Qualitative | Global | Environment and Health opioid/obesity | Yes | The motives for and welfare effects of environmental corporate social responsibility (CSR) based on experiences from Cholera/Malaria/Obesity/opioid crises |
| Sanyal and Neves | 2001 | Qualitative | Global | Environment and Health opioid/obesity | Yes | The Valdez Principles |
| Welker | 2009 | Qualitative | Indonesia | Environment and Health opioid/obesity | Yes | The corporate social responsibility industry, and environmental advocacy in Indonesia |
| Shaukat et al. | 2016 | Qualitative | Global | Environment and Health opioid/obesity | Yes | Board Attributes, Corporate Social Responsibility Strategy, and Corporate Environmental and Social Performance |

Table 2. *Cont.*

| Study | Year of Publication | Methodological Design | Setting | Focus | Funding | Key Objectives |
|---|---|---|---|---|---|---|
| Coussens and Harrison | 2007 | Qualitative | Global | Environment and Health/Spanish Flu/Cholera/Malaria | Yes | Global Environmental Health in the 21st Century |
| Málovics et al. | 2008 | Qualitative | Global | Environment and Health | Yes | The role of corporate social responsibility in strong sustainability |
| Kulczycka et al. | 2016 | Qualitative | Global | Environment and Health/Spanish Flu/Cholera/Malaria | Yes | Communication about social and environmental disclosure by large and small copper mining companies |
| Reinhardt and Stavins | 2010 | Qualitative | Global | Environment and Health | Yes | Corporate social responsibility, business strategy, and the environment |
| Chandler | 2020 | Qualitative | Global | Environment and Health/Spanish Flu/Cholera/Malaria | Yes | Reflecting on the need to include CSR principles in future legislative reforms |
| Kolk | 2016 | Qualitative | Global | Environment and Health | Yes | The environmental responsibility of international business |
| Alvarado-Herrera | 2017 | Qualitative | Global | Environment and Health/Spanish Flu/Cholera/Malaria | Yes | A scale for measuring consumer perceptions of corporate social responsibility following the sustainable development paradigm |
| Schönherr et al. | 2018 | Qualitative | Global | Environment and Health | Yes | How the Sustainable Development Goals (SDGs) as a global agenda may serve as a reference framework to support TNCs in improving their corporate social responsibility (CSR) engagement |
| Xia et al. | 2018 | Qualitative | Global | Environment and Health | Yes | Conceptualising the state of the art of corporate social responsibility (CSR) in the construction industry and its nexus to sustainable development |
| Givel | 2017 | Qualitative | Global | Environment and Health/Spanish Flu/Cholera/Malaria | Yes | The primary goal of the Responsible Care effort to change public concerns and opinion about chemical industry environmental and public health practices |
| Alon et al. | 2020 | Qualitative | Global | COVID | Yes | The Impact of COVID-19 on Gender Equality |

Table 2. *Cont.*

| Study | Year of Publication | Methodological Design | Setting | Focus | Funding | Key Objectives |
|---|---|---|---|---|---|---|
| Francis and Pegg | 2020 | Qualitative | Nigeria | COVID/Spanish Flu/Cholera | Yes | The challenges that one long running micro-scale development project has faced due to the COVID 19 disease outbreak and the closure of all schools in Rivers State, Nigeria |
| Williamson et al. | 2020 | Qualitative | Global | COVID | Yes | COVID-19 and experiences of moral injury in front-line key workers |
| Vaccaro et al. | 2020 | Qualitative | US | COVID | Yes | Practice Management During the COVID-19 Pandemic |
| Shingal | 2020 | Qualitative | Global | COVID/Spanish Flu/Cholera | Yes | Services trade and COVID-19 |
| Boone et al. | 2020 | Qualitative | Global | COVID | Yes | The socio-economic implications of the coronavirus and COVID-19 pandemic |
| Hevia and Neumeyer | 2020 | Qualitative | Global | COVID | Yes | A Conceptual Framework for Analyzing the Economic Impact of COVID-19 and its Policy Implication |
| Zeren and Hizarci | 2020 | Qualitative | Global | COVID | Yes | The Impact of COVID-19 Coronavirus on Stock Markets based on experiences from MES/Malaria |
| Cabral and Xu | 2020 | Qualitative | Global | COVID | Yes | Seller Reputation and Price Gouging: Evidence from the COVID-19 Pandemic |
| Delwin et al. | 2019 | Qualitatve | SubSaharan Africa | HIV-AIDS | Yes | Role of Multinationals in HIV-AIDS in Asian/SubSahara based on experiences from Cholera/Malaria |
| Dickson and Stevens | 2005 | Quantitative | South Africa | HIV-AIDS | Yes | Understanding the response of large South African companies to HIV/AIDS |
| Bendel | 2003 | Quantitative | Global South | HIV-AIDS | Yes | Response of large corporations to HIV/AIDS in Southern Africa based on experiences from Cholera/Malaria |
| Ntim | 2016 | Quantitative | subsaharan | HIV-AIDS | Yes | HIV/AIDS disclosures in Sub-Saharan Africa based on experiences from Cholera/Malaria |
| Delmas et al. | 2013 | Quantitative | Global | Environment and Health | Yes | Socially responsible investing |
| Annan-Diab | 2017 | Quantitative | US | Environment and Health | Yes | The importance of adopting an interdisciplinary approach to education for sustainable development based on experiences from Cholera/Malaria |

Table 2. Cont.

| Study | Year of Publication | Methodological Design | Setting | Focus | Funding | Key Objectives |
|---|---|---|---|---|---|---|
| Suárez-Cebador | 2018 | Quantitative | Portugal | Environment and Health | Yes | A model to measure sustainable development in the hotel industry |
| Chuang and Huang | 2018 | Quantitative | Taiwan | Environment and Health | Yes | The Effect of Environmental Corporate Social Responsibility on Environmental Performance and Business Competitiveness |
| Marco-Fondevila | 2018 | Quantitative | Spain | Environment and Health/COVID/Spanish Flu/Cholera | Yes | The determinants and empirical interrelations between accountability standards and environmental proactivity |
| López-Pérez | 2017 | Quantitative | South America | Environment and Health | Yes | Analysis of specific corporate social responsibility +CSR) training in sustainable development to boost the potential impact of CSR on shareholder value |
| Taylor et al. | 2018 | Quantitative | Global | Environment and Health | Yes | Benefits associated with voluntary disclosure of corporate social responsibility (CSR) activities |
| Osmani | 2019 | Quantitative | China | Environment and Health COVID/Spanish Flu/Cholera | Yes | Corporate Social Responsibility for Sustainable Development in China. Recent Evolution of CSR Concepts and Practice within Chinese Firms based on experiences from Cholera/Malaria |
| Dimmler | 2017 | Quantitative | South Africa | Environment and Health COVID/Spanish Flu/Cholera | Yes | Linking social determinants of health to corporate social responsibility: Extant criteria for the mining industry based on experiences from Cholera/Malaria |
| Senay and Landrigan | 2018 | Quantitative | US | Environment and Health COVID/Spanish Flu/Cholera | Yes | Assessment of environmental sustainability and corporate social responsibility reporting by large health care organizations |
| Albuquerque et al. | 2020 | Quantitative | US | COVID/Environment | Yes | How firms with high Environmental and Social (ES) ratings fare during the first quarter of 2020 compared to other firms |
| Shan and Tang | 2020 | Quantitative | China | COVID | Yes | The role of employee satisfaction in withstanding the public health shock |
| Laing | 2020 | Quantitative | Global | COVID | Yes | The economic impact of the Coronavirus 2019 (COVID-2019): Implications for the mining industry |

Table 2. *Cont.*

| Study | Year of Publication | Methodological Design | Setting | Focus | Funding | Key Objectives |
|---|---|---|---|---|---|---|
| Makridis and Hartley | 2020 | Quantitative | US | COVID | Yes | The Cost of COVID-19: A Rough Estimate of the 2020 US GDP Impact |
| Nuno-Fernandes | 2020 | Quantitative | Europe | COVID | Yes | Economic effects of coronavirus outbreak (COVID-19) on the world economy |
| Maital and Barzani | 2020 | Quantitative | Global | COVID | Yes | Global Economic Effects of COVID-19 |
| Barua | 2020 | Quantitative | Global | COVID | Yes | The Economic Implications of the Coronavirus (COVID-19) Pandemic |
| Johson et al. | 2010 | Qualitative | Global | Natural Disasters | Yes | Reasons why MNC engage in health-related CSR |
| Vian et al. | 2007 | Qualitative | Global | Global Health | Yes | How multinational pharmaceutical companies engage in CSR activities in the developing world |
| Soobaroyen and Ntim | 2013 | Qualitative | South Africa | HIV-AIDS COVID/Spanish Flu/Cholera | Yes | Global Reporting Initiative guidelines on HIV/AIDS to assess on whether corporations have adopted a substantive management strategy |
| Long | 2016 | Qualitative | Tanzania | HIV-AIDS COVID/Spanish Flu/Cholera | Yes | Role of PEPFAR Tanzania pin the national health sector's HIV/AIDS policy shift based on experiences from Cholera/Malaria |
| Gilbert | 2017 | Qualitative | South Africa | HIV-AIDS COVID/Spanish Flu/Cholera | Yes | Investigating HIV/AIDS intervention management by construction organizations in South Africa based on experiences from Cholera/Malaria |

## 3.2. Study Quality

To evaluate the quality of the studies, the Mixed Methods Appraisal Tool (MMAT) was applied as shown in Table 3. Pluye and Hong [10] explain that the MMAT tool helps to provide quality appraisal for quantitative, qualitative, and mixed methods to be included in systematic reviews. The score of the MMAR results in this case is presented in Table 3. As disclosed, scores for the selected studies ranged between 25% and 83%. In addition, 4% of the studies received 25% rating based on the MMAT criteria whereas 5% of the studies received 33.3%. Similarly, 13.5% studies received 50% while 38.5% received between 60 and 80%. The remainder of the studies received in excess of 80% on the MMAT tool.

The most frequent weaknesses related to lack of discussion on the reason for studying specific organizations, the influence of the organization on the research, and researcher influence in qualitative and mixed methods studies. There were also issues with lack of a clear description of the sampling process of respondents adopted by authors in quantitative studies and sub threshold rates for acceptable response or follow-up in non-randomized quantitative studies were also recorded as major weaknesses of the quantitative research. Most of the studies had support from funding agencies or organizations for whom the research outcome serves their interest. Thus, the influence of such organizations in the conduct of the research was not disclosed by the researchers.

## 3.3. Differences and Similarities between the Nature and Effect of COVID-19 and HIV-AIDS

Table 4 presents a comparative analysis of some of the key characteristics of the main epidemics that have influenced corporate social responsibility within the last couple of years. Ten main epidemics were noted from the extant literature. These were COVID-19, Spanish flu, HIV-AIDS, cholera, environmental pollution, malaria, MES, ebola, opioid, and obesity. Predictably, COVID-19 frequented in the studies most as a target for CSR. This was followed by HIV-AIDS and environmental health. The opioid and obesity pandemics have received the lowest concentration of CSR articles about them. These ten different epidemics have affected CSR in its current practice because they have attracted the attention of the international community and agencies such as the United Nations as well as multinational organizations. There were differences that were found among the ten epidemics and these differences and similarities equally affect CSR practice and even the enormity of commitment that is invested by companies on their related CSR [11,12]. The epidemics differ in terms of the scope of geographical coverage of infection. For example, COVID-19 is global but MES was restricted to the Middle East and parts of Asia. Even though malaria and cholera are global, most of the studies emerged from developing countries in Sub-Saharan Africa, South East Asia, South America, etc., and these are the places where most of the CSR activities are concentrated.

A similar observation was made about HIV-AIDS. It is a global pandemic but southern parts of Africa have received the highest concentration of studies and CSR resources from countries. The seasonal variation in the infection is also one of the sources of differences. In this case, COVID-19 and MES vary according to weather conditions while most of the others do not. The scale of public panic over COVID-19 has been enormous compared to the panic that greeted HIV-AIDS and MES [13–15]. In the case of COVID-19, MES, and the Spanish flu, the studies show that physical lockdowns were used to control infections. Together with cholera, isolations were also used to control infection rate. Even though HIV-AIDS had its own stigma, the scale of COVID-19 and Ebola were enormous. We found that obesity also belongs to this category of epidemics with some stigma. With ebola, MES, COVID-19, cholera, and the Spanish flu, mass gatherings were major sources of infections but there is the possibility of early detection and treatment for all the diseases with the exception of HIV-AIDS which can be moderated but not treated [16].

**Table 3.** MMAT assessment of quality of extracted articles for systematic review.

| Qualitative Research | Data sources relevant? | Data analysis process relevant? | Findings relate to context? | Findings relate to researchers' influence? | Clear description of the sampling process of respondents? | Support from funding agencies | % |
|---|---|---|---|---|---|---|---|
| Bowen et al. | Y | Y | Y | N | Y | N | 67% |
| Ramperasad | Y | Y | Y | N | Y | N | 67% |
| Ferreira | Y | Y | Y | N | Y | N | 67% |
| Bolton | Y | N | N | N | Y | N | 50% |
| Mah-ajan et al. | Y | Y | Y | Y | Y | N | 83% |
| Davis and Anderson | Y | Y | Y | N | Y | N | 67% |
| Dufee | Y | Y | Y | N | Y | N | 67% |
| Stadler | Y | Y | Y | N | Y | N | 67% |
| Rajak | Y | Y | Y | N | Y | N | 50% |
| Sharma and Kiran | Y | Y | Y | N | Y | N | 67% |
| Orlitzky et al. | Y | Y | Y | N | Y | N | 67% |
| Lyon and Maxwell | Y | Y | Y | N | Y | N | 67% |
| Sanyal and Neves | Y | Y | Y | N | Y | N | 67% |
| Welker | Y | Y | Y | N | Y | N | 67% |
| Shaukat et al. | Y | Y | Y | N | Y | N | 67% |
| Coussens and Harrison | Y | N | Y | N | N | N | 33% |
| Malovics et al. | Y | Y | Y | N | Y | N | 67% |
| Kulczycka et al. | Y | Y | Y | N | Y | N | 67% |
| Reinhardt and Stavins | Y | Y | N | N | Y | N | 50% |
| Chandler | Y | Y | Y | N | Y | N | 67% |
| Kolk | Y | Y | Y | N | Y | N | 67% |
| Alvarado-Herrera | Y | Y | Y | N | Y | N | 67% |
| Schönherr et al. | Y | Y | Y | N | Y | N | 67% |
| Xia et al. | Y | N | Y | N | Y | N | 67% |
| Givel | Y | N | N | N | Y | N | 33% |
| Alon et al. | Y | Y | Y | N | Y | N | 67% |
| Francis and Pegg | Y | Y | Y | N | Y | N | 67% |
| Williamson et al. | Y | Y | Y | N | Y | N | 67% |
| Vaccaro et al. | Y | Y | Y | Y | Y | N | 83% |
| Shingal | Y | Y | Y | N | Y | N | 67% |
| Boone et al. | Y | Y | Y | N | N | N | 50% |
| Hevia and Neumeyer | Y | N | N | N | N | N | 33% |
| Zeren and Hizarci | Y | Y | Y | N | Y | N | 67% |
| Cabral and Xu | Y | Y | Y | N | Y | N | 67% |
| Delwin et al. | Y | Y | Y | Y | Y | N | 83% |

| Quantitative Research | Clear description of the randomization? | Clear description of allocation or concealment? | Complete outcome data? | Low withdrawal/drop-out? |
|---|---|---|---|---|
| Dickson and Stevens | Y | Y | Y | Y |
| Bendel | Y | Y | Y | Y |
| Nitin | Y | Y | Y | Y |
| Delmas et al. | Y | Y | Y | Y |
| Annan-Diab | Y | Y | Y | Y |
| Suárez-Cebador | Y | Y | Y | Y |
| Chuang and Huang | Y | Y | Y | Y |
| Marco-Fondevila | Y | Y | N | Y |
| López-Pérez | Y | Y | Y | Y |
| Taylor et al. | Y | Y | Y | Y |
| Osmani | Y | Y | Y | Y |
| Dimmler | Y | Y | Y | Y |
| Senay and Landrigan | Y | Y | Y | Y |
| Albuquerque et al. | Y | Y | Y | Y |
| Shan and Tang | N | Y | N | Y |
| Laing | Y | Y | Y | Y |
| Makhdis and Hartley | Y | Y | Y | Y |
| Nuno-Fernandes | Y | Y | N | Y |
| Majlal and Barzani | Y | N | Y | Y |
| Barua | Y | Y | Y | Y |
| Johson et al. | Y | Y | N | N |
| Vian et al. | N | N | Y | Y |
| Soobaroyen and Nitim | Y | Y | Y | Y |
| Long | Y | Y | Y | Y |
| Gilbert | Y | Y | Y | Y |
| Gentilini | Y | Y | N | N |
| Lindgreen et al. | Y | Y | Y | Y |
| Amoako et al. | Y | Y | Y | Y |
| Makwara et al. | Y | Y | Y | Y |
| Flanagan and Whiteman | Y | Y | Y | Y |
| Utuk et al. | Y | Y | N | Y |
| Uduji et al. | Y | Y | Y | Y |

Table 3. Cont.

| Qualitative Research | Dickson and Stevens | Bendel | Ntim | Delmas et al. | Annan-Diab | Suárez-Cebador | Chuang and Huang | Marco-Fondevila | López-Pérez | Taylor et al. | Osmani | Dimmler | Senay and Landrigan | Albuquerque et al. | Shan and Tang | Laing | Makridis and Hartley | Nuno-Fernandes | Maital and Barzani | Barua | Johson et al. | Vian et al. | Soobaroyen and Ntim | Long | Gilbert | Gentilini | Lindgreen et al. | Amoako et al. | Makwara et al. | Flanagan and Whiteman | Utuk et al. | Uduji et al. |
|---|---|---|---|---|---|---|---|---|---|---|---|---|---|---|---|---|---|---|---|---|---|---|---|---|---|---|---|---|---|---|---|---|
| Reason for studying specific organizations | Y | N | Y | N | N | N | N | N | Y | N | N | Y | N | Y | N | Y | N | N | Y | Y | N | Y | Y | N | Y | Y | N | Y | N | N | Y | N |
| The influence of the organization on the research | N | N | N | N | N | N | N | N | N | N | N | N | N | N | N | N | N | N | N | N | N | N | N | N | N | N | N | N | N | N | N | N |
| Researcher influence in qualitative and mixed methods studies | N | N | N | N | N | N | N | N | N | N | N | N | N | N | N | N | N | N | N | N | N | N | N | N | N | N | N | N | N | N | N | N |
| Support from funding agencies | Y | Y | Y | N | Y | Y | N | Y | Y | N | Y | Y | N | Y | N | N | Y | Y | Y | N | N | N | Y | Y | Y | N | Y | Y | Y | Y | Y | Y |
| Total score (%) | 75% | 63% | 75% | 75% | 75% | 75% | 75% | 50% | 75% | 75% | 75% | 75% | 50% | 75% | 25% | 75% | 75% | 50% | 63% | 75% | 25% | 50% | 75% | 75% | 75% | 38% | 75% | 75% | 75% | 75% | 63% | 75% |

Key: Y = Yes, N = No.

Table 4. Differences and similarities between the global health pandemics that have influenced CSR.

| Variables | COVID-19 | Spanish Flu | HIV-AIDS | Cholera | Environmental Pollution | Malaria | MES | Ebola | Opioid | Obesity |
|---|---|---|---|---|---|---|---|---|---|---|
| Scope of geographical coverage of infection | All Continents/Countries | Asia/Europe/America | Mostly Sub-Saharan Africa | Underdeveloped countries | All Continents/Countries | Underdeveloped countries | Middle East | Africa | Developed Countries | Developed Countries |
| Scale of public panic reaction to disease | Very High | Very High | Very High | High | Low | High | High | High | Low | Low |
| Seasonal variation of infection | Yes | Yes | No | High | Low | High | High | High | Low | Low |
| Need for physical lockdowns to control infections | Yes | Yes | No | No | No | No | No | No | No | No |
| Isolation of patients to control infection | Yes | Yes | Yes | Yes | No | Yes | Yes | Yes | No | No |
| Scale of stigma associated with infection | High | High | Very High | None | None | None | High | Very High | High | High |
| Scale of conspiracy theories to explain infection | Yes | Yes | Yes | No | No | No | Yes | Yes | No | No |
| Effect of mass gathering on infections | Yes | Yes | No | Yes | No | Yes | Yes | Yes | No | No |
| Possibility of early detection and treatment | Yes | Yes | Yes | Yes | Yes | Yes | Yes | Yes | Yes | Yes |
| Effect of underlining conditions of criticality of illness | Yes | Yes | No | Yes | No | Yes | Yes | Yes | Yes | No |
| Age variation in infection rate | Elderly | Elderly | Youth | All | All | All | All | All | All | All |
| Gender variation in infection rate | Non | Non | Non | Non | Non | Non | Non | Non | Non | Non |
| Geographical concentration of highest rate of infection/deaths | Advanced/Emerging Countries | Advanced/Emerging Countries | Developing Countries | Developing Countries | All Continents/Countries | Developing Countries | Middle East | Africa | Advanced/Emerging Countries | Advanced/Emerging Countries |
| Scale of frontline deaths | Very High | Very High | Low | High | Low | High | High | High | Low | Low |
| Scale of direct impact of epidemic on socio-economic activities globally | Very High | Very High | High | Low | High | Low | High | High | Medium | Medium |
| Scale of direct impact of epidemic on cost to businesses globally | Very High | Very High | Very High | Low | High | Low | High | High | High | High |
| Scale of direct impact of epidemic on business revenue globally | Very High | Very High | Medium | Low | Medium | Low | Medium | Medium | Low | Low |
| Scale of use of inter-government regulations to control infection | Very High | Very High | High | Medium | High | Medium | Medium | High | Low | Low |
| Epidemic disruptions as cause of major employee layoffs | Very High | Very High | Medium | Low | Low | Low | Low | Low | Low | Low |

Table 4. Cont.

| Variables | COVID-19 | Spanish Flu | HIV-AIDS | Cholera | Environmental Pollution | Malaria | MES | Ebola | Opioid | Obesity |
|---|---|---|---|---|---|---|---|---|---|---|
| Cross border lockdowns to prevent spread of epidemics | Yes | Yes | No | No | No | No | Yes | Yes | No | No |
| Rate of infection among people | Very High | Very High | Low | High | Low | High | Very High | Very High | Low | Low |
| Mode of transmission of epidemic | Droplets | Droplets | Blood | Sanitation | Prolong Exposure | Sanitation | Droplets | Droplets | Habits | Habits |
| Intensity of CSR | Very High | Very High | Very High | Very High | Very High | Very High | Low | Low | Low | Low |
| Criticisms of CSR | Very High | Very High | Very High | Very High | Very High | Very High | Very High | Very High | Very High | Very High |

Other considerations that distinguish these epidemics include effect of underlining conditions of criticality of illness, age variation in infection rate, gender variation in infection rate, geographical concentration of highest rate of infection/deaths, and scale of frontline deaths. The rest of the differences and similarities include the scale of direct impact of epidemic on socio-economic activities globally, scale of direct impact of epidemic on cost to businesses globally, scale of direct impact of epidemic on business revenue globally, and scale of use of inter-government regulations to control infection [17]. Finally, differences and similarities also exist among the ten epidemics in terms of how the epidemic disruptions, cross border lockdowns to prevent spread of epidemics, rate of infection among people, mode of transmission of epidemic, intensity of CSR, and criticisms of CSR.

## 4. Discussion

### 4.1. Business Interest versus CRS in Response to the Spanish Flu

Reviewing the paper by Ntim [18], they contend that business organizations often claim that the main reason why they are involved in CSR is to support the society to overcome some of its critical challenges. However, the authors note that business organizations are driven into corporate social responsibility because it is an opportunity to minimize cost or improve revenue and less of an opportunity to support society. It is therefore important to look at some of the losses that are occassioned by epidemic outbreaks. According to Bolton [19], businesses began to support the fight against epidemics only after they estimate how much loss they can realistically avoid or how much revenue they can maximize. The events before corporate involvement in CSR during the 1919 Spanish flu is examined in Mahajan et al. [20]. The Spanish flu is important in this context because it closely compares to COVID-19 in terms of infections (500 million) and mortality (50 million) and its impact on macro and micro economic indicators that determines the survivability of business enterprises. This flu occurred at a time when the global economic system was emerging from the ashes of the WW1.

According to the Federal Reserve Bank of St. Louis and the Arkansas Gazette, popular merchants in Little Rock (Arkansas) reported 40–70% decline in business revenue and other retailers lost nearly two-thirds of their income. Despite the increase in the sales of drugs, bed, springs, and mattresses, thousands of irrecoverable goods were lost daily due to poor storage system or lack of it [21]. The negative effect of this influenza on businesses in Memphis (Tennessee) was even worse. The banks were unwilling to offer them overdrafts due to panic withdrawal. The Memphis Street Railway and the Cumberland Telephone Company redeployed half of their employees and that lead to a cut in production and services. On the 18th of October 1918, the "Tennessee Coal Mines" shut down its main operations unit causing fifty percent decline revenue over six months. Sanyal [22] and Welker [23] also reports that several mines throughout east Tennessee and southern Kentucky were closed down. The coalfield in Tennessee, which was one of the largest coal production hubs, had only 2% of its 500 employees available to work.

Typically, small and medium scale enterprises were the worst affected by the Spanish flu just as it is the case with COVID-19 as the latter were unable to keep up with some manufacturing schedule or to delayed trading until the market conditions improved. The worsening macro-economic indicators also laid a strong foundation for companies to support the fight to end the Spanish flu. Delmas et al. [24] reveal that the macroeconomic environment under the Spanish flu equally plummeted. In the US alone, the death toll led to a sharp decline in GDP by 1.5% and consumption by 2.1%. Both large and small scale businesses were affected by the sharp rise in inflation by 5% and interest rates by 13% by the end of the first six-months of the pandemic. It is worth noting that these indicators were already at their terrible levels due to WWI. Shaukat [25] also explains that by the time business organizations saw the need to be involved in halting the continuous spread of the Spanish flu, the stock returns had dropped by 7% and the safest government bonds had tumbled by 3.5%.

The trend in the US was not an isolated case because the entire global economic indicators were heading towards danger to the detriment of international merchants and cross border trade which was already under siege by the aftermath of WWI. Without prejudice to the growth in pharmaceutical, medical supplies, and healthcare, Barro et al. [26] explain that the Spanish flu reduced the global real GDP per capita by nearly 6%. Similarly, Correia et al. [27] report of an 18% decline in the US's manufacturing output. In Sydney, the sales volume fell between 25% and 40% while several hitherto large retailers folded up as a result of decline in foot traffic.

Faced with such challenges, business organizations had no option than to be involved in what they called CSR. Initially, large scale business merchants supported government through information dissemination and increased support to their affected employees. With time, a number of flourishing merchants opted to help pre-finance the manufacturing of vaccines in return for preferential trade treatments that had been rolled out by the governments. As the disease was subsiding, employment became one of the major CSR tools that companies rolled out to the extent that it was economically beneficial [28].

Idowu et al. [29] report that the aftermath of WWI had also created a large stock of veterans that were struggling to reintegrate into the society. Several merchants and larger corporations took advantage of the opportunities to reabsorb veterans into the labor market in return for government stimulus packages (tax exemptions, wage subsidy, rent subsidy, preferential supply contracts, special export and import licenses, etc.) were targeted at companies that could help solve some of the political problems created from WWI. In order to take advantage of government stimulus packages, large manufacturing companies re-absorbed returning veterans into the labor market as a form of corporate social responsibility. Malovics et al. [30] report that since the economic benefit that were to accrue to the enterprises inspired their decision to engage in this form of CSR, the selection of veterans also came with challenges. This is because business competed for veterans with professional training and physical capabilities that were suitable for their business operations to the detriment of veterans who suffered restraining disabilities during WWI.

*4.2. Business Interest versus CRS in Responding to Malaria and Cholera Outbreaks*

According to Reinhart and Stavins [31], an analysis of how companies responded to CSR with the onset of malaria and cholera pandemics indicates that these were also mostly inspired by the need to boost business revenue and minimize business cost. According to the World Economic Forum, malaria is bad for business. When the malaria crisis first emerged, several corporate employees unknowingly became agents for community transmission and this highly affected their businesses and the local economy [32].

The local economies lost due to deteriorated human capital, losses in savings, and investments and loss of tax revenues. In a survey conducted among companies in Sub-Saharan Africa, Central Asia, and South East Asia, the World Economic Forum reported that 72% of companies had suffered revenue losses and high cost as a result of malaria-led employee absenteeism, reduced production and productivity, and escalating benefit cost [33].

Overseas, UK businesses such as BHP Billiton, which owned Mozal Aluminum Smelter in Mozambique, lost 7000 employees and 13 expatriates' deaths in two years. The UK-based mining and metals company had investment of over US $1.4 billion at that time but the state of the malaria outbreak over two years made it difficult to recoup their investments. The company spent an estimated US $2.7 million to help control malaria-related illness, absenteeism, and treatment before the company resumed uninterrupted business. Even though these commitments are classified as corporate social responsibility intended to support society to meet its health crisis, Alvarado-Herrera et al. [34] argue that it was only through investment in the health of their workers that they could be guaranteed uninterrupted production cycle, minimize cost, and boost competitiveness.

This supports the work of Schönherr et al. [35] that it is through CSR for malaria that business organizations can scale back malaria to reduce malaria-related illness, deaths, expenditure, absenteeism, and even loss of staff. In some of the worst affected cholera countries in the world such as Zambia, Mozambique, Ghana, etc., companies often use their resources and infrastructure to secure external funding, scale up interventions which may have taken a long time to come, but being a good corporate citizen in a time of epidemic is the only way to strengthen business reputation and obtain self-perpetuating social legitimacy for the future [36].

For example, the M2030 was introduced by the Asia Pacific Leaders Malaria Alliance (APLMA) as a forum to harness and inspire CSR among concerned enterprises. Its stated objective was to unite businesses, consumers, and health organizations towards the elimination of malaria in Asia and Pacific. Within a year of commencement of operations, many companies became attracted to the M2030 and the idea to support the funding of malaria programs [37].

However, a lot of companies also enrolled into the program because M2030 as an inter-governmental initiative, permitted partner companies to use the M2030 brand for campaigns, and even rebrand some of its products and services to enhance their sales. Many of the companies therefore saw this opportunity more as a cause-related marketing strategy instead of a humanitarian gesture to society, hence the rush to enroll in this coordinated CSR program [38]. Not surprisingly, companies that did not see much economic benefit from the M2030 later became dormant members. Most of the critics of the M2030 CSR project still believe that it is avenue for the benefit of businesses to boost their corporate reputation. A recent concern by Chaung and Huang [39] gives credence to this factor when they assert that the success of the M2030 project and the continuous support from firms is contingent on the M2030 brands ability to help drive sales and customer retention.

The cholera outbreak is one of the major epidemics that has always attracted CSR activities due to its effect on business cost and business revenue. Marco-Fondevila et al. [40] explain that cost and revenue considerations have persistently informed business intentions to engage CSR right from the outbreak of the Asiatic "cholera" which broke out in 1832. According to Alon et al. [41], the Asiatic cholera was believed to have originated from India but moved westwards through Eurasia, Europe, and eventually the United States with citizens put on edge. Predictably, citizens along cities where the pandemic arrived left the city in haste as doctors pressed for public announcements to alert households of the debilitating effect of the ranging pandemic.

Significantly, Albuquerque [42] asserts that public health boards and mayors were initially hesitant to release timely information due in part to the influence of large business organizations, prominent bankers, and merchants that had bankrolled the politicians into office for fear of loss of business, revenues, trade deals, and excessively huge cost as a result of the panic. It is documented in Ozil and Arun [43] that even when the pandemic was at its highest peak, hotels wrote to local newspapers to run notices that their premises were free of cholera and open to business in disregard of public health recommendations. "The American Hotel," the Evening Post dutifully reported, "neither has been nor will be closed." Yet, as the fear eventually unfolded, CSR was used as the key strategy to recoup losses. Besides the drying up of merchandize, the epidemic changed even the personal lifestyle of the rich merchants and their spouses had to bake breads themselves due to the closure of city shops [44]. The famous Pearl Street goods market and city dwellers withdrew their savings to the chagrin of banks that had run out of liquidity.

More recent outbreaks of cholera amidst business losses and CSR interventions further supports the idea that business organizations are more focused on the benefits derived from them [45]. For example, in 2017, MTN Zambia spent more than half a million Kwacha to procure 300 bins, 60 vests, towels, hand sanitizers, soaps, and other equipment to help curb the cholera outbreak in Lusaka. Even though all of these materials were bought on the open market, a lot of money was spent to rebrand them with MTN symbols and promotional messages.

A news commentary in Gentilini [46] criticized MTN for commercializing the epidemic situation extensive promotion of MNT through a non-commensurable donation. This reaction was due to the fact that within two months, the whole country had been painted with the yellow MNT drums and symbols, drawing public criticisms, earning them free publicity that would have cost them more money than the cost of the donation if they had paid for the public spaces. One newspaper sarcastically reported that the outbreak of the yellow epidemic (in reference to MNT colors) was more than the cholera outbreak.

The Zimnat Group did the same thing when cholera broke out in Zimbabwe in September 2018 [47]. Over three months, the company donated 20,000 L of water to several locations including Budirio 5D Current Shopping Centre in Harare in tanks that were hilariously branded in the company's green colors to boost their prominence during the epidemic time. The intimidating green presence across the length and breadth of the capital city attracted several criticisms from the press for attempting to commercialize the pandemic.

Another way CSR comes under the cover of business promotion during an epidemic is how Kia Motors and LG Electronics (both Korean owned companies) have partnered Korea-based International Vaccine Institute (IVI) to provide an emergency cholera vaccination program in Malawi and Ethiopia, respectively [48]. On the face of it, these multinational giants seek to improve quality of life through such interventions without disclosing the business opportunities it creates for them. However, the IVI is a United Nations initiative based in Korea and stimulates partnership with companies for humanitarian purposes by offering them several incentives to promote their businesses. For their support for the vaccine program, KIA and LG Electronics benefit through access to high global networking of UN agencies and governments [49]. They also get support in the form of connectivity with stakeholders, its tools, resources and trainings, local network support in 85 countries and more importantly, the moral authority, knowledge, and experience of the United Nations which can facilitate access to major international and national level contracts.

### 4.3. Business Interest versus CSR Response to HIV-AIDS

In Vaccaro et al. [50], it is reported that support for private sector (NGOs) involvement in the fight against HIV-AIDS was started by non-business groups such as Family Health International. These initial efforts were not classified as CSR since they did not emanate from corporate enterprises. Due to lack of funding, most of these non-business organizations focused their HIV-AIDS intervention on data collection and analysis, individual risk assessment, prevention and cure education, impact assessment of HIV/AIDS on specific industries, and development of proposals to guide workplace prevention and care. Frequent engagement with these NGOs stimulated corporate interest to start their own programs through CSR [51].

Just as it is with other forms of public health concerns, some critics of HIV-AIDS-related CSR believe that business organizations use the epidemic platform to consolidate their importance, minimize cost, and optimize potential business opportunities created by the epidemic. According to Ferreira [52], several business opportunities are inherent in the pandemics that enterprises can explore, and HIV-AIDS is one of those with high business interest and this can be procured through CSR. The interest of MNCs in HIV-AIDS-related CSR, emerged crystalized as the global advocacy for HIV-AIDS intensified in the early 1980s. At this point in time, the pandemic was largely concentrated in Sub-Saharan Africa [53] before growing to every part of the world.

The early signals of the catastrophic effect of HIV-AIDS to disrupt a wide range of socio-economic and corporate activities notwithstanding, serious documentation of HIV-AID-related CSR programs started in the late 1990s [54]. At this point in history, the ominous or devastating effect of the pandemic on human resources and economic development had become entrenched across continents [55]. With exponential increase in the number of infected persons across industries and countries, a global alarm was sounded by the International Labour Organization (ILO) in 1990, to highlight the epidemiological influence of HIV-AIDS on individuals, households, workforce, employers, and organizations [56].

The ILO subsequently engaged several enterprises to begin incorporating appropriate strategies to control the threat posed by the HIV-AIDS pandemic to decent work, productivity, and national development [57]. As documented by the World Health Organisation [58], this initial effort formed the basic documentary framework for discussions at the Special High-Level Meeting on HIV/AIDS and the World of Work in Geneva in 2000. To gain a deeper attention of business enterprises to invest their resources into HIV-AIDS-related CSR, the International Labour Organization (ILO) and the United National Development Program (UNDP) released a joint document that provided statistical evidence of how business were going to suffer (due to labor shortages) if the pandemic persist [59]. Classified data from thirteen African countries, Thailand, and Haiti collected from the United Nations Population Division were analyzed with the e ILO-POPILO software [60]. Based on the ILO assessment, business became conscious of the fact that rapid increase in HIV-AIDS infection among the 20–49 years bracket was significantly altering the age and sex distribution of the labor force and that could affect enterprise production [61].

Three main problems were identified by enterprises of this persistence, hence the need to join the fight against HIV-AIDS through CSR. Firstly, high HIV-AIDS-related deaths were pushing children or less experienced people into the labor force. Secondly, experienced employees with HIV-AIDS withdrew from the labor force early and thirdly elderly people had to be retained in the labor force due to rising economic dependency due to the early death of younger employees [62].

In 2001, 17 eminent and visionary companies founded the Global Business Council on HIV/AIDS. In the work of Harvey [63], this initiative added the needed global impetus to place HIV-AIDS at the center of corporate solidarity and responsibility. Harvey [63] again posits that the Global Business Council on HIV-AIDS collaborated with the UNDP, the Prince of Wales Business Leaders Forum, and Nelson Mandela Foundation to develop a business response to confront HIV-AIDS head-on in mainly developing countries [63]. The Global Business Council (GBC) developed a broad range of CSR strategies i.e., public information strategies for its members and others. It also set up the annual award for business excellence to recognize the contribution of businesses to the HIV-AIDS pandemic. In 2002, the Global Business Council participated in the UN General Assembly Special Session on AIDS (UNGASS). It used the forum to expand the need for high level business response to HIV-AIDS among prominent business leaders and international policy-makers. Its frequent publications on HIV-AIDS and other health-related crisis continue to inspire new business responses to global health crisis including the HIV/AIDS pandemic [64].

A major success of the GBC is that 46% of businesses in the US got involved in some kind of HIV/AIDS philanthropy across the globe. However, critics of the Global Business Council on HIV, which has since changed to the GBCHealth, believe that the companies have benefited from HIV-AIDS more than the communities. Firstly, the decision to appoint the then World Bank president James Wolfenson as the chairperson of the club of companies instead of a technical person with practical experience in humanitarian issues was the first indication that the interest was about creating business opportunities through HIV-AIDS-related CSR other than supporting society [65].

When the club was formed, it developed 6 key approaches to work but critics argue that five of them are just focused on the benefits that the businesses will extract from their undertaking rather than the support for communities and affected individuals. The first priority of the group was to convene and connect businesses, governments, multilaterals, and civil society while the second is to represents businesses in driving the creation of high-impact partnerships-business-to-business and business-to-government [66]. The third goal of the group is to provide recognition and visibility to companies while the fourth is to represent business in key global health settings. The last objective stated by the group is to provide guidance to companies on their workplace and corporate social investment initiatives. Faced with these objectives, and guiding principles, it becomes difficult for one to clearly accept the previously held notion that patients and affected communities are more important in the quest to fight HIV-AIDS than the personal interest of the companies. The analyzed studies also present specific MNC interventions in HIV-AIDS through corporate social responsibility but the twin-face of an organization as using such platforms to promote their interest is also evidently shown [67].

To support the claim that businesses that get involved with HIV-AID-related CSR were more interested in protecting their interest rather than society, Makwara et al. [67] again highlight the case of Daimler Chrysler, De Beers, Nestle, Johnson and Johnson, Coca-Cola and Unilever, Proctor and Gamble who were among the companies that first started HIV-AIDS-related CSR in Kenya and South Africa [68]. These companies only conducted research on the association between HIV-AID- related CSR (prevention and treatment of HIV-AIDS) and the company's balance sheet [69]. These research studies confirmed the need to be involved in HIV-AIDS related CSR in order to protect the firm's greatest resources (human resources). Nestle went further to simulate how employee work productivity differs between infected employees with company supported medication and those without company supported medication.

These companies were alarmed by the potential high level of absenteeism, frequent sick leave, poor organizational citizenship behaviors, and even death that permanently terminates the work relationship. The companies understood the potential loss of revenue, customers, and the high cost that they were confronted with if the situation should persist and solicited the support of the media to help eradicate HIV-AIDS [70].

Significantly, the media accepted the partnership from major companies because they benefited from the publicity and promotional budgets of the corporate enterprises. With this knowledge, several individual organizations began to navigate company specific approaches and mechanisms to incorporate HIV-AIDS programs into its corporate social responsibility budget to support affected employees, community, and country.

Adegbite et al. [71] reechoes this when they say that these initial CSR initiatives to manage the threat of HIV-AIDS in the early part of the 1990s were largely focused on how companies could protect their employees from acquiring the HIV-AIDS virus and prevent avoidable intra-organizational spread of the pandemic

Even though HIV-AIDS-related CSR entered a different phase in the late 1990s, the effect of business interest over societal interest increased [72]. For instance, Coca-Cola partnered with UNAIDS to provide extraordinary support against the HIV/AIDS fight in Africa [73]. This collaboration was the first and largest private sector initiative of a major global brand to implement a systematic philanthropic and corporate citizenship program with a specific focus on HIV-AID in Africa [74]. This initiative allowed Coca-Cola to focus beyond the employees living with AIDs and bring the larger community in focus, support infrastructure to support patients, use its wide range distribution channels to market HIV-AIDS related resources, while strengthening its human resource policies to ensure greater involvement in the fight against HIV/AIDS [75]. However, this massive involvement of Coca-Cola in HIV-AIDS came at a time when the company was facing severe backlash in South Africa and other parts of the content.

It is recalled that in 1982, black workers led a boycott of Coca-Cola products in protest against low wages, pension funds, and the depleted bargaining power of workers union. Since then, several critics have referred to Coca-Cola as a conduit of economic support for white South Africa and its apartheid system. International friends of South Africa such as Tennessee State, Penn State, and Compton College in California, even established a "Coke Free Campus" while the Georgia Coalition led a series of protests to move Coca-Cola out of South Africa [76]. At that time, Coca-Cola rolled out massive support to improve housing and education for black South Africans and sell 30% of shares in bottler and 50% of canning operations to native South Africans but these were rejected. It was within this time that the HIV-AIDS prevalence rate escalated in Southern Africa and Coca-Cola seized the opportunity of CSR to hold on to its stay in South Africa [77].

Again, in 2015, it came to light that Coca-Cola had influenced research by the Global Energy Balance Network to promote research findings that blamed obesity on lack of exercises and not on reducing the intake of calories. This was deliberately engineered to deceive the public of the impact of the excessive sugar content of Coca-Cola in the spread of obesity and type 2 diabetes. This happened at the time Coca-Cola had just announced major humanitarian support for a series of health crises across the globe [78].

The CSR effort of the Corporate Council on Africa (CCA) is also addressed by Kurland [79]. Corporate Council on Africa (CCA) is a leading business association of American enterprises that connects business interest in Africa. The group formed two lobby groups i.e., a Task Force on AIDS in Africa and the Coalition for AIDS Relief in Africa that brings together major pharmaceutical companies, such as Abbott Laboratories, Bristol-Myers Squibb, Pfizer, etc., to lobby Congress on how the President's Emergency Plan for AIDS Relief (PEPFAR funding) can benefit business interests in Africa. Since its inception, the Corporate Council on Africa has released periodic timely reports to support concerned enterprises to standardize their HIV-AIDS-related corporate social responsibility programs.

The main advantage of the mode of operation of the Corporate Council on Africa is that it partners high profile companies including Ford Motors, Coca-Cola, Boeing, Microsoft, etc. to work through local groups and governments to design, develop, and implement culturally sensitive strategies to combat HIV/AIDS among the African workforce [80]. The CCA also has its critics on the genuineness of the humanitarian endeavors that it engages it. For example, Shingal [81] explains that even though the CCA considers itself a non-profit making enterprise, its main objective as describe by the council is to promote business and investment between the United States and the nations of Africa which are all profitable ventures. The first three of its key goals equally gives credence to the fact that CSR is a pathway to consolidating business interest for its members other than the society. For example, the first goal of this enterprise is to work closely with governments, multilateral groups, and businesses to improve Africa's trade and investment climate and to raise the profile of Africa in the U.S. business community. According to the CCA, its most important goal is to support member companies to increase their investment in and trade with the nations of Africa. Thus, CSR is therefore one of the ways by which they can have access to the African market [82].

The role of the banking sector in incorporating HIV-AIDS-related programs in their CSR activities is also well documented by Nicola et al. [83]. For example, in 2003, the Standard Chartered Bank launched the "Living with HIV" project to support the global fight against the HIV-AIDS epidemic. Through this program, the bank trained staff volunteers as advocates (Living with HIV Champions) to handle HIV/AIDS-related issues within and outside the organization [84]. By 2017, the Standard Chartered Bank had provided HIV-AIDS education to more than 75,000 employees. Currently, the bank has an active HIV-AIDS community education program across the globe. This program has trained, empowered, and resourced more than 3 million individuals and organizations (particularly in Africa, Asia, and South America) to support [85].

In the work of Coussens and Harrison [86], they point out that unlike COVID-19, HIV-AIDS-related CSR in Asia did not start early, relative to the case in Africa. However, as the disease swept across Asia, corporate enterprises became aware of its debilitating effect. To this end, most notable Asian companies have also scaled up their effort to support HIV-AIDS-related programs. In India, for example, companies such as Tata Tea Ltd., Larsen & Toubro, Modicare Foundation, Aditya Birla Group, Apollo Tyres, SAIL, and Bajaj Auto etc., have been actively involved in supporting HIV-AIDS advocacy. Despite the initial set back, companies in South East Asia have many encouraging examples of public-private led CSR partnerships supporting promotional activities [87]. The main CSR activities include promoting HIV/AIDS prevention, support, and care initiatives. In the Asia Pacific region, in particular, many companies have the UNDP's Regional HIV and Development Programme through donations and other forms of support [88].

Again, in India, the Steel Authority of India Ltd. (SAIL) started the SAIL AIDS Control Program (SACP) to create local awareness and support community advocacy programs through sponsorship [89]. It has partnered with India's National AIDS Control Organization (NACO) and other inter-sectorial collaborations to school an AIDS education programme, family health awareness campaign, safe blood and blood products, and establish voluntary counseling and testing center.

It has also supported the annual World AIDS Day Celebrations as well as initiating exhibition and displays counseling and guidance and AIDS Art Centers. Johnson and Johnson is another important partner in the global fight against the HIV-AIDS pandemic in all forms as part of its role in attacking neglected tropical diseases (NTD). Over three decades, the company has established global partnerships in Asia and Africa [90]. To date, Johnson and Johnson has committed to HIV-AIDS partnership programs in 25 African countries (Kenya, Swaziland, Botswana, Cameroon, Zambia, Senegal, Liberia, Zimbabwe, Somalia, Malawi, Morocco, Cape Verde, DRC, South Africa, Sudan, Namibia, Mozambique, Eritrea, Tanzania, Ethiopia, Egypt, Nigeria, Ghana, Sierra Leone, Rwanda, Uganda) [91].

In these countries, it partners with different national and International NGOs to intervene in mainly HIV/AIDS anti-stigmatization advocacy and capacity building of HIV-AIDS advocacy groups and foot soldiers. Even in the case of Johnson and Johnson, these interventions are not without criticism as to being a tool to rebuild its damaged reputation. By the end of 2018, Johnson and Johnson had been implicated in 500 opioid-related cases. It is one of the companies blamed for the escalation of the opioid epidemic in the United States. Beside problems such as foreign bribery accusations, consumer fraud settlements, illegal marketing, and product recalls, J & J faced public criticisms for its role in the manufacture and sale of the cancer-causing baby powder scandals which affected its corporate reputation [92]. Faced with this crisis which directly affects human life and social goals, many critics see their effort at CSR as an attempt to clear up their battered image to remain competitive in business and not to support society as they claim to be doing.

### 4.4. Business Interest versus CSR Response to Environmental Health

The effort of private companies in solving environmental health crises through CSR is one of the often criticized efforts of corporate enterprises. This is because they are perceived to be the direct agents of environmental pollution hence and only put up CSR as a smokescreen to deceive the public into believing that they are concerned about the environment. Three selected studies indicates that the Carson's 1962 bestseller "silent spring" was a watershed moment that brought environmental health and CSR to the fore [93]. This publication raised a new level of social consciousness among corporate enterprises and explained the inextricable linkage between pollution and public health [94]. These explanations influenced the rise of environmental advocates, some of whom had long begun navigating their own path to hold businesses accountable for the impact of their operations on the environment.

Gaylord Nelson, a junior senator from Wisconsin must also be commended for catalyzing the aspirations of earth day in 1970 which ultimately led to the establishment of the Environmental Protection Agency in the US and the subsequent enactment of several pro-environment laws [95]. These laws have protected millions of men, women, and children from diseases and death as averted the extinction of hundreds of species.

In the late 1990s, environment-led CSR became a source of competitive advantage as businesses engaged in different pro-environment activities to catch the eyes of an informed public and or avoid stringent government regulations on pollution. The United Nations used the Earth Summit in Rio de Janeiro (1992) and Johannesburg (2002) to define a comprehensive vision for sustainable and eco-friendly development. Even before the Johannesburg Summit in 2002, some corporate enterprises that participated in the World Economic Forum in 2000 had accepted to partner the UN to set up the United Nations Global Compact (UNGC) at the behest of the then Secretary General (Kofi Annan) of the United Nations [96]. The UNGC was to serve as a common vehicle to diffuse shared values and principles of sustainable development to give a human face to the global market order. In July 2000, the UNGC was launched between the UN and 24 enterprises. The UNGC began to insert human rights, social and environmental responsibility values into the corporate operations to guarantee better healthcare for global public as enterprises rapidly altered their production processes [97]. The UNGC also helped to fill the environmental governance gap of the time.

Its most significant achievement is that it defined ten principles and values to guide corporate pro-environment behavior [98]. Secondly, it formulated guidelines on the mechanisms by which the ten principles and values can be incorporated into a company's operational strategies, working procedures and programs and policies to help create a long term corporate culture of integrity that prioritizes the health and wellbeing of society [99]. While the United Nations Global Compact was not CSR- specific tool, the ten principles it proposed played a major role in bringing social responsibility and environmental engagements to the fore of industrialization and development at the beginning of the 21st Century. The adoption of the United National Millennium Development Goals subsequent to the adopting of the Millennium Declaration in 2000 was another milestone in aligning environmental health and corporate social responsibility [100]. For fifteen years, the MDGs set the international agenda for CSR and environmental health even though it was not a CSR specific intervention project. Through the help of the UNDP, the MDG was presented to corporate enterprises as a key framework for the UN's private sector cooperation on responsible enterprise [101]. By the end of 2015, environmental health concerns had become the most dominant health-related crisis shaping contemporary CSR across the globe.

However, critics of the UNGC believe that it used the offices of the United Nations to tacitly endorse companies that were destroying the environment while contributing huge sums of money to support the UNGC. For example, it is believed that the UNGC lacked effective monitoring and enforcement of the provisions, hence failed to hold companies accountable. On the contrary, these corporations misused their affiliation to the UNGC for public relations and economic gains under the guise of humanitarian concern. This phenomenon was christened "bluewashing" [102].

This explains why informal networks emerged to counter how corporations enrolled under the UNGC used their membership and supposed participation in philanthropic and charity-based activities of the UN as an excuse and an entry door to increase corporate influence upon international organizations. Some of these network groups that emerged to remove the veil of "bluewashed" UNGC members include the Global Compact Critics, the Alliance for a Corporate-Free UN which was led by Corpwatch, Peter Utting (deputy director of UNRISD), Maude Barlow (adviser to the President of the United Nations General Assembly), and David Andrews (adviser on Food Policy and Sustainable Development). Some leaders of Paragua's Ayoreo tribe protested the membership of Yaguarete Porá in the UNGC. The Yaguarete Porá was a Brazilian ranching company which had illegally occupied and destroyed Ayoreo's forests, and also concealing the presence of unknown tribesmen living in the forest. Another source of worry in the discharge of environment-led CSR is that while the environmental health crisis raged, opioid and obesity persisted contemporaneously but did not attract their attention since it provided minimal business opportunities to them [102].

Microsoft is one of the best examples of CSR with environmental health focus. The company's CSR agenda targets the regulation of energy and water consumption, waste reduction and recycling, carbon emissions and sustainable sourcing. Microsoft also supports local communities, educates and empowers workers at Microsoft. Microsoft also provides health and wellness programs for families and other benefactors. Through the Microsoft CARES and Microsoft Ergonomics Programs, Microsoft seeks to empower and engage employees, competitors, collaborators, and the larger society to monitor and adhere environment-related CSR principles [103]. This notwithstanding, Microsoft has had its fair share of criticisms as far as the environment is concern.

The studies in relation to environmental-led CSR offer insight into the influential role of environmental factors in global advocacy and multinational enterprises decision making. According to McQueen [104], a dominant feature that has shaped contemporary corporate social responsibility since 2000 is environmental concern. Environmental concern is not an end in itself, but its consequential health effects is viewed as a form of environmental pandemic or climate change pandemic. Since the 1970s, environmental researchers have recognized that climate change, and other health stressors (both natural and man-made), can exert high influence on human health and disease in various ways but intense epidemiological reconnaissance of the crisis took time to mature.

Beyond environmental damage, the effect of climate change on health determinants such as safe drinking water, sufficient food, clean air, secure shelter, outbreak of vaccine-preventable diseases is well documented in several studies. The persistent outbreak or reports of drug-resistant pathogens and other multiple humanitarian health crises were directly traced to climate change and environmental pollution. Since the 2000s, renewed global effort has focused largely on soliciting a broad base of industrial support to transform the mechanism for tackling environmental health risks. The role of corporate institutions in actualizing this objective is the reason why environmental health promotion and prevention has become a central theme in todays' corporate social responsibility policies [105]. However, over time, many advocacy groups including the United Nations have become disillusioned by the attempt to lower the ambition of the 2015 Paris Agreement by powerful nations with the tacit support of powerful multinationals [76]. There is the belief that environmental lethargy is growing rapidly among the top echelon of society while potential environmental led catastrophes persist. This growing pathological state of sleepiness, deep unresponsiveness, and inactivity has irked concerned citizens and environmental advocacy groups to rise up to demand greater action for the protection of the planet and its people.

According to the New South Wales State Archives & Records [106], the poignant social, cultural, and environmental advocacy of the 1970s has re-emerged as fresh and frustrated Millennials persistently refusing to settle for verbal platitudes of environmental care. Millions of such people have constituted themselves into very vibrant and sometimes violent groups who take to the streets to protest and demand a new paradigm in environmental health protection by large multinationals. Fortunately, the social and digital media have become common meeting grounds through which these discussions, protests, strikes, mobilizations, and sentiments are brought to the attention of the global audience. This has never before united concerned global citizenry and catalyzed a generation to join together to take on the environmental health challenges with the greatest possible firmness.

*4.5. Business Interest versus CSR Response to COVID-19*

A review of the selected literature again points to the fact that the next major health-related factor that can potentially shape the future of corporate social responsibility is COVID-19. Unlike HIV-AIDS and environmental health concerns, COVID-19 has gathered global advocacy within six months and its impact in the corridors of global power has been immense. This is largely because COVID-19 possesses the same if not more of the disruptive effect of HIV-AIDS and environmental health. The epidemic broke out in December 2019, as a novel corona virus in Wuhan in the Hubei province of central China [107]. At the onset, it was thought to be a domestic problem in China and its pathogenic and contagious character was not very clear even to the World Health Organization. However, overtime, the virus has spread across almost every country in the world with unfathomable momentum.

By the end of 2020, nearly 100,000,000 infections and 2,200,000 deaths had been recorded. The largest numbers of infections have occurred in the US, Brazil, India, UK, France, Spain, Germany, Russia, Canada, France, etc. In the absence of a known vaccine, political authorities in different countries have implemented several "draconian" or "non-routine" measures to break the viral chain despite the ramifying effect of such measures on economic activities and corporate stability.

For the corporate sector, some of these measures have become disruptive as they were unanticipated. The measures include stay at home orders, total lockdown of cities, closure of businesses, limits on nonessential businesses and business travels, social distances between two persons and group of persons, limit on public gatherings, closure of schools, continuous education on virus prevention measures, compulsory temperature monitoring, and quarantine of high-risk and sick persons [108]. As explained in [109], in the short term, several areas of COVID-19 are of CSR interest to corporate organizations. For example, with schools closed, companies must design working practices that enable parents to adequately spend time with their kids. They have to rank business travels to eliminate non-essential ones and provide support and for frontline workers. Enterprises must also redesign office work space to accommodate social distance requirements and reorient a new organizational culture on public health practices [110].

Even in Ghana and other less affected countries for example, the government has set up a national emergency fund that receives donations from corporate organizations. At the same time, the private sector has also set up a parallel support system under its own control to build isolation hospitals to support government initiatives. In India, the private sector has taken the responsibility to provide food support programs to worst affected by lockdowns and redeployed. This is in addition to all manners of humanitarian supports, donations in kind and in cash, transport services, food distribution, etc., for other vulnerable members of the society [111]. Direct corporate interventions in COVID-19 are well documented in the studies as well. For example, Starbucks and other telecom companies have embraced the Keep Americans Connected agenda where they are currently supporting working professionals to remain connected from remote locations [112]. The effect of COVID-19 on CSR also requires companies to guarantee financial security to the most vulnerable in the midst of business closures, reduced hours of work in response to the pandemic. A case in point is Lululemon. Despite been temporarily shut, Lululemon stores in North America indicated its willingness to continue paying employees and provide access to a pay relief fund [113]. Similarly, Microsoft has committed to paying its hourly workers their regular pay despite the dip in the demand for their services [114].

Walmart, Apple, and the Olive Garden on the other hand have updated sick-leave policies to ensure that their most vulnerable workers are adequately supported and covered. The Wall Street Journal believes that small business may suffer significant loss of business confidence as a result of COVID-19. It has therefore initiated advocacy for larger enterprises to support such SMEs through the difficult times [115]. Major enterprises such as Amazon have embraced this initiative as a form of corporate social responsibility. Amazon has set up a $5 million relief fund to support SMEs in their vicinity. Google has also pledged $1 million to support "pandemic-hit" SMEs in Mountain View, California where it operates [116]. The President, CEO, and top management personnel of United Airlines Company have decided to forego their salary to ensure uninterrupted business operations and safeguard the salaries of lower level employees. LVHM holdings has also converted a facility to quickly produce hand sanitizers for free distribution to French hospitals while Tottenham Hotspur Stadium has installed equipment to operate drive-through COVID-19 testing and swabbing for NHS staff, families, and their dependents. In this way, enterprises are creatively adapting to the pandemic to further their brand in the long run while caring for people in the current climate.

There are those who believe that business organizations involved in CSR during the COVID-19 are again employing the same mind game that characterized involvement in the United Nations Global Compact. The voluntary actions require significant outlay of resources which are non-existing when production and companies have closed down. It is believed therefore that these voluntary investments entail economic benefit for the companies and are designed to align with the objectives of investors/shareholders as profit seeking agents. For example, in North America, companies were willing to continue to pay employees when their companies were forced to close because of the benefit from the Payroll Protection Plan by the U.S. government [117]. This plan provides loans to businesses that can be forgiven (i.e., the loans can be converted to grants), hence companies do not need to repay if they maintain a certain percentage of their employees. Walmart, Apple, the Olive Garden, and Lululemon belong to this category of companies that stand the chance to benefit from the Payroll Protection Plan. Moreover, according to Verma and Gustafsson [118], the real benefit of CSR strategies are economic more than social. There are motivational benefits for employees and clients that lead to better hiring opportunities and greater market shares; cost reductions and increases in efficiency and productivity; increased competitiveness; access to sources of external financing and capital under more optimal conditions; limitation and greater control of corporate risks; and generating a reputation and long-term competitive advantages.

Gostin and Wiley [119] espouse the innate relationship between corporate social responsibility and branding. According to Zeren and Hizarci [85], how enterprises use CSR to respond to the changing phases of COVID-19 can influence their brand image which is needed in the post epidemic reconstruction of firms. Through CSR, the values of honesty, dedication, and community support can authenticate the brand value of companies in uncontrollable times. According to Daniels [120], companies that support or work with NGOs and other charities on COVID-19 can foster strong social relationships through genuine and mutually beneficial care. It offers enterprises the opportunity to build new relationships and better communication engagement.

In this case, COVID-19 can provide the CSR and business community teams with the opportunity to re-think and re-structure plans to place community needs at the top of their conversations. In some countries also, practices that qualify for CSR activities are being redefined under COVID-19 with strict guidelines. For example, the government of India has instructed that corporate contributions made towards the PM care fund will be regarded as CSR whereas contributions given to the prime ministers fund will not qualify for CSR donation. Thus, in this way, CSR contribution can significantly affect corporate tax assessment and access to other state support systems available to companies that are actively involved in one form of CSR or the other.

In the midst of this challenge, the effect of COVID-19 on the global economy poses one of the greatest threats to corporate involvement in CSR. At the end of April 2020, an estimated amount of nearly $17 trillion worth of the global business income and businesses had been wiped away by COVID-19 and $2.5 trillion was needed to reboot economies. The effect has been widespread including airlines, cruise ships, hospitality, manufacturing, and many other industries. COVID-19 has therefore assailed business organizations with unprecedented dangers of running at a loss, depleting capital retentions, inability to meet recurring debts and tax obligations, loss of an entire workforce and even customer base. Additionally, there is a strong association between capital market and public health and with the capital market roiled by COVID-19, there is the need for a revolutionary definition of corporate citizenship in this crisis time that balances voluntary support for society against the dwindling economic fortunes of corporate enterprises.

According to Bartik et al. [121], a major corporate social responsibility issue that assail enterprises under COVID-19 is navigating salary adjustments, furlough, redundancies, continuous payment of wages and salary for sick and stay at home staff, support and replacement of dead staff, and unanticipated absenteeism. Enterprises must also deal with disinfection of business offices; restructure business hours, partitioning shared office spaces among others [48]. The process of returning to a full-time work schedule has also been fraught with several challenges that have corporate social responsibility implications. In the UK, for example, the biggest trade unions are intransigent about allowing their members to work under the current conditions unless government and employers agree on a nationwide health and safety revolution to protect their members against the debilitating effect of the COVID-19 pandemic.

Alluding to the fringe interest in employer commitment to employee health and safety measures in a free market, these unions have reiterated the need for radical overhauled and stepping up of health and safety inspection and facilities at the workplace until they back the government's effort to ease, and eventually end, the lockdown [122]. Other employee unions are equally demanding for employers to draw up and publish rejuvenated risk assessments that thoroughly clearly outline the specific measures to ensure a safe work environment for employees. Finally, there is also the demand for government to impose hefty punishment on rogue employers and state investment into more frequent health and safety inspections of workplaces.

While contributing financially and emotionally to reduce social burden of COVID-19, there is a moral obligation of enterprises to discard extreme free-market ideologies that prioritizes profit at the expense of safety of employees. The call for a radical overhaul of health and safety measures in enterprises is now urgent more than ever before. There is a moral obligation for enterprises to reform current risk assessments and cooperate more deeply with state agencies and industry collaborators to invest in the health and safety inspections at the world place [123]. Thus, with COVID-19, business organizations must recognize the need to ensure a balance between profit, people, and the planet since their economic growth depends on it. To that extent, CSR can be the game changer among various corporate strategies that creates unrivalled competitive advantage in uncontested market spaces for businesses to flourish. To this end, CSR strategies that focus on overcoming the effects of global healthcare crises must be of major concern to all enterprises because of their catastrophic effects on the very survival of firms if not nipped in the bud. Since workplace health and safety issues will not be the same after the sweeping effect of COVID-19, CSR strategies must be proactive to endure other unknown pandemics with equal capacity to disrupt business operations. These new CSR strategies must be capable of addressing the new frontiers in workplace health and safety (new normal) that have emerged [124]. There is the need for consistent research to retrace previous steps and strategies adopted to manage historical crisis of this magnitude. COVID-19-related CSR must therefore aim at alleviating mental and psychological wellbeing of its employees to embrace the wide range of changes that may occur. For example, work from home and social distancing measures vitally reduce the spread of the virus but have a negative influence of emotional wellbeing of employees [80]. Thus, leading corporations must support mental and emotional wellbeing of their staff. Moreover, navigating salary adjustments, furlough, redundancies, continuous payment of wages and salary for sick and stay at home staff, support and replacement of dead staff, and unanticipated absenteeism are just a few of the challenges that assail corporate organizations and these require a CSR response.

Companies must create innovative and regular activities to educate their stakeholders to become more committed to safeguarding future enterprise-based defense mechanism needed to diagnose, protect, treat, and rehabilitate victims and those threatened by pandemics and other emergencies that affect the stability of an organization to reduce its cost and protect revenue [83].

COVID-19 has shown that even though individual enterprise contingency plans are necessary, to fight the economic effects of pandemics, they are not sufficient by themselves. COVID-19 must teach enterprises that they operate in a complex, uncertain, and intertwined economic environment and pandemics spare no one. Companies must design CSR strategies with each other as collaborators and not necessarily competitors. This is because most of the lone ranger and disconnected CSR strategies paraded by enterprises to fight COVID-19 have not shown much resilience under COVID-19. For most companies, their existing strategies lack systematic integration and standardized performance metrics to measure their outcomes, usability efficiency, performance, and suitability which makes it difficult to determine their success or failure as effective CSR tools in the management of a pandemic [125].

Going forward, there is the need for group of firms to develop multi-agency and multi-disciplinary decision making and evaluation processes through collaborative networks. Already the idea and benefits of collaborative networks as a business strategy to mitigate the effect of catastrophic health and environmental crisis on business enterprises is gaining grounds in many different industries in the quest to respond positively to a changing business environment, and the healthcare sector is no exception. In China, for example, the biotech, medtech, and pharmaceutical clusters have accentuated effort to promote greater environmental health security through self-regulating and collaborative network of environmentally responsible behaviors, programs, and standards. These industry-led initiatives have engendered greater public support, renewed political commitment from top leaders and elicited heavy government subsidies for the industry among others. According to [126], nowadays, more and more enterprises are aware and motivated to adhere to collaborative platforms as business enablers, allowing groups of companies to improve their offer and competitiveness. This is because today's firms must not only see themselves as competitors but as collaborators of the same goal when it comes to managing risks such as COVID-19 through shared burden. To that extent, collaborative can help groups of enterprises to develop a multi-tier system of organizations to supplement each other's competencies to be well equipped to handle the complexities of modern healthcare issues in an innovative, efficient, and effective manner than individual firms [127].

Collaborative efforts in the fight against COVID-19 can give firms the opportunity to enjoy the vast awareness, credibility, and the brand equity that single firms find lacking in operations. Owing to their sizable budgets and greater scale of operations, collaborative firms are poised to have easier access to funds to undertake strategic programs. They will be more equipped with the necessary resources that single firms may find hard to acquire [128]. Additionally, inimitable assets like a steadfast reputation for process rigor and quality response to market opportunities might turn out to be critical for sustaining a competitive edge in crowded therapy markets. Such intangible assets could be more easily accruable to collaborative firms because of their vast portfolios and long track records of market presence and innovation [129]. These collaborative CSR strategies may lead to accumulation of different perspectives on a variety of topical issues affecting CSR practice by quickly sharing knowledge and effectively using 'Wisdom of the corporate Crowds'. With time this, "Ideas Bank" can grow and become a warehouse with a variety of cases that can be grouped together and searched simultaneously by individual enterprises and others who need them. The next step will be to develop he mechanism to regularize the forums and develop a good publishing format and start publishing these rich case discussions, either a part of a journal or in another citable online format in public domains.

## 5. Conclusions

The objective of the study was to explore how enterprises are able to balance their business and social needs through CSR during pandemic situations. Firstly, the studies show that pandemics have similar characteristics that stimulate the business decision to get involved through CSR. Through CSR, business enterprises can strengthen societal pillars to better understand and withstand the shock of debilitating pandemics throughout history. The studies show that pandemics such as the Spanish flu, malaria, cholera, HIV-AIDS, environmental health, and COVID-19 created economic opportunities by themselves for business organizations as well. In instances where these economic opportunities were not obvious, the CSR strategies employed by business organizations were targeted at reducing the cost of the effect of the pandemics and maximizing any revenue potential. Through the various interventions to support their employees that were affected directly or indirectly by the pandemic, business organizations were actually protecting or building up their stock of human capital which is the greatest resource of every organization.

Secondly, the reviews have proven that the impact of COVID-19 on business enterprise has been unique, unprecedented, and may be endless. With new strains and new waves emerging unabated, COVID-19 is peerless when it comes to global health crises that have posed the biggest challenge to the CSR of firms. The momentum of infections across the globe and the seasonal wave with various mutated strains makes it difficult to predict the future of COVID-19 and range of business disruptions with clarity and certainty. This notwithstanding business organizations can seize the opportunities created by COVID-19 to develop better risk management strategies, bolster their brand image to obtain social legitimacy, and redesign their supply chains to enhance efficiency.

Our study contributes in two ways to advancing the theories of corporate social responsibility. Firstly, our study contributes to the emerging field of "evolutionary theory of corporate social responsibility" that emerged from Darwin's analogy that the most adaptive species are the fittest. In this case, we contend that only adaptive enterprises that are fit can survive COVID-19 and other pandemics irrespective of how much funds they invest in CSR. These are the enterprises who earliest in time see the risks posed by COVID-19 and similar pandemics on business operations. These enterprises have the systems to see things clearly and weigh them justly. They then apply their experience to succeed, not merely because they have an innate power but because the impact of COVID-19 is so rapid and the accompanying competition so fierce that the enterprise that makes a late start is left out and can seldom overtake others. Evolutionary theory of CSR teaches enterprises to develop CSR strategies that go beyond simply designing plans to mitigate damages when crises such as COVID-19 occur. Instead, CSR must include the development of a robust and continuous information sensing system that constantly feed enterprises with complete, timely correct, relevant updates on potential changes in the environment that threaten business stability.

The study also contributes to advancing the frontiers of behavior theory of CSR. Behavioral CSR theorists have stoked a new controversy in their analysis of the impact of COVID-19 on CSR. They argue that COVID-19 CSR-related reactions and interventions are only transient and will not necessarily lead to positive organizational outcomes. They contend that CSR positive outcomes will occur only if CSR is continuously embedded within the organizational structure and strategy. Thus, an enterprise that seeks to boost their economic fortunes through extended CSR during COVID-19 may find their actions mired in chaos and confusion.

Typical of academic studies, a number of limitations may affect the results of this research. For example, the studies were taken from only ten databases and supplemented with three additional sources. This implies that all other studies outside these sources were ignored. The small sample size of articles studied may limit the findings of this research. Relatedly, the strict inclusive and exclusive criteria used to select articles means that other articles with potentially useful information were deemed lower-quality, downgraded, and disregarded. Further, the methodological limitations of the parent studies (particularly, regarding the sampling strategies of reviewed materials in the case of primary studies) limits the findings of the research. This is because most of these studies did not clearly indicate how participants in the studies were recruited and sampled and that may limit the transferability of the findings of this research. Even in the case of the secondary research-based studies, the authors themselves have disclosed limitations regarding the process of sampling the studies which further limits any analysis made from them.

This study included only articles published in the English language and the coverage of the final set of admitted articles did not equally cover all the geographical areas of the world. This limits the generalizability of the findings to other contexts. This review is primarily a tangential contribution to the overall fight against COVID-19 from an organization point of view. Future research must relook at the proposed compulsory unemployment insurance and their ability in ameliorating the effect of future pandemics. This study requires more primary-based information that can be simulated to understand the different scenarios of effectiveness based on historical records and projections into the future.

**Author Contributions:** Conceptualization, H.A.A. and T.M.; Data curation, L.Z.; Formal analysis, H.A.A. and X.X.; Funding acquisition, L.Z.; Investigation, L.Z., X.X. and T.M.; Methodology, H.A.A. and X.X.; Project administration, X.X.; Supervision, L.Z.; Visualization, T.M.; Writing—original draft, H.A.A. and T.M.; Writing—review & editing, H.A.A. All authors have read and agreed to the published version of the manuscript.

**Funding:** This research was funded by the National Natural Science Foundation of China (71904066), the Social science application research project of Jiangsu Province (19SYB-095, 20SHD002), the Universities' Philosophy and Social Science Researches in Jiangsu Province (2019SJA1884) for their support for this project.

**Informed Consent Statement:** Not applicable.

**Data Availability Statement:** The data for this research is held by the authors and will be made available upon reasonable request.

**Acknowledgments:** The authors deeply appreciate the support of the staff and fellows of the Center for Health and Public Policy Research at the Jiangsu University. The support of the postdoctoral fellows at the School of Management is also highly appreciated. Officer in departments of the Provincial Administration of Jiangsu Province are also acknowledged for their diverse service toward the collection of accurate data for the research.

**Conflicts of Interest:** The authors declare no conflict of interest. The funders had no role in the design of the study; in the collection, analyses, or interpretation of data; in the writing of the manuscript, or in the decision to publish the results.

## References

1. Roy, D.A. Trends in global corporate social responsibility practices: The case of Sub-Saharan Africa. *Int. J. Civ. Soc.* **2010**, *8*, 64.
2. Johnson, B.R.; Connolly, E.; Carter, T.S. Corporate social responsibility: The role of Fortune 100 companies in domestic and international natural disasters. *Corp. Soc. Responsib. Environ. Manag.* **2011**, *18*, 352–369. [CrossRef]
3. Auld, G.; Bernstein, S.; Cashore, B. The new corporate social responsibility. *Annu. Rev. Environ. Resour.* **2008**, *33*, 413–435. [CrossRef]
4. Toward an Understanding of Corporate Social Responsibility: Theory and Field Experimental Evidence. Available online: https://www.nber.org/papers/w26222 (accessed on 8 April 2021).
5. Lindgreen, A.; Swaen, V.; Campbell, T.T. Corporate social responsibility practices in developing and transitional countries: Botswana and Malawi. *J. Bus. Ethics* **2009**, *90*, 429–440. [CrossRef]
6. Amoako, G.; Dartey-Baah, K.; Owusu-Frimpong, N.; Kebreti, C. Corporate Social Responsibility: Perspectives of Foreign and Local Oil Marketing Companies in Ghana. *Communicatio* **2019**, *45*, 67–92. [CrossRef]
7. Vian, T.; McCoy, K.; Richards, S.C.; Connelly, P.; Feeley, F. Corporate social responsibility in global health: The Pfizer Global Health Fellows international volunteering program. *Hum. Resour. Plan.* **2007**, *30*, 30.
8. Livingston, E.; Desai, A.; Berkwits, M. Sourcing personal protective equipment during the COVID-19 pandemic. *JAMA* **2020**, *323*, 1912–1914. [CrossRef]
9. D'Aprile, G.; Mannarini, T. Corporate social responsibility: A psychosocial multidimensional construct. *J. Glob. Responsib.* **2012**, *3*, 48–65. [CrossRef]
10. Pluye, P.; Hong, Q.N. Combining the power of stories and the power of numbers: Mixed methods research and mixed studies reviews. *Annu. Rev. Public Health* **2014**, *35*, 29–45. [CrossRef]
11. Flanagan, W.; Whiteman, G. "AIDS is Not a Business": A Study in Global Corporate Responsibility–Securing Access to Low-cost HIV Medications. *J. Bus. Ethics* **2007**, *73*, 65–75. [CrossRef]
12. Bowen, P.; Allen, Y.; Edwards, P.; Cattell, K.; Simbayi, L. Guidelines for effective workplace HIV/AIDS intervention management by construction firms. *Constr. Manag. Econ.* **2014**, *32*, 362–381. [CrossRef]
13. Dickinson, D.; Stevens, M. Understanding the response of large South African companies to HIV/AIDS. *Sahara-J J. Soc. Asp. Hiv Aids* **2005**, *2*, 286–295. [CrossRef] [PubMed]
14. Utuk, I.G.; Osungbade, K.O.; Obembe, T.A.; Adewole, D.A.; Oladoyin, V.O. Stigmatising attitudes towards co-workers with HIV in the workplace of a metropolitan state, Southwestern Nigeria. *Open Aids J.* **2017**, *11*, 67. [CrossRef]
15. Rampersad, R. HIV and AIDS in South Africa: A social and moral responsibility in shaping organisational action. *Corp. Ownersh. Control* **2013**, *928*, 10.
16. *United Nations Joint Programme of Support on HIV/AIDS 2016–2018*; UN Headquarters: New York, NY, USA, 2016.
17. Uduji, J.I.; Okolo-Obasi, E.N.; Asongu, S.A. Multinational oil companies in Nigeria and corporate social responsibility in the HIV/AIDS response in host communities. *Local Environ.* **2019**, *24*, 393–416. [CrossRef]
18. Davis, G.F.; Anderson, P.J. Social movements and failed institutionalization: Corporate (non) response to the AIDS epidemic. In *The Sage Handbook of Organizational Institutionalism*; SAGE Publications Ltd.: Newbury Park, CA, USA, 2008; pp. 371–388.
19. Ntim, C.G. Corporate governance, corporate health accounting, and firm value: The case of HIV/AIDS disclosures in Sub-Saharan Africa. *Int. J. Account.* **2016**, *51*, 155–216. [CrossRef]
20. Bolton, P.L. Corporate responses to HIV/AIDS: Experience and leadership from South Africa. *Bus. Soc. Rev.* **2008**, *113*, 277–300. [CrossRef]
21. Mahajan, A.P.; Colvin, M.; Rudatsikira, J.-B.; Ettl, D. An overview of HIV/AIDS workplace policies and programmes in southern Africa. *Aids* **2007**, *21*, S31–S39. [CrossRef] [PubMed]
22. Sanyal, R.N.; Neves, J.S. The Valdez principles: Implications for corporate social responsibility. *J. Bus. Ethics* **1991**, *10*, 883–890. [CrossRef]
23. Welker, M.A. "Corporate security begins in the community": Mining, the corporate social responsibility industry, and environmental advocacy in Indonesia. *Cult. Anthropol.* **2009**, *24*, 142–179. [CrossRef]
24. Delmas, M.A.; Etzion, D.; Nairn-Birch, N. Triangulating environmental performance: What do corporate social responsibility ratings really capture? *Acad. Manag. Perspect.* **2013**, *27*, 255–267. [CrossRef]

25. Shaukat, A.; Qiu, Y.; Trojanowski, G. Board attributes, corporate social responsibility strategy, and corporate environmental and social performance. *J. Bus. Ethics* **2016**, *135*, 569–585. [CrossRef]
26. The Coronavirus and the Great Influenza Pandemic: Lessons from the "Spanish Flu" for the Coronavirus's Potential Effects on Mortality and Economic Activity. Available online: https://www.nber.org/papers/w26866 (accessed on 8 April 2021).
27. Correia, S.; Luck, S.; Verner, E. *Pandemics Depress the Economy, Public Health Interventions Do Not: Evidence from the 1918 Flu*; March, Unpublished Manuscript; Social Science Electronic Publishing Inc.: Rochester, NY, USA, 2020.
28. Kuo, L.; Yeh, C.C.; Yu, H.C. Disclosure of corporate social responsibility and environmental management: Evidence from China. *Corp. Soc. Responsib. Environ. Manag.* **2012**, *19*, 273–287. [CrossRef]
29. Idowu, S.O.; Capaldi, N.; Zu, L.; Gupta, A.D. *Encyclopedia of Corporate Social Responsibility*; Springer: Berlin/Heidelberg, Germany, 2013; Volume 2.
30. Málovics, G.; Csigéné, N.N.; Kraus, S. The role of corporate social responsibility in strong sustainability. *J. Socio Econ.* **2008**, *37*, 907–918. [CrossRef]
31. Reinhardt, F.L.; Stavins, R.N. Corporate social responsibility, business strategy, and the environment. *Oxf. Rev. Econ. Policy* **2010**, *26*, 164–181. [CrossRef]
32. Chandler, D.M.C. Achieving Sustainable Drug Development through CSR: Possibility or Utopia. In *Bioeconomy for Sustainable Development*; Springer: Berlin/Heidelberg, Germany, 2020; pp. 303–319.
33. Kolk, A. The social responsibility of international business: From ethics and the environment to CSR and sustainable development. *J. World Bus.* **2016**, *51*, 23–34. [CrossRef]
34. Alvarado-Herrera, A.; Bigne, E.; Aldas-Manzano, J.; Curras-Perez, R. A scale for measuring consumer perceptions of corporate social responsibility following the sustainable development paradigm. *J. Bus. Ethics* **2017**, *140*, 243–262. [CrossRef]
35. Schönherr, N.; Findler, F.; Martinuzzi, A. Exploring the interface of CSR and the sustainable development goals. *Transnatl. Corp.* **2017**, *24*, 33–47.
36. Xia, B.; Olanipekun, A.; Chen, Q.; Xie, L.; Liu, Y. Conceptualising the state of the art of corporate social responsibility (CSR) in the construction industry and its nexus to sustainable development. *J. Clean. Prod.* **2018**, *195*, 340–353. [CrossRef]
37. Annan-Diab, F.; Molinari, C. Interdisciplinarity: Practical approach to advancing education for sustainability and for the Sustainable Development Goals. *Int. J. Manag. Educ.* **2017**, *15*, 73–83. [CrossRef]
38. MSuárez, C.; Rubio-Romero, J.C.; Pinto-Contreiras, J.; Gemar, G. A model to measure sustainable development in the hotel industry: A comparative study. *Corp. Soc. Responsib. Environ. Manag.* **2018**, *25*, 722–732.
39. Chuang, S.-P.; Huang, S.-J. The effect of environmental corporate social responsibility on environmental performance and business competitiveness: The mediation of green information technology capital. *J. Bus. Ethics* **2018**, *150*, 991–1009. [CrossRef]
40. Marco-Fondevila, M.; Abadía, J.M.M.; Scarpellini, S. CSR and green economy: Determinants and correlation of firms' sustainable development. *Corp. Soc. Responsib. Environ. Manag.* **2018**, *25*, 756–771. [CrossRef]
41. The Impact of COVID-19 on Gender Equality. Available online: https://www.nber.org/papers/w26947 (accessed on 8 April 2021).
42. Love in the Time of Covid-19: The Resiliency of Environmental and Social Stocks. Available online: https://ideas.repec.org/p/cpr/ceprdp/14661.html (accessed on 8 April 2021).
43. Ozili, P.K.; Arun, T. *Spillover of COVID-19: Impact on the Global Economy*; Social Science Electronic Publishing Inc.: Rochester, NY, USA, 2020. [CrossRef]
44. Shan, C.; Tang, D.Y. *The Value of Employee Satisfaction in Disastrous Times: Evidence from Covid-19*; Social Science Electronic Publishing Inc.: Rochester, NY, USA, 2020; No 3560919. [CrossRef]
45. Francis, N.N.; Pegg, S. Socially distanced school-based nutrition program feeding under COVID 19 in the rural Niger Delta. *Extr. Ind. Soc.* **2020**, *7*, 576–579.
46. Social Protection and Jobs Responses to COVID-19: A Real-Time Review of Country Measures. Live Document. Available online: http://www.ugogentilini.net/wp-content/uploads/2020/03/global-review-of-social-protection-responsesto-COVID-19-2.pdf (accessed on 21 December 2020).
47. The Economic Ripple Effects of COVID-19. Available online: https://pubdocs.worldbank.org/en/366061585780198787/slides-wb-apr12020.pdf (accessed on 8 April 2021).
48. Williamson, V.; Murphy, D.; Greenberg, N. COVID-19 and experiences of moral injury in front-line key workers. *Occup. Med.* **2020**, *70*, 317–319. [CrossRef]
49. Laing, T. The economic impact of the Coronavirus 2019 (Covid-2019): Implications for the mining industry. *Extr. Ind. Soc.* **2020**, *7*, 580–582. [PubMed]
50. The Cost of COVID-19: A Rough Estimate of the 2020 US GDP Impact. Available online: https://www.mercatus.org/publications/covid-19-policy-brief-series/cost-covid-19-rough-estimate-2020-us-gdp-impact (accessed on 8 April 2021).
51. Vaccaro, A.R.; Getz, C.L.; Cohen, B.E.; Cole, B.J.; Donnally, C.J., III. Practice Management during the COVID-19 Pandemic. *J. Am. Acad. Orthop. Surg.* **2020**, *28*, 464–470. [CrossRef]
52. Ferreira, L. Access to affordable HIV/AIDS drugs: The human rights obligations of multinational pharmaceutical corporations. *L. Rev.* **2002**, *71*, 1133.
53. Waking up to Risk: Corporate Responses to HIV/AIDS in the Workplace. Available online: https://data.unaids.org/publications/irc-pub06/jc968-wakinguptorisk_en.pdf (accessed on 8 April 2021).

54. Long, C.A. New institutional formation in the intersection of Tanzanian decentralization and HIV/AIDS interventions. *J. East. Afr. Stud.* **2017**, *11*, 692–713. [CrossRef]
55. Gilbert, G.; Cattell, K.; Edwards, P.; Bowen, P. A sequential mixed methods research approach to investigating HIV/AIDS intervention management by construction organisations in South Africa. *Acta Structilia* **2017**, *24*, 27–52. [CrossRef]
56. Dunfee, T.W. Do firms with unique competencies for rescuing victims of human catastrophes have special obligations? Corporate responsibility and the AIDS catastrophe in Sub-Saharan Africa. *Bus. Ethics Q.* **2006**, *16*, 185–210. [CrossRef] [PubMed]
57. Sharma, A.; Kiran, R. Corporate social responsibility initiatives of major companies of India with focus on health, education and environment. *Afr. J. Basic Appl. Sci.* **2012**, *4*, 95–105.
58. World Health Organization. Foundation for Innovative New Diagnostics, WHO Working Group on HIV Incidence Assays: Meeting Report, Boston, MA, USA, 20–26 February 2016. Available online: https://apps.who.int/iris/handle/10665/254868 (accessed on 8 April 2021).
59. López-Pérez, M.E.; Melero, I.; Sesé, F.J. Does specific CSR training for managers impact shareholder value? Implications for education in sustainable development. *Corp. Soc. Responsib. Environ. Manag.* **2017**, *24*, 435–448. [CrossRef]
60. Taylor, J.; Vithayathil, J.; Yim, D. Are corporate social responsibility (CSR) initiatives such as sustainable development and environmental policies value enhancing or window dressing? *Corp. Soc. Responsib. Environ. Manag.* **2018**, *25*, 971–980. [CrossRef]
61. Osmani, A. Corporate Social Responsibility for Sustainable Development in China. Recent Evolution of CSR Concepts and Practice within Chinese Firms. Ph.D. Thesis, Università Ca'Foscari Venezia, Venice, Italy, 2019.
62. Barua, S. *Understanding Coronanomics: The Economic Implications of the Coronavirus (COVID-19) Pandemic*; Social Science Electronic Publishing Inc.: Rochester, NY, USA, 2020. [CrossRef]
63. Harvey, D. *Anti-Capitalist Politics in the Time of COVID-19*; Jacobin: New York, NY, USA, 2020.
64. Clark, M.; Hertel, G.; Hirschi, A.; Kunze, F.; Shockley, K.; Shoss, M. *COVID-19: Implications for Research and Practice in Industrial and Organizational Psychology Cort W*; Rudolph Saint Louis University Blake Allan Purdue University: Saint Louis, MI, USA, 2020.
65. Jennejohn, M.; Nyarko, J.; Talley, E.L. *COVID-19 as a Force Majeure in Corporate Transactions*; Social Science Electronic Publishing Inc.: Rochester, NY, USA, 2020. [CrossRef]
66. Ishak, S.; Omar, A.R.C.; Osman, L.H. *Sympathy and Benevolence of Business Entities: Evidence during the COVID-19 Pandemic Outbreak*; Social Science Electronic Publishing Inc.: Rochester, NY, USA, 2020. [CrossRef]
67. Makwara, T.; Mutambara, M.; Magagula-Hlatjwako, S. A comparative literature review survey of employee HIV and AIDS-related corporate social responsibility (CSR) practices in small, micro and medium enterprises (SMMEs) in Zimbabwe and South Africa. *Probl. Perspect. Manag.* **2019**, *2*, 339–347. [CrossRef]
68. Stadler, J. AIDS ads: Make a commercial, make a difference? Corporate social responsibility and the media. *Continuum* **2004**, *18*, 591–610. [CrossRef]
69. Rajak, D. 'HIV/AIDS is our business': The moral economy of treatment in a transnational mining company. *J. R. Anthropol. Inst.* **2010**, *16*, 551–571. [CrossRef]
70. Soobaroyen, T.; Ntim, C.G. Social and environmental accounting as symbolic and substantive means of legitimation: The case of HIV/AIDS reporting in South Africa. *Account. Forum* **2013**, *2*, 92–109. [CrossRef]
71. Adegbite, A.; Amiolemen, S.O.; Ologeh, I.O.; Oyefuga, I. Sustainable development policy and corporate social responsibility in business organisations in Nigeria. *J. Sustain. Dev.* **2012**, *5*, 83–89. [CrossRef]
72. Tuodolo, F. Corporate social responsibility: Between civil society and the oil industry in the developing world. *Acme Int. E J. Crit. Geogr.* **2009**, *8*, 530–541.
73. Jenkins, H.; Yakovleva, N. Corporate social responsibility in the mining industry: Exploring trends in social and environmental disclosure. *J. Clean. Prod.* **2006**, *14*, 271–284. [CrossRef]
74. Orlitzky, M.; Siegel, D.S.; Waldman, D.A. Strategic corporate social responsibility and environmental sustainability. *Bus. Soc.* **2011**, *50*, 6–27. [CrossRef]
75. Lyon, T.P.; Maxwell, J.W. Corporate social responsibility and the environment: A theoretical perspective. *Rev. Environ. Econ. Policy* **2008**, *2*, 240–260. [CrossRef]
76. Dimmler, L. Linking social determinants of health to corporate social responsibility: Extant criteria for the mining industry. *Extr. Ind. Soc.* **2017**, *4*, 216–226. [CrossRef]
77. Senay, E.; Landrigan, P.J. Assessment of environmental sustainability and corporate social responsibility reporting by large health care organizations. *JAMA Netw. Open* **2018**, *1*, e180975. [CrossRef] [PubMed]
78. Givel, M. Motivation of chemical industry social responsibility through Responsible Care. *Health Policy* **2007**, *81*, 85–92. [CrossRef]
79. Kurland, N.B.; Baucus, M.; Steckler, E. *Business and Society in the Age of COVID-19*; Business and Society Review; Wiley-Blackwell: Hoboken, NJ, USA, 2020.
80. Maital, S.; Barzani, E. *The Global Economic Impact of COVID-19: A Summary of Research*; Samuel Neaman Institute for National Policy Research, Technion: Haifa, Israel, 2020.
81. Shingal, A. Services trade and COVID-19. In *Forthcoming VoxEU CEPR Policy Portal Column*; World Bank Research Working Paper; World Bank: New York, NY, USA, 2020.
82. Boone, L.; Haugh, D.; Pain, N.; Salins, V. Tackling the fallout from COVID-19. In *Economics in the Time of COVID-19*; CEPR Press: London, UK, 2020; p. 37.

83. Nicola, M.; Alsafi, Z.; Sohrabi, C.; Kerwan, A.; Al-Jabir, A.; Iosifidis, C.; Agha, M.; Agha, R. The socio-economic implications of the coronavirus and COVID-19 pandemic: A review. *Int. J. Surg.* **2020**, *78*, 185–193. [CrossRef]
84. Hevia, C.; Neumeyer, A. A Conceptual Framework for Analyzing the Economic Impact of COVID-19 and its Policy Implications. *Undp. Lac. Covid-19 Policy Doc. Ser.* **2020**, *1*, 29.
85. Zeren, F.; Hizarci, A. The Impact of COVID-19 Coronavirus on Stock Markets: Evidence from Selected Countries. *Muhasebe Finans İncelemeleri Derg.* **2020**, *3*, 78–84. [CrossRef]
86. Coussens, C.; Harrison, M. *Global Environmental Health in the 21st Century: From Governmental Regulation to Corporate Social Responsibility: Workshop Summary*; National Academies Press: Washington, DC, USA, 2007.
87. Cabral, L.; Xu, L. *Seller Reputation and Price Gouging: Evidence from the COVID-19 Pandemic*; Mimeo Inc.: New York, NY, USA, 2020.
88. Fernandes, N. *Economic Effects of Coronavirus Outbreak (COVID-19) on the World Economy*; Social Science Electronic Publishing Inc.: Rochester, NY, USA, 2020.
89. Barro, R.J. *Non-Pharmaceutical Interventions and Mortality in U.S. Cities*; NBER Working Paper No. 27049; National Bureau of Economic Research: Cambridge, MA, USA, 2020.
90. Bootsma, M.; Ferguson, N. The Effect of Public Health Measures on the 1918 Influenza Pandemic in U.S. Cities. *Proc. Natl. Acad. Sci. USA* **2007**, *104*, 7588–7593. [CrossRef] [PubMed]
91. Butlin, M.W. *A Preliminary Annual Database 1900/01 to 1973/74*; RBA Research Discussion Paper No 7701; Reserve Bank of Australia's Research Department: Sydney, Australia, 1977.
92. Caley, P.; Philp, D.J.; McCracken, K. Quantifying Social Distancing Arising from Pandemic Influenza. *J. R. Soc. Interface* **2008**, *5*, 631–639. [CrossRef]
93. Liu, Y.; Lee, J.M.; Lee, C. The challenges and opportunities of a global health crisis: The management and business implications of COVID-19 from an Asian perspective. *J. Asia Bus. Stud.* **2020**, *19*, 277–297.
94. Cheng, W.; Carlin, P.; Carroll, J.; Gupta, S.; Rojas, F.L.; Montenovo, L.; Nguyen, T.D.; Schmutte, I.M.; Scrivner, O.; Simon, K.I.; et al. *Back to Business and (re) Employing Workers? Labor Market Activity during State COVID-19 Reopenings*; National Bureau of Economic Research: Cambridge, MA, USA, 2020.
95. Parker, L.D. The COVID-19 office in transition: Cost, efficiency and the social responsibility business case. *Account. Audit. Account. J.* **2020**, *13*, 21–29. [CrossRef]
96. Profit with Purpose: The Role of Business in Achieving Sustainable Development. Available online: https://www.iied.org/profit-purpose-role-business-achieving-sustainabledevelopment (accessed on 18 December 2020).
97. Curson, P.; McCracken, K. An Australian Perspective of the 1918–1919 Influenza Pandemic. *NSW Public Health Bull.* **2014**, *17*, 103–107.
98. Economic Effects of the Spanish Flu Bulletin. Available online: https://www.rba.gov.au/publications/bulletin/2020/jun/economic-effects-of-the-spanish-flu.html (accessed on 9 April 2021).
99. Forster, C. Australian Unemployment 1900–1940. *Econ. Rec.* **1965**, *41*, 426–450. [CrossRef]
100. Garrett, T.A. Economic Effects of the 1918 Influenza Pandemic: Implications for a Modern-Day Pandemic. *Fed. Reserve Bank St. Louis Rev.* **2008**, *90*, 75–93.
101. Hatchett, R.J.; Mecher, C.E.; Lipsitch, M. Public Health Interventions and Epidemic Intensity during the 1918 Influenza Pandemic. *Proc. Natl. Acad. Sci. USA* **2007**, *104*, 7582–7587. [CrossRef]
102. Keogh-Brown, M.R.; Wren-Lewis, S.; Edmunds, W.J.; Beutels, P.; Smith, R.D. The Possible Macroeconomic Impact on the UK of an Influenza Pandemic. *Health Econ.* **2010**, *19*, 1345–1360. [CrossRef] [PubMed]
103. Markel, H.; Lipman, H.B.; Navarro, J.A.; Sloan, A.; Michalsen, J.R.; Stern, A.M.; Cetron, M.S. Nonpharmaceutical Interventions Implemented by US Cities During the 1918–1919 Influenza Pandemic. *J. Am. Med. Assoc.* **2007**, *298*, 644–654. [CrossRef]
104. McQueen, H. The 'Spanish' Influenza Pandemic in Australia, 1912–1919. In *Social Policy in Australia–Some Perspectives 1901–1975*; Roe, J., Ed.; Cassell Australia: Stanmore, NSW, Australia, 1976; pp. 131–147.
105. Defining Moments: Influenza Pandemic. 2020. Available online: https://www.nma.gov.au/defining-moments/resources/influenza-pandemic (accessed on 9 April 2021).
106. Pneumonic Influenza (Spanish Flu). 1919. Available online: https://www.records.nsw.gov.au/archives/collections-and-research/guides-and-indexes/stories/pneumonic-influenza-1919 (accessed on 13 January 2021).
107. Rinaldi, G.; Lilley, A.; Lilley, M. *Public Health Interventions and Economic Growth: Revisiting the Spanish Flu Evidence*. Harvard University Economics Department and Harvard Business School; Havard University: Boston, MA, USA, 2020; unpublished manuscript.
108. Fooks, G.; Gilmore, A.; Collin, J.; Holden, C.; Lee, K. The limits of corporate social responsibility: Techniques of neutralization, stakeholder management and political CSR. *J. Bus. Ethics* **2013**, *112*, 283–299. [CrossRef]
109. Wirth, H.; Kulczycka, J.; Hausner, J.; Koński, M. Corporate Social Responsibility: Communication about social and environmental disclosure by large and small copper mining companies. *Resour. Policy* **2016**, *49*, 53–60. [CrossRef]
110. Donthu, N.; Gustafsson, A. Effects of COVID-19 on business and research. *J. Bus. Res.* **2020**, *117*, 284–289. [CrossRef] [PubMed]
111. Craven, M.; Liu, L.; Mysore, M.; Wilson, M. *COVID-19: Implications for Business*; McKinsey & Company: New York, NY, USA, 2020.
112. Amankwah-Amoah, J.; Khan, Z.; Wood, G. COVID-19 and business failures: The paradoxes of experience, scale, and scope for theory and practice. *Eur. Manag. J.* **2021**, *39*, 179–184. [CrossRef]
113. Krishnamurthy, S. The future of business education: A commentary in the shadow of the Covid-19 pandemic. *J. Bus. Res.* **2020**, *117*, 1–5. [CrossRef]

114. Bansal, P.; Grewatsch, S.; Sharma, G. How COVID-19 informs business sustainability research: It's time for a systems perspective. *J. Manag. Stud.* **2021**, *58*, 602–606. [CrossRef]
115. Haines, K.J.; Berney, S. Physiotherapists during COVID-19: Usual business, in unusual times. *J. Physiother.* **2020**, *66*, 67. [CrossRef]
116. Bartik, A.W.; Bertrand, M.; Cullen, Z.; Glaeser, E.L.; Luca, M.; Stanton, C. The impact of COVID-19 on small business outcomes and expectations. *PNAS* **2020**, *117*, 17656–17666. [CrossRef]
117. Brammer, S.; Branicki, L.; Linnenluecke, M.K. COVID-19, Societalization, and the Future of Business in Society. *Acad. Manag. Perspect.* **2020**, *34*, 493–507. [CrossRef]
118. Verma, S.; Gustafsson, A. Investigating the emerging COVID-19 research trends in the field of business and management: A bibliometric analysis approach. *J. Bus. Res.* **2020**, *118*, 253–261. [CrossRef]
119. Gostin, L.O.; Wiley, L.F. Governmental public health powers during the COVID-19 pandemic: Stay-at-home orders, business closures, and travel restrictions. *JAMA* **2020**, *323*, 2137–2138. [CrossRef]
120. Daniels, M.J.; Cohen, M.G.; Bavry, A.A.; Kumbhani, D.J. Reperfusion of ST-segment–elevation myocardial infarction in the COVID-19 era: Business as usual? *Circulation* **2020**, *141*, 1948–1950. [CrossRef]
121. Bartik, A.W.; Bertrand, M.; Cullen, Z.B.; Glaeser, E.L.; Luca, M.; Stanton, C.T. How are small businesses adjusting to COVID-19? Early evidence from a survey. *Natl. Bur. Econ. Res.* **2020**. [CrossRef]
122. Czeisler, M.É.; Tynan, M.A.; Howard, M.E.; Honeycutt, S.; Fulmer, E.B.; Kidder, D.P.; Robbins, R.; Barger, L.K.; Facer-Childs, E.R.; Baldwin, G.; et al. Public attitudes, behaviors, and beliefs related to COVID-19, stay-at-home orders, nonessential business closures, and public health guidance—United States, New York City, and Los Angeles, 5–12 May 2020. *MMWR* **2020**, *69*, 751. [CrossRef] [PubMed]
123. de Caro, F.; Hirschmann, T.M.; Verdonk, P. Returning to orthopaedic business as usual after COVID-19: Strategies and options. *Knee Surg. Sports Traumatol. Arthrosc.* **2020**, *28*, 1699–1704. [CrossRef]
124. Balla-Elliott, D.; Cullen, Z.B.; Glaeser, E.L.; Luca, M.; Stanton, C.T. Business reopening decisions and demand forecasts during the COVID-19 pandemic. *Natl. Bur. Econ. Res.* **2020**. [CrossRef]
125. Hasanat, M.W.; Hoque, A.; Shikha, F.A.; Anwar, M.; Hamid, A.B.; Tat, H.H. The impact of coronavirus (COVID-19) on e-business in Malaysia. *Asian J. Multidiscip. Stud.* **2020**, *3*, 85–90.
126. Akpan, I.J.; Udoh, E.A.; Adebisi, B. Small business awareness and adoption of state-of-the-art technologies in emerging and developing markets, and lessons from the COVID-19 pandemic. *J. Small Bus. Entrep.* **2020**, *25*, 1–8. [CrossRef]
127. Verbeke, A.; Yuan, W. A few implications of the covid-19 pandemic for international business strategy research. *J. Manag. stud.* **2021**, *58*, 597–601. [CrossRef]
128. Worlds: Business and Networks during COVID-19. Available online: https://www.tandfonline.com/doi/full/10.1080/14660970.2020.1782719 (accessed on 9 April 2021).
129. Commonwealth Bureau of Census and Statistics, Canberra Official Year Book of the Commonwealth of Australia. Available online: https://www.nature.com/articles/134049c0 (accessed on 9 April 2021).

MDPI
St. Alban-Anlage 66
4052 Basel
Switzerland
www.mdpi.com

*Healthcare* Editorial Office
E-mail: healthcare@mdpi.com
www.mdpi.com/journal/healthcare

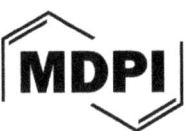

Disclaimer/Publisher's Note: The statements, opinions and data contained in all publications are solely those of the individual author(s) and contributor(s) and not of MDPI and/or the editor(s). MDPI and/or the editor(s) disclaim responsibility for any injury to people or property resulting from any ideas, methods, instructions or products referred to in the content.

www.ingramcontent.com/pod-product-compliance
Lightning Source LLC
LaVergne TN
LVHW070747100526
838202LV00013B/1325

*9 7 8 3 7 2 5 8 0 2 8 9 0*